ORAL PSYCHOPHYSIOLOGY

Stress, Pain, and Behavior in Dental Care

Ilana Eli

ORAL PSYCHOPHYSIOLOGY

Stress, Pain, and Behavior in Dental Care

CRC

CRC Press
Boca Raton Ann Arbor London Tokyo

Library of Congress Cataloging-in-Publication Data

Eli, Ilana
Oral psychophysiology: stress, pain, and behavior in dental care / Ilana Eli
p. cm.
Includes bibilographical references and index.
ISBN 0-8493-0159-9
1. Dentistry—Psychological aspects. 2. Dental care—Psychological aspects. 3. Medicine, Psychosomatic. 4. Psychophysiology. I. Title.
[DNLM: 1. Dental Care—methods. 2. Dental Care—psychology. 3. Dentist—Patient Relations. 4. Pain—psychology. 5. Stress, Psychology. WU 29 E420]
RK53.E63 1992
617.6′001′9—dc20
DNLM/DLC
for Library of Congress 91-29350
CIP

Direct all inquiries to CRC Press, Inc., 2000 Corporate Blvd., N.W., Boca Raton, Florida, 33431.

International Standard Book Number 0-8493-0159-9

Library of Congress Card Number 91-29350
Printed in the United States 1 2 3 4 5 6 7 8 9 0
Printed on acid-free paper

To Pazit, Rosa, and Leon —
the most important people in my life.
I. E.

PREFACE

Until recently, dentistry was perceived as a technical profession. Dental curricula paid utmost attention to the acquisition of technical skills, judging the quality of dental treatment on the basis of technical competence, accuracy and biocompatibility. Treatment failure due to patient behavior (e.g., avoidance of or restlessness during treatment, lack of compliance with preventive regiments) was blamed on the patient and considered beyond the dentist's responsibility. Approaches to managing patient behavior were considered appropriate for the treatment of children but were rather unfamiliar in the treatment of adults.

This view is rapidly changing. As in other fields of medicine, dental professionals have started to accept that the patient's behavior is crucial to the eventual outcome of the treatment, and that emotions and cognitions play a major role in all its stages.

Today, the dental profession accepts, as the dentist's responsibility, the handling of behavioral dysfunctions that relate to the oral cavity. Being a good dentist means not only producing a fine, accurate restoration, but also establishing a positive rapport with the anxious patient. It also means realizing that many of the apparently "physiological" symptoms (e.g., excessive gagging reflex, atypical odontalgia) may harbor hidden psychological aspects which should be addressed; the so-called field of "oral psychophysiology" is rapidly expanding.

Psychophysiology is a relatively new discipline. It is only during the last few decades that the concept by which "emotions and motives cannot be conceptualized by either physiology or psychology alone" was generally accepted.[1] The discipline of psychophysiology deals basically with manipulation of behavioral events and recording of physiological variables, such as the relationship between psychological states (fear, anxiety, depression) and physiological correlates (EEG, electrodermal activity).[2] Its numerous applications also include the monitoring of physiological reactions while undergoing severe stress.[3]

Giddon[4] pointed out that the general definition of psychophysiology includes the oral cavity, and deals also with the effect of stress on different oral structures. In this respect Giddon referred to three main questions:

1. What determines the stressfulness of a particular situation for a given individual?
2. What are the mediators or pathways to alteration in organ function and consequent damage?
3. What determines which particular organ will be affected?

These questions cover numerous issues. They refer to the issue of stress in the dental situation, as well as to its immediate and long-term effects on oral health. After all, although the physiological effect of stress is usually measured by direct physiological variables (e.g., salivary fluid), it also harbors multiple, less-direct, long-term effects (e.g., neglecting dental care due to fear or anxiety).

This book summarizes some of the psychophysiological aspects of dental care. Section 1 relates to concepts of stress and pain, with special emphasis placed on the dental situation. What is stress? What is so unique about dental treatment that makes it so stress-inflicting? What are the psychological aspects of acute and chronic pain? These are some of the questions covered in this first section.

These are broad subjects and include endless sources of literature. Therefore, only those points were chosen which would be especially important to the dental practitioner, and they are presented in a clinically pertinent way. For example, in Chapter 3, no effort is made to cover the complex anatomical and physiological aspects of pain transferance, but rather it is related to the various psychological (cognitive, emotional) aspects of the pain experience.

Section 2 concerns different behavioral aspects of dental treatment, including specific oro-related behavioral dysfunctions (fear, anxiety, and phobia; excessive gagging reflex; orofacial pain). Special attention is given to the specific problems of elderly dental patients, including possible problems in adapting to dentures. The effects of stress on physiological conditions in the oral cavity (i.e., on the salivary fluid, on soft and hard tissues) and on stress-related behavior, such as syncope or inability to achieve proper local anesthesia, are discussed.

Possible treatment modalities for patients who find it difficult to cope with the various aspects of dental care are summarized in Section 3. The different treatment methods include modalities from both the behavioral and pharmaceutical disciplines.

It is impossible to present accurate prescriptions of how to treat the different oro-related behavioral dysfunctions. Modes of behavior modification, as well as deep sedation or general anesthesia, can be used in any of the described situations. This is the main reason why no detailed treatment suggestions are included at the end of each chapter in Section 2. Dealing with possible treatment modalities in a concentrated manner gives the reader a better overview of the possible treatments and enables better choice of an appropriate mode for each case.

No book can completely cover all the complex psychophysiological aspects of dental care. During the process of writing, I had to decide which aspects of this huge subject to discuss in detail, which to mention briefly, and which to omit. The decision was often difficult and I might have chosen incorrectly in some of the issues. Many psychological aspects may seem lacking in the eyes of the professional psychologist, just as many physiological issues are probably lacking as far as the professional physiologist is concerned.

Although many of the issues covered herein are common for both children and adults, no specific references to child behavioral problems are made; these subjects are widely covered by the pedodontic literature. This book is aimed primarily at dentists, experts in various treatment specialities (prosthodontics, endodontics, periodontics, etc.) who encounter a "problematic" adult patient. These patients require more than the usual, familiar, manual skills and are often a source of stress and frustration to the dentist. The book presents a holistic approach to the understanding and treatment of these patients. It is my intention that, by understanding some of the underlying principles of the patient's behavior, the clinician will be able to create a better interpersonal relationship, prevent some problems, and solve others.

REFERENCES

1. **Ax, A. F.,** Editorial, *Psychophysiology*, 1, 1, 1964.
2. **Stern, J. A.,** Toward a definition of psychophysiology, *Psychophysiology*, 1, 90, 1964.
3. **Darrow, C. W.,** Psychophysiology yesterday, today and tomorrow, *Psychophysiology*, 1, 4, 1964.
4. **Giddon, D. B.,** Psychophysiology of the oral cavity, *J. Dent. Res.* (Supplement to No. 6), 45, 1627, 1966.

THE AUTHOR

Dr. Ilana Eli, DMD, is a Senior Lecturer at the Maurice and Gabriela Goldschleger School of Dental Medicine, Tel Aviv University, Tel Aviv, Israel.

Dr. Eli graduated in 1976 from the Hebrew University in Jerusalem and has since been working in the fields of operative dentistry and the treatment of patients with various oro-related behavioral dysfunctions.

At present, Dr. Eli serves as President of the Israeli Division of the International Association of Dental Research (IADR); she is an active member of the IADR and The International Association for Clinical and Experimental Hypnosis.

Dr. Eli has published over 45 scientific papers in the fields of behavioral sciences and operative dentistry, and she has presented over 50 papers at international meetings all over the world. Dr. Eli holds several international patents for newly developed oral diagnostic techniques.

ACKNOWLEDGMENTS

Writing a book is a long process. The encouragement and help of many people made this book possible. Dr. Moris Kleinhauz, a senior psychiatrist, colleague, and friend, was the first to introduce me to the complex problem of oro-related behavioral dysfunctions. It was his initiative to establish, more than 10 years ago, the Clinic of Oral Psychophysiology at the School of Dental Medicine, Tel Aviv University. Together, we have since treated hundreds of patents. Dr. Kleinhauz's ideas shaped the clinical principles of the Clinic operation and its multidisciplinary approach. I will always be grateful for his tutorship and guidance.

Special thanks to Dr. Arie Shifman, whose "computer-like" memory supplied me with many literature sources, for constructive criticism of the text; to Dr. Mark Littner for excellent comments on the subject of glossodynia; and to my friends Dr. Mel Rosenberg and Dr. Ervin Weiss for encouragement and support.

Aside from the mere writing of the text, publishing a book requires editorial assistance. This was carried out with utmost devotion and skill by Ms. Rita Lazar.

TABLE OF CONTENTS

SECTION I

STRESS AND PAIN IN DENTAL CARE

Chapter 1

WHAT IS STRESS?

Stress is a general term that has continually changed meanings over the past several decades. It is both a stimulus and a reaction, and includes both physiological and psychological components.[1]

Selye,[2] the pioneer on stress research, defined stress as "the nonspecific response of the body to any demand made upon it..." and described it as a "general adaptation syndrome", i.e., a nonspecific means by which the body defends itself against damage caused by a noxious stimulus. This syndrome includes the physiological secretion of the pituitary hormones that activates the cortex of the adrenal glands. Moreover, regardless of the "stressor" (the stimulus that results in the individual's stress reaction, be it wound, hunger, or psychological assault), the body responds with the same nonspecific type of reaction.

Singer and Davidson[3] referred to the confusing term "nonspecific" and noted that while each stressor causes some specific reactions (e.g., edema in the case of a broken leg, gastrointestinal reactions to food poisoning), they also include anonymous, nonspecific reactions of the whole organism (e.g., increased output of adrenal cortical steroids) which are not dependent on the nature of the stimulus. This nonspecific response is the same whether the "stressor" is physical (a wound) or psychological (an anxiety-arousing situation).

A complete distinction between the two factors is impossible: each physical assault carries subjective psychological meanings which can be stressful to the individual (e.g., fear of death or fear of losing control). Similarly, a psychological stressor, such as an anxiety-arousing situation, threatens the individual's integrity in much the same way as a physiological stimulus.

Lazarus[1] defined stress as a "circumstance external to a person which makes unusual or extraordinary demands on him, or threatens him in *some* way..." (emphasis added). Since people may react to the same situation differently, stress is thus "the responses or reactions of the person rather than the situation producing them."

Levine and Scotch[4] pointed out that various situations are not objectively stressful, but are socially or psychologically defined as such by individuals in terms of social and cultural norms. If a person perceives a given situation to be disturbing or threatening and is unable to mobilize personal or social resources to handle it, his energy is concentrated on dealing with the disturbance. This preoccupation has been defined as a stressful condition.[5]

Perception is therefore basic in causing a stressful condition. This, of course, varies from individual to individual. A situation which is natural to one person (e.g., lecturing before an audience) can be highly stressful to another. Furthermore, interpretation of the threat is crucial.[6] A person may be calm in a situation where his/her superiority is accepted (e.g., lecturing in front of undergraduate students), but experience stress in an apparently similar situation, where knowledge and authority can be threatened (e.g., lecturing in a scientific meeting).

I. THE STRESS RESPONSE

An individual's responses and reactions to the stress-producing situation, referred to as the stress response, fall into four main categories:[7,8]

1. Physiological changes — increase in heart rate, elevation of blood pressure, changes in galvanic skin response, increase in respiration, etc.
2. Behavioral effects — fear, anxiety, anger, depression, guilt, etc.
3. Motor changes — tremor, increase in muscle tension, particular facial expressions, etc.
4. Changes in cognitive functioning — distortive unproductive thinking, indecisiveness, and impaired perception, judgment, and problem solving skills.

It is not important whether the agent or situation causing stress is pleasant or unpleasant. What does matter is the intensity of the demand for readjustment made on the individual,[9] which impairs normal functioning by binding up energy to restore the disrupted homeostasis.[4]

II. THE CONCEPT OF THREAT[1,7]

The term *threat*, introduced by Lazarus, expresses the condition of a person confronted with a stimulus which that person defines as endangering physically and/or psychologically. He defined threat as "the anticipation of harm of some kind."

The anticipated harm can be physical (pain, injury), psychological (failure, loss of control), or interpersonal (shame, loss of the respect of others), but in all cases it threatens the basic needs, goals, or motives of the individual. Threat has, therefore, two main variables: it is anticipatory or future-oriented, and it is brought about by cognitive processes involving perception, learning, memory, judgment, and thought.

A. ANTICIPATION

The anticipation of a future, bound-to-happen harm is a powerful stress-provoking stimulus. The anticipated threat can be actual or subjective — the very expectation of harm, real or imaginary, triggers the stress response.

Thus, Lazarus makes a distinction between the threat stimulus (the stimulus which provokes stress) and actual harmful occurrences defined as "confrontation with harm." According to this distinction, while threat concerns cues of imminent harm, confrontation refers to the actual occurrence of the anticipated event. Each of these factors can, separately or concomitantly, result in a stress response.

In situations related to dentistry, physiological stress reactions can be brought about entirely by the anticipation of a perceived-as-harmful experience, e.g., a local anesthetic injection. Mere anticipation of the injection was found to result in as much stress as the actual penetration of the needle, as measured by the level of hydrocortisone in the blood.[10]

B. COGNITIVE PROCESSES

For threat to occur, an evaluation must be made of the situation. This evaluation, called threat appraisal, involves a person's knowledge, beliefs, and feelings. It is not the simple perception of the situation that is important, but the personal judgment, ideas, and expectations. We know how profoundly different patients are, and how differently they behave when facing a similar threatening situation (e.g., a tooth extraction). Such differences originate from individual variations in threat appraisal and coping resources.

In situations of actual confrontation with harm, the appraisal of threat is affected not only by the potency of the stimulus, but also by the resources at the individual's disposal to counter or avoid the harm. It is the balance between the harm-producing stimulus and the counter-harm resources which eventually affects threat appraisal. When the balance favors the former, threat is increased; when it favors the latter, threat is reduced.

C. INTENSITY OF STIMULUS

Generally, the stronger the stimulus and the more intense the cues of danger, the higher the evidence of threat. In cases of immediate danger, threat appraisal increases in direct relation to its intensity. For example, a patient who is usually calm during routine dental treatments can experience stress when facing surgical extraction.

D. TIME

Threat is also significantly affected by the factor of time. When the anticipated danger is bound to happen in the distant future, the degree of threat is relatively low. As the event approaches and can no longer be easily put out of mind, threat appraisal gradually gains in strength.

Thus, dental patients with an impending appointment were found to be more anxious than those who were not facing treatment.[11] Furthermore, anxiety was found to increase as treatment approached and decrease dramatically afterwards.[12]

The two variables, power and imminence of the harm-producing stimulus, are closely related. While a weak stimulus can sometimes be overlooked when time prior to confrontation is short, a strong stimulus can cause a reaction even when the time of confrontation is far ahead. The relevant dental examples include patients who make an appointment for a stress-provoking procedure (e.g., tooth extraction) and cancel as time approaches. In others, the very thought of treatment is so stressful that they avoid the dental encounter altogether (see also Chapter 4).

III. VARIABLES OF THREAT APPRAISAL[1,7]

A. CONTROL VS. HELPLESSNESS

Generally, an individual's conception of his own power to master the situation is an important factor in threat appraisal. Situations that can be mastered are usually less threatening than those which make one feel helpless in the face of a superior power. It is the feeling of power rather than the actual power that is important. The very knowledge that such control is possible is usually sufficent to relieve threat, and no further *real* control is necessary.

Another factor which increases the feeling of helplessness is ambiguity. An unclear, vague stimulus, carrying unknown anticipated harm, usually provokes a stronger feeling of danger than a known threat.

The aspect of helplessness is especially relevant in the dental situation, where the patient lies in the dental chair, submitting to unfamiliar threatening procedures with no ability to react or terminate the treatment (see Chapter 2).

B. PERSONALITY

The interpretation of a situation as threatening is also influenced by the individual's motives. Situations are appraised as threatening when related to goals that are considered important. This varies among individuals. For example, some students facing an important examination may show less evidence of threat than others due to less motivation to succeed.[13]

C. ENVIRONMENTAL

Family support, physical conditions, and socioeconomic level also enhance or reduce threat appraisal. Threat appraisal is affected not only by objective environmental factors but also by subjective beliefs about these factors. An individual who *believes* he/she can count on a supportive social environment will appraise a stimulus as less threatening than a person with a pessimistic, helpless outlook. Those who believe that the environment is hostile and dangerous and that they are powerless to manipulate it successfully, often see threat in situations others do not. Egocentricity, distrust, pessimism, anxiety, and resentment increase threat appraisal, while optimism and belief in one's own masterfulness decrease it.

In the dental situation the patient's perception of self-control is significantly correlated with anxiety towards treatment. Highly anxious patients report a greater decrease in the extent of their control as the dental appointment approaches than those with low anxiety, suggesting that anxiety is related to notions of self-efficacy and self-control.[14,15]

IV. COPING WITH STRESS

When confronting stress, each person consolidates his/her own coping strategies and reaction patterns depending on individual motives, ego resources, coping dispositions, situational constraints, and viability of alternative coping actions. The most important coping reaction patterns include direct action tendencies (attack and avoidance), defensive reappraisals — maneuvers in which the individual deceives himself about the actual conditions of threat (denial and rationalization), and anxiety reaction patterns.[7]

A. ATTACK

Attack is an action aimed at preventing "anticipated harm by means of assault on the agent of harm."[7] It may be simple or complex, physical or verbal, subtle or obvious, depending on one's personality and situational constraints in the form of social norms and pressures.

Attack is often accompanied by anger, indicating that the person is threatened or frustrated. Such frustration (often stemming from the patient's own feeling of failure for not being able to face treatment) may be shifted to the dentist and expressed verbally (e.g., "All dentists are butchers..."; "I simply hate dentists..."). Social constraints often prevent clear expression of anger, especially when the patient faces actual treatment and feels dependent on the dentist, but may be expressed unconsciously in nonverbal signs.

B. AVOIDANCE

Avoidant coping is sometimes used by dental patients through cognitive strategies, such as distraction ("not thinking about bad feelings or unpleasant things"),[16] but is often expressed by total or partial avoidance of treatment. While avoidant coping through distractive thoughts before, during, and after dental treatment is associated with low self-ratings of anxiety,[16] total avoidance is usually associated with high dental anxiety. This is probably one of the most popular reactions to threat appraisal in the dental situation and is dealt with in detail in Chapter 4.

C. DEFENSIVE-REAPPRAISAL PATTERNS

Occasionally, an individual chooses to avoid coping directly with a threatening situation, activating defense mechanisms instead. These include denial ("there's nothing wrong with my teeth, they are perfectly all right"), rationalization ("there is no point in treating my teeth, they will all fall out anyway"), or isolation ("I have more important things to do at this stage of my life").

D. ANXIETY REACTION PATTERNS

In many cases in which threat is appraised, there is a general feeling of anxiety with an unclear definition of its source. Anxiety usually indicates ambiguous threat, whether it derives from a normal appraisal of anticipated harm (e.g., pain of dental treatment), or from secondary meanings subconsciously related to the specific stimulus (e.g., symbolic meaning of the dental situation). It can lead to avoidance, attack, or defensive reappraisal patterns, or it can remain a general undefined feeling of anxiety.

E. STRATEGIES USED BY PATIENTS

The strategies used by patients facing treatment depend highly on individual factors. Wong and Kaloupek[16] have shown several coping strategies exhibited by patients during dental treatment: avoidant ("I was not thinking about bad feelings or unpleasant things"), cognitive ("I was thinking that this is not pleasant but is necessary for my health"), behavioral ("I was trying to find out about what was going to happen next"), focus problem ("I was focusing on the treatment procedure"), emotional ("I was focusing on how I felt"), and unfocused ("I was not thinking about anything"). According to the study, the avoidant strategy is generally associated with low self-ratings of anxiety and is the most frequently endorsed overall.

Chaves and Brown[17] reported that in a sample of patients undergoing extractions 44% used spontaneous cognitive strategies, mostly attention diversion (refocusing on something other than the stressful situation). Of the patients, 37% catastrophized, engaging in cognitive activity which exaggerated the fearful aspects of their experience (most of them involving nonimagery negative thoughts). The study showed that the tendency to catastrophize is associated with personal variables, such as past dental experience, high trait anxiety, and external locus of control. It is also associated with higher stress levels during the dental procedure than the stress experienced by those who used cognitive coping to minimize pain and stress.

Generally, a person can also cope with stress through various self-presentational strategies.[18] These include defensive strategies, such as "self-handicapping" in which the patient has a ready explanation for potential failure, thus reducing the threat to self-esteem.[19] In the dental setting, the self-preservational strategies may be expressed by conditions such as an excessive gagging reflex ("...I cannot receive treatment because I gag at any attempt"; see also Chapter 5). Self-serving explanations[20] ("...I do not have the time/money necessary for treatment"); self-deception ("...everything is just fine, I do not need the treatment"); or self-extending strategies which manifest excessive self-confidence in spite of the stress may also be part of a self-preservational strategy.

V. SUMMARY

The term "stress" is generally used to express both the stimuli and the responses associated with stressful conditions. While stress as a stimulus involves circumstances external to a person which present demands that are objectively or subjectively perceived as threatening, stress as a response involves the arsenal of physiological, behavioral, and cognitive responses aimed at restoring the disrupted homeostasis.

The magnitude in which a certain stimulus may be potentially stress-inflicting is affected largely by the individual's threat appraisal of a particular situation. This is determined by stimulus-dependent factors (intensity of the stimulus, time prior to the anticipated exposure, etc.), cognitive processes (anticipation of harm, control vs. helplessness, etc.), personality variables, and environmental factors.

A stressful stimulus is usually associated with a future, bound-to-happen harm; something unpleasant, better to be avoided. It evokes unpleasant physiological, behavioral, and cognitive responses, and involves individual coping mechanisms aimed at confronting the anticipated threat. In spite of its generally accepted unpleasantness, it is important to remember that some degree of stress is essential for everyday life, for the complete lack of stress is death.[9]

REFERENCES

1. **Lazarus, R. S.,** *Patterns of Adjustment and Human Effectiveness*, McGraw-Hill, New York, 1969.
2. **Selye, H.,** *The Stress of Life*, McGraw-Hill, New York, 1956.
3. **Singer, J. E. and Davidson, L. M.,** Specificity and stress research, in *Dynamics of Stress*, Appley, M. H. and Trumbull, R., Eds., Plenum Press, New York, 1986.
4. **Levine, S. and Scotch, N. A.,** *Social Stress*, Aldine, Chicago, 1970.
5. **Scott, R. and Howard, A.,** Models of stress, in *Social Stress*, Levine, S. and Scotch, N. A., Eds., Aldine, Chicago, 1970.
6. **May, R.,** *The Meaning of Anxiety*, W. W. Norton, New York, 1977.
7. **Lazarus, R. S.,** *Psychological Stress and the Coping System*, McGraw-Hill, New York, 1966, 465.
8. **Cattell, R. B. and Scheier, I. H.,** *The Meaning and Measurement of Neuroticism and Anxiety*, Ronald, New York, 1961.
9. **Selye, H.,** *Stress Without Distress*, Hodd & Stoughton, London, 1974.
10. **Shannon, I. L. and Isbell, G. M.,** Stress in Dental Patients: Effect of Local Anesthetic Procedures, Tech. Rep. No. SAM-TDR-63-29, U. S. Air Force School of Aerospace Medicine, Brooks Air Force Base, Texas, 1963.
11. **Corah, N. L. and Salmonson, R. J.,** Psychologic response to a simulated dental procedure as a function of proximity to an actual dental appointment, *J. Dent. Res.*, 49, 438, 1970.
12. **Bernstein, D. A. and Kleinknecht, R. A.,** Multiple approaches to the reduction of dental fear, *J. Behav. Ther. Exp. Psychiatry*, 13, 287, 1982.
13. **Mahl, G. F.,** Anxiety, HCl secretion and peptic ulcer etiology, *Psychosom. Med.*, 11, 30, 1949.
14. **Kent, G.,** Self-efficacious control over reported physiological, cognitive and behavioural symptoms of dental anxiety, *Behav. Res. Ther.*, 25, 341, 1987.
15. **Kent, G. and Gibbons, R.,** Self-efficacy and the control of anxious cognitions, *J. Behav. Ther. Exp. Psychiatry*, 18, 33, 1987.
16. **Wong, M. and Kaloupek, D. G.,** Coping with dental treatment: The potential impact of situational demands, *J. Behav. Med.*, 9, 579, 1986.

17. **Chaves, J. F. and Brown J. M.,** Spontaneous cognitive strategies for the control of clinical pain and stress, *J. Behav. Med.*, 10, 263, 1987.
18. **Laux, L.,** A self-presentational view of coping with stress, in *Dynamics of Stress*, Appley, M. H. and Trumbull, R., Eds., Plenum Press, New York, 1986.
19. **Jones, E. E. and Berglas, S.,** Control of attributions about the self through self-handicapping strategies: the appeal of alcohol and the role of underachievement, *Personality Soc. Psychol. Bull.*, 4, 200, 1978.
20. **Schlenker, B. R. and Leary, M. R.,** Social anxiety and self-presentation: a conceptualization and model, *Psychol. Bull.*, 92, 641, 1982.

Chapter 2

STRESS AND THE DENTAL SITUATION

Stress is closely associated with the dental situation. Treatment involves both physiological stimuli (pain-inflicting procedures, possible damage to tissues, etc.) as well as psychological aspects which may cause the patient to judge the situation as a threat to his/her physical and mental well-being (anticipation of pain, physical closeness to an authoritative figure, etc.).[1]

During the late 1960s, visiting the dentist was ranked fourth among the situations feared most among Americans (after snakes, heights, and storms).[2] Today, the prevalence of moderate to high dental fear is estimated about 204 per 1000 people (making it more fearful than illness, enclosures, storms, and being alone).[3]

To understand why stress is so closely related to dental treatment, various aspects of the dental situation and its meaning to the patient are discussed.

I. CONFLICT AND DENTAL TREATMENT

Stress may be caused not only by a direct threat, but also by the simultaneous presence of two incompatible tendencies which create a conflict. Conflict is an important parameter, since it often makes threat inevitable. Two major patterns of conflict[4] are especially applicable to the dental situation.

A. AVOIDANCE-AVOIDANCE CONFLICT

An avoidance-avoidance conflict usually involves two negative stimuli, each causing threat appraisal. The patient wishes to avoid both stimuli; however, the avoidance of one inevitably confronts him with the other.

Avoidance-avoidance conflict in the dental situation occurs when the fear of treatment opposes the fear of pain caused by the pathologic condition. In such cases, the final pattern of behavior relies on the relative strength of the stimuli. If fear of treatment is greater than fear of pain (e.g., from a sore tooth), treatment is avoided, resulting in further neglect. However, if pain becomes greater than fear of actual treatment, professional help is obtained.

The avoidance-avoidance conflict of anxious dental patients is often expressed by a relatively long duration from the initial onset of pain until professional help is sought. This time is significantly longer in patients suffering from so-called "dental phobia" compared to a control group. While patients without dental fear usually seek treatment after 3 days of pain, the "dental phobics" wait about 17 days.[5]

As in other avoidance-avoidance conflicts, a phenomenon of "vacillation" is likely to occur in the dental situation.[4] It is caused by the increasing strength of each stimulus the closer one gets to it. An individual approaching a negative stimulus finds it increasingly threatening and tends to retreat or withdraw. As a consequence, the individual comes closer to the other stimulus and finds it, in turn, increasing in threat appraisal. Thus, a fearful dental patient will make an appointment when pain becomes severe. As the actual appointment approaches, however, the greater the fear of the dental encounter and the greater the probability of cancellation.

Another important feature of the avoidance-avoidance conflict is an attempt to leave the conflict situation, i.e., to run away physically, or by regressing or fantasizing. Anxious patients often choose avoidance as a way of escaping the situation, using defensive reappraisals (denial, rationalization, etc.) to cope with the stress involved (see also Chapter 4).

B. APPROACH-AVOIDANCE CONFLICT

The approach-avoidance conflict is where the individual is presented with a stimulus which is both repulsive and attractive. Dental treatment is often associated with an unpleasant necessity which, nevertheless, carries with it some positive recompensation (nice healthy teeth). It is the relative strength of each stimulus that finally determines avoidance or cooperation regardless of the fear. The desire for a healthy mouth can be a powerful incentive for some patients in spite of their dental anxiety.[6,7]

II. THE ORAL CAVITY AND PERSONALITY DEVELOPMENT

To understand the psychodynamic significance of the oral cavity, some aspects of the human personality should be noted. From the psychological point of view, personality concerns the psychological properties or traits that influence one's actions in various situations. It is not how others react to the person (like or dislike, pleasant or unpleasant, etc.), but how the person himself reacts, and what motivates his actions that is important.[8]

The oral cavity is an important element at various stages of life according to different theories of personality development. Freud's[9] psychosexual theory of personality divided psychological development into three stages according to the parts of the body which release sexual energy (libido): the oral stage (first year), the anal stage (second and third years), and the genital stage (starting around the third or fourth year). Occasionally, some libidinal energy fixates in one of the early stages (oral or anal), a fixation which will influence the personality throughout life.

The mouth is the first zone of pleasure and satisfaction in the newborn, not only through its organic role as a supplier of nutrition, but also as an erogenous zone which provides sexual pleasure. Sucking, licking, and exploring objects with the lips, tongue, and gums are major activities at this age. If, at the oral stage, the child is prevented from sucking or made to feel anxious about it, an oral fixation may result. Fixation at this stage results in an adult who continues to discharge considerable amounts of libidinal energy through the oral cavity and creates a personality, defined by Freud, as "an oral character." These individuals retain personality characteristics typical to the oral stage, such as passive dependence on others (similar to the child who at this stage passively receives satisfaction of all needs from the mother), expressing verbal aggression, and preoccupation with the oral cavity. Freud suggested that even in normal individuals who have successfully passed to the genital stage of development, some sexual activity (e.g., kissing) remains fixed with the oral cavity.

Later theorists of human personality believed that Freud exaggerated the importance of the early years in the development of personality and regarded the personality as too firmly fixed in this short first period. They argued that further changes occur in puberty, middle, and later life. However, the importance of the oral cavity throughout life remains undisputed.

Erikson[10] expanded the Freudian description of psychosexual stages to include the social meanings that accompany each stage. The importance of the oral cavity to the newborn during the oral stage lies not only in the distraction of sexual energy, but also affects mutual contact with the mother who nourishes the infant, thus stimulating the oral cavity. According to Erikson, what characterizes the oral stage is a social conflict of trust vs. mistrust. The child completely relies on his mother to respond to biological needs (nutrition). Therefore, the mother's behavior at this stage affects the trust (or mistrust) the child develops towards the social environment in later life.

Piaget[11,12] was one of the first to stress the importance of cognitive processes in personality development. He divided the stages of child development into the sensorimotor stage (from birth to 2 years) and the conceptual level (after 2 years). During the first stage, the child acquires knowledge of the environment through concrete sensorimotor activities. At this stage the oral cavity acts as one of the first organs of perception for the infant (sucking, exploring objects through the mouth, repeating actions which produce interesting results, solving simple problems, trial-and-error experimentation, etc.). The conceptual level includes the development of more complex images and concepts, such as the symbolic meaning of things, the ability to reason without the manipulation of concrete objects, etc.

The early theories of personality pay little attention to the impact of environment and learning processes. However, it is now clear that these processes play a significant role in shaping our lives. Social interactions are crucial in shaping the human personality and are essential for normal, everyday existence. Reinforcement learning, vicarious learning from models, and imitation are some of the processes that shape one's reactions to the various situations faced during life (including the dental situation).

III. THE COMPLEX ROLE OF THE ORAL CAVITY

Different organs in the body have separate and usually highly specific roles. The oral cavity is one of those unique organs that provides complex physiological, psychological, and social functions vital to human existence.[13] Its importance extends beyond its actual size or apparent function. Although relatively small, the orofacial area is represented in the cerebral cortex by a proportionally large area[14] (Figures 1 and 2).

According to the holistic-dynamic theory presented by Maslow,[15] the human personality is made up of complex specifications (behaviors, thoughts, perceptions, impulses) with a common unity, function, or purpose. Motivation is affected by the whole individual rather than only part (e.g., a hungry person has changes not only in his/her gastrointestinal tract, but also in perception, memory, emotion, etc.).

To explain the complexity of human behavior, Maslow developed a hierarchy of needs that have to be fulfilled:

1. Physiological — most basic, vital for survival (e.g., nutrition)
2. Safety — protection against threat or danger
3. Belongingness — affection and love
4. Esteem — desire for self-respect, self-esteem, and for the esteem of others
5. Self-actualization — self-fulfillment, reaching one's full potential

Maslow claimed that human needs have to be satisfied according to their relative hierarchy strength. The first, most prepotent, are the physiological needs. If these are not satisfied, all others become nonexistent or pushed into the background. Thus, the chronically and extremely hungry person concentrates only on obtaining food even at the expense of safety. In such situations, the person tends to think that, if only food is "granted", he/she will be happy and will never want anything more. Freedom, love, and respect may all be waved aside as useless.

Once the physiological needs are fulfilled, the individual can begin to fulfill safety needs (dealing with threat or danger). If unfulfilled, safety needs can be just as dominating as physiological needs. When both the physiological and safety needs are fairly well gratified, love, belongingness, and affection will emerge, taking over the center of motivation. The person who previously thought of nothing but food or safety will now long for relationships with others, for a place in a group, and for achievements. Once this is satisfied, the individual turns energy to achieve adequacy, reputation, prestige, status, recognition, attention, importance, and appreciation (esteem needs). And finally, some may still have an urge to achieve something more, to fulfill their potential. This is the highest degree of human need — the need for self-actualization. Maslow also added the need for esthetics which, although unclear, plays an important role for some individuals.

The oral cavity plays a significant part at each of those need levels.[16] The most basic and crucial role of the oral cavity is to fulfill the survival functions (physiological and safety needs) of the human organism. From the moment of

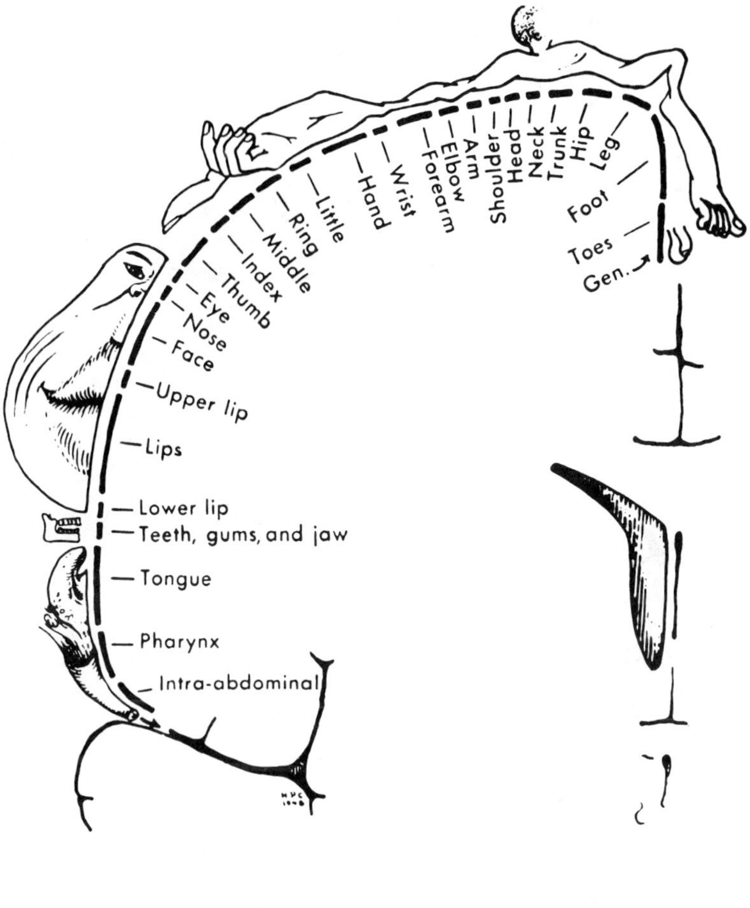

FIGURE 1. Sensory homunculus drawn overlying a cross section of the hemisphere in proportion to the extent of sensory cortex devoted to it. The length of the underlying block lines indicates the comparative extent of each representation. (From Penfield, W. and Rasmussen, T., *The Cerebral Cortex of Man: A Clinical Study of Localization of Function*, 1957, 44, with permission.)

birth until death the oral cavity provides the organism with the most basic needs essential for survival — the functions of nutrition and respiration. Damage caused to the region blocking the airway or hindering the administration of food presents the organism with an immediate existential danger. Maintaining the health and integrity of the oral cavity are, therefore, crucial for existence and safety.

The oral cavity also carries indirect connotations of protection against threat or danger. In man, as in other animals, teeth are still considered weapons,[17] although the existence of superior artificial weapons makes them no longer

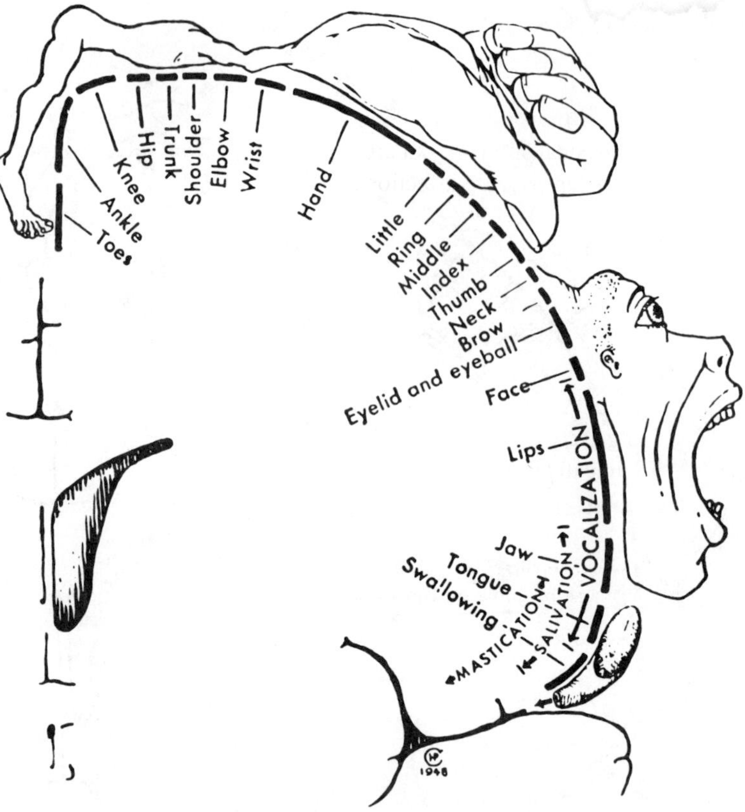

FIGURE 2. Motor homunculus drawn overlying a cross section of the hemisphere in proportion to the extent of sensory cortex devoted to it. The length of the underlying block lines indicates the comparative extent of each representation. (From Penfield, W. and Rasmussen, T., *The Cerebral Cortex of Man: A Clinical Study of Localization of Function*, 1957, 57, with permission.)

vital for this purpose; however, observations do show that when one is under stress, the teeth are sharpened. Every[18] has shown complex and precise mandibular movements in man which stimulate sharpening of the teeth for use as weapons (bite) or tools (separate, hold, and speak).

In the survival functions of the oral cavity, Dworkin et al.[16] also included communication and sexual activity. Speech and facial expressions are common and efficient means of communication. In society, cooperative behavior is necessary for survival. Man needs to be part of a society, both physically and psychologically. Verbal and nonverbal communication, through speech, facial expressions, and body gestures, are vital to our existence. Furthermore, the face and mouth play an important role in sexual attraction, essential for the survival of the species. It is a significant source of gratification and reinforcement of sexual behaviors (kissing, oro-genital activity), a pleasure which encourages the repetition of sexual acts and increases the opportunities for reproduction.

Fulfillment of the socialization needs (love, belonging, and esteem) is also closely related to the oral cavity. Speech and communication are not only important for physical survival, but are basic for achieving stable relationships with others who can provide affection and belongingness. Communication is crucial in order to fit in most of the professional framework of modern society, an interface which is one of the common ways leading to development of self-esteem and the esteem of others. Thwarting of these needs leads to feelings of inferiority, weakness, and helplessness, whereas satisfaction creates a positive feeling of usefulness and a place in society.[15]

In addition, expressions of self-actualization are carried out through the oral cavity (philosophy, poetry, and song). Even more manual self-actualization skills (painting, sculpturing, playing an instrument) are also dependent on verbal communication skills.

Undoubtedly, the more vague esthetic needs, even though not so clearly defined, are also significantly affected by the appearance of the oral region.[13] Although the definition of beauty changes periodically, and varies from society to society, the mouth and face are generally central features in creating the impression of attractiveness.[16]

IV. THE COMPLEX NATURE OF THE DENTAL SITUATION

The dental situation is unique in many respects. It involves environmental and psychodynamic factors which increase threat appraisal and result in stress response.

A. ENVIRONMENTAL FACTORS

1. Imminence of Physical Harm

Dental treatment is basically restorative in nature and inflicts a feeling of immediate physical threat. In most cases, treatment involves surgical procedures by which the affected tissue is removed and artificially restored. Procedures such as drilling, boring, cutting, pulling, striking, and agitating are the "bread and butter" of routine dental treatment and create a stimulus of immediate physical harm.

Although pain is no longer an unavoidable companion in modern dentistry, many dental patients (especially the anxious ones) are still troubled by the possibility of severe pain while in the dental chair.[19] Components of physical threat,[20] fear of pain and mutilation (e.g., tissue damage),[21] have been found to be closely related to dental fear. Threat appraisal can vary from procedure to procedure according to the relative strength of the stimulus involved (e.g., prophylactic treatment vs. surgical extraction),[19,22] but is present (to some degrees) with most dental treatment encounters.

2. Physical Closeness

There are accepted social distances preserved during social contacts with others.[23,24] Hall[23] distinguished between four distal zones typical to most social contacts:

1. The "public distance" (12 feet or more) is for formal contacts, i.e., appearance before an audience, or the distance that automatically surrounds an important public figure. At this distance, speech is loud and much of the nonverbal communication is transmitted by gestures and body language rather than by facial expressions.

2. The "social distance" (4 to 12 feet) is suitable for communication with associates or individuals with whom we are vaguely familiar. Intimate visual details of the face are not perceived and there is no direct physical contact.

3. The "personal distance" (1 to 4 feet) where the finer details of the face, skin, eyes, and teeth are perceived. This zone is for closer, everyday contacts. Direct physical contact is possible ("arm's length" distance) but is not usual. Subjects of personal interest and involvement can be discussed without voice elevation.

4. The "intimate distance" (up to 1 foot) is usually for close relationships (lovemaking, comforting, and/or protecting). Physical contact, or the possibility of it, is present in the situational context and the individuals involved are acutely aware of this. Heat and odor from each other are clearly detectable. Sight is often distorted and the smell, sound, and feel of the partner's breath combine to signal unmistakable involvement with each other.

The tendency to preserve accepted social distances originates from early developmental instincts whereby animals mark and preserve their territory. An invasion of such territory is interpreted as aggression. In humans, aggression is often expressed by bringing one's face close to that of one's opponent (invasion of intimate distance). In crowded conditions, such as in an elevator, subway, or bus, where one is forced to invade the intimate distance of others, the basic tactic is to stand still and avoid direct eye contact. If touching is unavoidable, muscles in the affected areas are strained due to social taboos about relaxing and enjoying bodily contact with strangers.[23] Total and mutual looking are also significantly affected by distance. There is usually more mutual looking at longer distances than at shorter distances.[25]

In the dental situation, the patient's intimate space is constantly invaded. The sense of smell, close vision of the dentist's face, and sensation of his body heat and breath are involved. Dentists (and their assistants) hold their face close to that of the patient, with an intense, direct look for the duration of the treatment. Such closeness can pose a direct threat to one's privacy and cause threat appraisal.

Furthermore, during treatment, the patient experiences a prolonged, unavoidable, intimate contact between his/her face and a "stranger." Many find it difficult to relax under these conditions and react with increased tension of head and neck muscles.

3. Long Duration Encounters

Effects of stress are cumulative. The longer its duration (continuous, cyclic, or episodic) the higher the possibility of exhaustion.[26,27]

During our lifetime, we experience many encounters with members of the medical profession. In a generally healthy individual, these encounters are usually sporadic and short. The situation, however, is different for dental treatment, where the actual "confrontation with harm" lasts for a relatively long time. Even a simple routine dental procedure, such as an amalgam restoration, requires one to submit to the hands of the dentist for 30 min or more. Other procedures may take significantly more time. This relatively long duration of the "harm-producing" stimulus increases the amount of energy needed for the coping process and increases threat appraisal and stress response.

4. Life-Long Commitment

Unfortunately, dentistry is a medical discipline which cannot provide a definite cure to the involved pathology. The dental practitioner can usually provide only restorative and preventive means that reduce the prevalence of disease but cannot prevent it completely.

The dental patient is presented with a life-long commitment, which involves significant effort and sacrifice (routine oral hygiene, change of cariogenic diet, routine examinations in the dental office) but with only relative compensation. This is often frustrating and unsatisfactory. Frustration, caused by the inability to achieve the expected goal (no caries or periodontal disease until death), carries with it feelings of aggression towards the "responsible" figure or procedure (dentist, dental treatment, preserving oral hygiene, etc.). Reactions like "How come you found three new holes?…I have been brushing my teeth every day just as you told me." are common expressions of anger known to each practitioner.

B. PSYCHODYNAMIC FACTORS

1. Anticipation

The dentist's waiting room is a classic anticipatory setting whereby the patient is exposed to voices, smells, and atmosphere of the forthcoming treatment. Such anticipation usually leads to an increased threat appraisal and stress response.

The duration of the warning period, which elapses prior to a noxious stimulation (e.g., electric shock), has a significant effect on the subject's stress response.[28] Mittwoch et al.[28] suggested that when treatment is to be given immediately, it is best to keep the warning period brief and not lengthen it beyond 30 s. This suggestion is, however, only seldom fulfilled in the dental office.

Patients often expect more intense sensations and greater discomfort than they are likely to experience. For most, it is the anticipation rather than the experience of treatment itself which is stressful.[29]

While anticipating the dental treatment, the patient is often confronted with an avoidance-avoidance conflict, contributing further to threat appraisal. At this stage, the patient still holds the option to "retreat," namely, cope with the threatening stimulus through avoidance (leave before treatment). The resolution of an avoidance-avoidance conflict makes threat basically inevitable (threat of the anticipated treatment vs. that of the pain caused by neglect of treatment). Coping with the conflict involves some of the patient's energy, increasing threat appraisal, and stress response.

2. Loss of Control

Conditions which carry notions of helplessness are, as a rule, more threatening than situations that can be manipulated and controlled. Unfortunately, the dental situation bears many such aspects.

The very nature of the dental situation is based on the patient being in a supine position, with no ability to follow or observe the procedures that are being carried out. One or more figures lean towards the patient, holding unfamiliar instruments and/or materials. The patient's mouth is kept opened and the body is immobilized by the supine position and the dentist's instructions. Clearly, both verbal and nonverbal communications with the surrounding people are severely handicapped. The combination of an inability to observe and an inability to react creates a strong feeling of helplessness. Fear, anxiety, and apprehension are not easily expressed, leading to frustration in front of the uncontrolled stimulus.

An additional threat factor may be the lack of information and uncertainty regarding the anticipated procedures. The dentist, who is often concerned mainly with the technical aspects of treatment, occasionally neglects to inform and/or prepare the patient before a new procedure is used. Even a routine, unexpected use of a triple syringe causes some patients to jump with apprehension.

The importance attributed to personal control varies among patients. In a review concerning the relationship between stress and personal control over aversive stimuli, Averil[30] distinguished between three main types of personal control: behavioral (direct action on the environment), cognitive (the interpretation of events), and decisional (having a choice among alternative courses of action). Each type of control is related to stress in a complex fashion, sometimes increasing it, sometimes reducing it, and sometimes having no influence at all.

The relationship of personal control to stress is primarily a function of the meaning of the control response for the individual. In the dental setting, patients most at risk for an aversive dental experience are those who have a need to control but feel a loss of control while in the dental chair.[31]

Generally, lack of knowledge regarding the treatment contributes to the feeling of helplessness and control loss. Tullman et al.[32] have shown that uncertainty increased the anxiety in new dental patients even though they were told that no actual treatment would be carried out during the initial visit.

The feeling of helplessness is sometimes enhanced by the common assumption that some dental procedures, such as root canal treatment and tooth extraction, cannot be interrupted once started. This increasingly threatens the patient's feeling of autonomy and mastery over the situation. Fears of suffocation, aspiration, and vomiting may result from this threat.

3. Intrabody Penetration

Since the oral cavity bears multiple sexual connotations, penetration into the oral cavity is sometimes regarded as an invasion of the inner, intimate parts of the body. Although social tendency exists to conceal the inner parts of the oral cavity in public (covering the mouth during laughing or yawning),[33] this erogenous zone usually remains uncovered.

Patients occasionally express shame with regard to showing their oral cavity even to the dentist. The feeling may originate from shame of a neglected oral status ("...You have never seen such a horrible mouth before"); fear of rejection due to bad breath, or subconscious conflicts connected with the shame of exposing the intimate inner parts.

During dental treatment, the oral cavity is penetrated with sharp, threatening instruments. Aside from an immediate physical threat, this penetration can pose an additional threatening stimulus due to the symbolic meaning of the procedure.

V. LEARNED RESPONSES

The concepts and coping strategies of the various life events are continually affected by learning processes. Personality is both a product of inner, hereditary, and developmental forces and a function of outside environmental stimuli, social interactions, and social roles. Part of our behavior results from an extensive history of earlier life events fixed firmly in our conscious and subconscious mind.

A basic term in understanding learned responses is habit, defined as "...consistently recurring responses to a particular stimulus..."[34] Most learned habits are adaptive, i.e., they serve biological or acquired needs to avoid injury, pain, or discomfort (a child learns to recoil from fire, thus preventing pain and injury). However, some habits are unadaptive; their effects are unfavorable to the well-being of the individual (e.g., a person fears dental treatment and avoids encounters with the dentist, resulting in impaired oral status).

For a learned behavior to develop, exposure to the stimulus in question must occur, resulting in a response pattern. A basic principle is the process of reinforcement. Pavlov,[35] in his early research, demonstrated how the bond between a stimulus and a response is strengthened by supplying a positive reinforcement, e.g., food. It has been suggested that a similar process occurs in the acquisition of learned behavior by humans.

A major intent of reinforcement learning is that we learn the actions which produce reward or reduce punishment. When one is exposed to a response-producing stimulus which has been reinforced in some way, the response pattern is incorporated in the inventory of behavior. The source of reinforcement can be external (food) or internal (satisfaction, self-esteem), positive (pleasant) or negative (pain), and always acts as a strengthening process to the new (or existing) responses caused by the stimulus.

New behaviors can be acquired or modified by direct and/or indirect learning.

A. DIRECT LEARNING AND DENTAL CARE

1. Classical (Respondent) Conditioning

Basically, respondent behavior is the way one reacts to the environment.[36] It includes involuntary, autonomic responses (salivating, sweating) and emotional responses (fear, anxiety, anger). For conditioning to occur, two stimuli have to exist concomitantly. In 1920, Watson and Raynor[37] induced a rat phobia in a young child by exposing him to the animal concomitantly with a loud voice. The stimulus of noise and a white furry rat were presented to the child at the same time. As a consequence, the child developed fear and anxiety toward furry objects resembling the white rat which was initially associated with the threatening noise.

A similar conditioning pattern shapes human behavior in various aspects of everyday life. It can cause a fear of driving when screeching of car brakes is associated with a former accident; it can result in claustrophobia when a closed room is associated with some former scary incident; and it can cause aversive emotional response towards the physician and his setting (assistants, instruments) when the patient has had a former unpleasant experience in a physician's office.[36]

The dental setting provides various opportunities for negative operant conditioning. Many apprehensive patients quote an aversive encounter with a dentist as the first reason for their anxiety.[38-43] The stimulus varies from patient to patient, but the most common is pain associated with dental treatment. Although acute pain during dental treatment can be avoided in most cases, there are still many adults who have experienced it during dental treatment in the past. The old drilling instruments, together with treatment without proper local anesthesia, have created many phobic victims. Similarly, the authoritative educational approach, popular earlier in this century, by which the child was forced to obey his parents and submit to treatment in spite of his anxiety, have left us with numerous adults for whom dental treatment is seen as a major threat.

Even with the modern treatment methods and the more open approach to patients characteristic of dentistry today, in some instances the initial dental encounter can be traumatic and stress-inflicting. Stress may be caused by the fear of pain associated with the needle penetration, fear of the vibrations of the drill, or fear of loss of control. If untreated this may lead to classic negative conditioning, resulting in behavioral dysfunctions (e.g., anxiety, fear, avoidance) related to the dental situation (see also Chapter 4).

2. Operant (Instrumental) Conditioning

Operant behaviors include those which have an effect on one's environment (walking, crying, etc.) and are modified or maintained by the consequences that follow them. Operant or instrumental conditioning is a learning situation whereby certain events or consequences are made conditional on specified behaviors.[36] Positive and negative reinforcement, biofeedback, extinction, and punishment are methods of operant conditioning (see also Chapter 10).

A dental practitioner who acts without perseverance toward an apprehensive patient only serves to reinforce the negative behavior, thereby increasing the patient's fear. Reactions of impatience toward the "difficult to handle" patient, associated with unconscious punishment (treatment applied in an abrupt, harsh manner), reinforces the negative behavior of the patient, leading to further threat appraisal and anxiety.

Processes of operant conditioning serve as means to shape one's behavior in various situations throughout life. Beliefs, customs, and goals may be learned through operant conditioning. Some learning (especially that relevant to dentistry) is based on negative reinforcement — something painful, uncomfortable or fearful that is to be avoided. Learning of this type includes escape (to flee from an unpleasant situation once the individual is in the situation) and avoidance learning (to avoid or to prevent the unpleasant situation before it occurs). These two types of learning are usually linked together; one must first learn to escape before learning to avoid the situation in the future.[4] A patient who has learned to perceive the dental situation as painful, fearful, and threatening will develop ways to escape treatment while in the dental chair (e.g., developing a gagging reflex which prevents treatment; see Chapter 5) or to just avoid treatment.

B. INDIRECT LEARNING

An experience does not necessarily have to occur directly to an individual for learning to take place. Learning can be a result of observation. Since, the reward or punishment is not direct in such cases, they are defined as vicarious. One sees what happens to another and, presumably, assumes that one's own fate would be similar in the same situation.[44-46]

Vicarious learning, or modeling, is based on principles of imitation and identification with the model figure, in many instances a parent. Whiting[47] suggested that a child learns various roles by watching parents, without necessarily wanting to perform them. The child learns the adult patterns of conduct, and even if not used immediately, they are available if and when needed.

Thus, a child who accompanies his/her mother to the dentist and watches her apprehension may imitate this behavior later when facing dental treatment. Kleinknecht et al.[39] implicated the role of vicarious arousal and classical conditioning through exposure to the aversive reactions of family and friends or the mass media.

The effect of parental attitudes toward dental treatment does not necessarily have to be carried out by direct imitation of the model's behavior. It may also be by identification with the parent who is constantly complaining about the pain (caused by the teeth or the treatment). Identification with the "suffering" model creates a negative stimulus which causes dental treatment to be held as a threatening event to be avoided.

Vicarious learning can also be carried out through indirect suggestions of the models. Shoben and Borland[48] proposed that parents who suffer traumatic experiences involving the facial area, with dentists or physicians, become emotionally sensitized and communicate fears to their children. When a mother, bringing her child to the dentist, reassures in a trembling voice that "...there is no reason to worry...it will not hurt at all..." the nonverbal suggestion may often be the reverse and cause threat appraisal. Indeed, a direct relationship between the mother's anxiety and the child's behavior has been reported[49-53] (see also Chapter 4).

Indirect, vicarious learning is carried out not only by parents, but by the social environment as well. A classmate who returns from dental surgery with horrifying stories about the treatment can serve as a negative stimulus to his friends.

VI. COGNITIVE PROCESSES

Human behavior and physiological states are also affected by cognitive processes such as thoughts, attitudes, and beliefs.[36,54-57] People act in certain ways because they believe they should or must act this way; their emotions are caused and controlled by thinking; their attitudes towards a certain situation (denial, anger, guilt, acceptance, etc.) influence both their psychological and physiological reactions.

In other words, sensing, feeling, moving, and thinking are not experienced in isolation. If an individual senses something (e.g., pain during dental treatment) there is a tendency, at the same time, to do something about it (clench fists, groan), to have a feeling about it (dislike, hate), and to think about it (remember previous encounters, imagine what damage it caused).[54]

Cognitive processes are involved during dental situations just as in other situations in life. Attitudes, beliefs, expectations, and anticipations connected with dental treatment affect the final behavior of the patient. A patient arriving for treatment expecting it to cause pain or suffering is more prone to experience pain than the patient who does not anticipate pain.[58] Unfortunately, many people expect pain to be involved with treatment in some way.[59] Thus, dental care becomes linked to pain and suffering so that a strong cognitive set exists before the person even arrives for treatment. Under this condition, even the most benign acts of the dentist may be perceived as painful.

If the patient arrives with an initial attitude of anger towards "those dentists who have ruined my mouth," it is highly probable that there will be a reaction of anger and mistrust toward the dentist and to any suggested treatment procedures. The image of the treatment as causing damage to tissues ("...It was only a small hole...Why do I feel such a huge cavity?"); or damage to the esthetic appearance ("My teeth were much brighter before the dentist put on the crowns.") increases threat appraisal in many cases.

VII. DENTIST-PATIENT INTERPERSONAL RELATIONSHIP

Medical treatment is team work; it includes a close interpersonal interaction between the patient and the medical staff. Creating a proper doctor-patient relationship is directly related to the patient's compliance and success of treatment.

Basically, three types of doctor-patient relationships are possible:[60] the active-passive relationship, in which the doctor assumes full responsibility for the patient while the patient is not reacting (e.g., in treating an unconscious patient); the guidance-cooperation model, in which the physician advises, directs, and instructs the patient, expecting the patient to carry out the given instructions; and the mutual cooperation model, in which the patient is a full partner in taking responsibility for his/her health.

Dental treatment is a medical discipline requiring a lifelong interaction with the dentist and imposing constant demands for cooperation from the patient (e.g., preserving oral hygiene, periodic examinations). Its success, therefore, is based on developing proper patient-dentist interpersonal relationships which will enable mutual trust.

The dental profession is also unique in that the dentist usually works alone,[61] often independent of colleagues or professionals who can critically judge his work. While the average physician is part of a network (hospitals, specialists, and medical technologists),[62] the professional relationships of many dentists are almost exclusively with their patients.[63] The patients are those who provide the dentist with most of the professional feedback and esteem needed. Therefore, proper interpersonal relationships are as important to the dentist as they are to patients.

A. THE DENTIST'S PERSONALITY, ATTITUDES, AND BEHAVIOR

Whether the patient develops apprehension, or cooperation and trust, toward dental treatment is highly dependent on the attitudes, personality, and behavior of the dentist. Patients who are satisfied with their dentist's interpersonal skills are more likely to follow instructions and less likely to cancel appointments,[64] whereas patients who have a negative image of the dental profession are less likely to show up for preventive examinations.[65]

Fear and anxiety towards dental treatment often originate from an earlier aversive encounter with a dentist. The negative experience need not stem from pain or physical injury, but can be caused by the dentist's failure to establish a proper interpersonal relationship with the patient. Patients suffering from a high level of anxiety regarding dental treatment often recall "impersonal, noncaring, disinterested, or cold" behavior from the dentist.[66] Similarly, a high percentage of patients quote personal qualities as the most important when choosing and being satisfied with a dentist.[67,68]

The way in which patients perceive their dentist's behavior is significantly related to their satisfaction.[69,70] The patient-perceived dentist behaviors most associated with patient satisfaction are those portraying empathy, friendliness, and a calm and competent image to the patient.[70] Patients rate much more positively those dentists who interact with patients in a positive, active manner than those who do not communicate.[71] Patients usually seek competence and interpersonal and communication skills from their dentists.[72] The ideal dentist is one who possesses a pleasant, friendly, understanding, and supportive personality and who has the ability to put patients at ease.[73-75]

As in all other disciplines where people relate to each other, satisfaction or dissatisfaction with the another's personality is most highly affected by personal reasons. Some patients are pleased with a dentist who acts in a permissive way and lets them participate in the various stages of the treatment. To others, such an approach can inflict feelings of indecisiveness and lack of confidence, and a more authoritative approach would be advisable. For example, in one study, permissive behavior of dental students toward their child patients led to the children being uncooperative.[76]

When the dentist's personality and behavior match those of the patient, it is highly probable that a firm, healthy interpersonal relationship will develop. Ayer[77] suggested that dentists select their patients (and patients their dentists) on the basis of mutually shared values. However, the effect of a personal accord between dentist and patient occasionally is disadvantageous to the latter. Health care professionals prefer to spend more time and are more successful with patients who are similar to themselves and share their values.[78,79] Dentists who are generally of a high socioeconomic level would be expected to relate well with high-status patients.[74] Indeed, some dentists reported negative stereotypes of patients from a low educational and economic background.[80] Concomitantly, patients who were well motivated and cooperative (qualities valued by most dentists) were found to receive better care as measured by the quality of their dental restorations.[81]

Furthermore, a dentist's conception about himself, his profession, and his patients is profoundly affected by the long course of professional socialization in dentistry. The average dental student tends to be pragmatic, conforming, conservative, with a considerable interest in earning money and prestige.[82] Sherlock and Morris[83,84] found that among dental students, professional ethics declined steadily throughout their education, while cynicism increased, especially during the clinical years. Vinton[85] reported that dental school graduates place less value on interpersonal communication and more value on personal interests and goals. Similarly, Moody et al.[86] and Eli and Shuval[87] and Eli[88,89] reported the increasing cynicism of students during dental school.

This process can be attributed, in part, to the failure of the faculty in dental schools to provide students with the people-oriented traits that are important to the profession.[89] Israeli as well as American dental students criticize their faculty and quote improper or degrading behavior,[90] lack of interest in students,[91] lack of helpfulness to students,[92] and lack of "humane" traits[89] as some of the problems. Medical students express patterns of classic modeling with regard to the most idealistic and most cynical professional norms.[93] Accordingly, there may be a basis to the suggestion raised by MacKenzie[94] that there is a relationship between criticism of the faculty by students and the negative change in their attitudes and tendencies. The future professionals become influenced (even if unwillingly and unconsciously) by their role models in their perceptions of the chosen profession.

Although some evidence exists that the growing cynicism of the young professionals may be situational in nature,[86,88,95] the negative tendencies of the professional helper's perceptions work, in many cases, against their motivation to help others.[79] This fact should be a cause of concern, as unchecked patient management problems will transfer to and adversely affect the dentist's future professional practice.[96]

B. THE PATIENT'S PERSONALITY, ATTITUDES, AND BEHAVIOR

Just as the dentist's behavior, attitudes, and personality affect interpersonal relationships with patients, so does the patient's. As previously mentioned, health professionals (dentists included) tend to devote more time and relate better to patients with whom they feel closer.[67,78-81] Apprehension, mistrust, and/or dissatisfaction on the part of the patient have been reported as unpleasant and stress-inflicting to the dentist.[97-101] Conversely, high motivation and cooperation from the patient are valued by most dentists.[81]

Thus, it is probable that highly cooperative, relaxed patients, with pleasant personalities and relatively high socioeconomic status, will be preferred by the dentist and may even obtain better treatment.[81] These patients are likely to communicate easily with the dentist on an intellectual level, to understand and properly carry out instructions, and accept suggestions as to necessary treatment. Proper interpersonal relationships will provide the dentist with the desired feedback and esteem and increase his/her willingness to further provide the best treatment possible.

The apprehensive, mistrustful, and uncooperative patient causes increased stress and decreased motivation on behalf of the dentist to "invest time" in the patient. Instead of devoting extra attention to these patients, in order to gain their trust and compliance, many dentists tend to revoke the need for special care. It is easier to put the blame on the patient ("...He simply does not understand my instructions," "I cannot carry on with the treatment if you are so tense and restless") than to try and cope in the often unfamiliar fields of communication and behavior management. Thus, some of those patients most in need of dental care are most rejected and neglected by the professional community.

Cheney[102] suggested a model for the interrelationship between patient and dentist based on a personality assessment of the patient with regard to the parameter of "locus of control" — a belief held by people as to being in control of what happens to them. People with an external locus of control believe that whatever happens is a result of luck, fate, chance, or some powerful other being. They are unlikely to change their beliefs and behavior. In a study by Duke and Cohen,[103] "poor" patients were found to be significantly more external than "good" patients. The "poor" patients were uncooperative, did not follow the dentist's instructions, missed appointments, and generally appeared to be non-self monitors. Their feeling is that dental home care is useless, due to the "bad teeth" they now have. This causes them to ignore instructions and rely (as in other fields in life) on external factors such as fate, heredity, etc.

On the other hand, people with an internal locus of control believe that they are in control of what happens to them and that they are responsible for what happens (i.e., their oral disease). They accept responsibility for proper oral care and will usually be cooperative patients who collaborate to preserve their oral hygiene[103,104] and follow instructions to the letter.

C. COMMUNICATION SKILLS

Communication is the "magic" word by which we often explain our success, or lack of it, in dealing with interpersonal problems. Although dentistry is considered to be basically a technically oriented profession, the dentist's communication patterns have a significant influence on the behavior of their patients[76,105] and play an important role in coping with the patient's anxiety.[72,106]

Dworkin et al.[16] defined three critical stages essential for effective communication: attention, comprehension, and acceptance. For effective communication, it is necessary for the message to be received (seen, heard, or felt), understood, and accepted by the listener. If failure occurs in one of the stages, proper communication will not take place. The communication skills of both the dentist and the patient determine whether the transmitted message will succeed in grasping the patient's attention and whether it will be understood and accepted.

The dental situation does not generally favor mutual communication. The dentist is often seen as a person carrying a one-way conversation, while the patient is unable to participate because of the instruments and materials which are in his mouth.[107]

Communication is a *two-way street*. It is not enough for the dentist just to transmit messages to the patient. Receiving the patient's verbal and nonverbal messages is equally important in developing a rapport and a positive interpersonal relationship. If the dentist fails to receive and/or relate to messages of distress from the patient, this can lead to mistrust, anger, and further anxiety and avoidance. Understanding of and relating to the patient's stress and anxiety serve as an initial way to establish mutual trust and compliance.

The communication skills of both parties are important. The dentist transmits messages to the patient, but must also be sensitive to the messages transmitted back. It is helpful if the patient can send his messages in a clear, understandable manner, admit his/her apprehension, and pinpoint its source (fear of pain, injection, drill, etc.). It is more complicated if the patient fails to admit his feelings (even to himself) and appears cooperative, while his body language transmits opposite messages.

1. Verbal Communication

Verbal communication is the most common source of sending and receiving information. People communicate through talking and expressing syllables ("…a-ha.…oh…" etc.).

Too often we simply listen to the words without understanding what is really being said. For example "…How much longer will it take?…" can mean that the patient is in a hurry, but can also transmit the indirect message that he/she is tense and anxious to terminate the treatment. If the dentist answers only to the superficial aspect of the question ("another 10 minutes") and does not refer to its deeper possible meanings, an indirect message of misunderstanding and/or lack of acceptance of the patient's feelings is transmitted.

To establish proper interpersonal relationships, it is the dentist's responsibility to be attentive, to show understanding, and to accept the real messages of the patient, beyond the limits of the apparently clear verbal communication. A better understanding of the patient and more attention paid to the nonverbal signs are essential in this respect.

2. Nonverbal Communication

Verbal communication generally implies sharing cognitive tasks and problems, whereas the nonverbal aspects of the conversation have a greater impact on the emotional aspect of the relationship.[74] Emotions, such as friendship, assertiveness, and dominance, are reported to depend more on nonverbal than verbal behavior.[108,109]

Nonverbal communication in health care interactions primarily involves the cues of emotion through facial expressions, body posture and movements, and voice tone and inflections. The physician's ability to read emotions conveyed through the nonverbal channel, as well as his ability to express his own emotions through nonverbal communication, was found to positively correlate with patient satisfaction.[110,111]

The face, a powerful channel of expression, is a rich and reliable source of information about how one feels.[112] There are distinct, characteristic facial expressions that accompany acute painful experiences[113,114] that can be overlooked by the dentist. During treatment, the dentist's eyes are concentrated in the small, confined work area, a fact which often causes neglect of nonverbal signs from the patient. Since the patient's mouth is blocked, nonverbal communication is the only way messages can be transmitted to the environment. Lowering the brow with the skin drawn in tightly around closed eyes,[113,114] clenching the fists, and/or flexing or extending the feet or palms are clear signs of tension, apprehension, or pain.

3. Development of Mutual Trust

Mutual trust is a fundamental aspect of any proper interpersonal relationship. It is especially crucial in medical situations in which the patient submits himself to the hands of the doctor, often without a clear understanding of the procedures involved. Lack of trust enhances feelings of helplessness and increases threat appraisal and stress response.

Mutual trust is usually established after several visits during which both the patient and the dentist observe one another. Interpersonal communication skills, verbal and nonverbal messages, play a major role in this process. A patient who is apprehensive has to gain the reassurance that the apprehension is understood and accepted; similarly a patient who fears losing control must gain the confidence that the situation can be mastered through agreed–upon signs, and treatment will really cease when the sign is given.

Friedman et al.[115] described the doctor/patient relationship as a pyramid. The building starts with initial communication during which the doctor projects attitudes, warmth, interest, and aloofness and collects information while the patient projects feelings and expresses his dental needs, experience, and expectations. Gradually, as oral examination and treatment commence, mutual trust is established allowing complex dental procedures to be performed.

VIII. ENVIRONMENTAL FACTORS

A. SOCIAL LEARNING

All life events are influenced by the social setting in which they occur. When in the presence of others, our thoughts, feelings, and actions are, to some degree, guided by them. Several social variables play a role in defining dental treatment as a stressful situation.

1. Cultural Factors

Profound differences exist among societies in many aspects. Hall[23] described how accepted social and personal distances vary in the cross-cultural context. What is acceptable in one culture is often unacceptable in another. Similarly, there are broad cultural differences in dental behaviors, attitudes, and methods of treatment of oral disease.

Kiyak,[116,117] and Price and Kiyak,[118] reported the cultural differences in the way people view dental esthetics and good oral hygiene in general. For example, among low-income citizens of Seattle, Caucasian patients were better informed about the causes and consequences of dental disease, but were less likely to perform appropriate health care behaviors than Pacific Asians. Asians were more concerned about the esthetic and social consequences of poor oral health and more likely to describe pain as an outcome of dental disease.[116]

Domoto et al.[119] studied dental patients in Japan and reported some differences between the behavior of Japanese and American patients. Although the prevalence of dental fear in Japan appears to be higher than among the American population, and although the Japanese show a higher tendency to delay appointments because of fear, they were found less likely to cancel once the appointment was made, due to their strong sense of obligation to authority figures.

With respect to actual dental treatment, international comparisons of dental health reveal significant differences among different communities. For example, a much higher proportion of adult patients in New Zealand wear full dentures than comparable groups in other countries with similar levels of dental disease. While the European tradition is oriented towards the preservation of the natural dentition, in Australia and New Zealand there is a tendency towards extraction of teeth and fitting of dentures.[120]

The concept of pain and pain reaction is affected by cultural factors as well. Zborowski[121] pointed out several paths of reaction to pain among different ethnic groups in the U.S. (see Chapter 3).

2. Socioeconomic Factors

Dental treatment usually involves considerable expense. But the effect of social class and status is beyond pure financial significance. Awareness of the need of dental care, as well as awareness of health and esthetics in general, change among different socioeconomic groups.

Parents of high socioeconomic status cite professional competence as a reason for their satisfaction with the dentist, whereas parents of low socioeconomic status state a positive relationship between their child and the dentist as being most important.[122] Furthermore, patients of high socioeconomic status expect their "ideal dentist" to be, first of all, skillful and only later, friendly and informative. Patients of low socioeconomic status quote reassurance and friendliness as most important with professional skill rated lower.[123]

Although the negative perception of patients of low socioeconomic status as being less interested in dental care than in material things was found to be incorrect,[80] this is still a common public and professional view. Such stereotypes can affect actual patient care. Those who feel that their problems are not appreciated or understood may eventually act in the way which is expected.[74]

3. Family Factors

The family, as the most basic social group, has an enormous impact on attitudes toward dental care. Parents serve as initial models for behavior to the developing child. Their attitude and behavior towards dental treatment affects the future behavior and attitudes of the child. Anxious mothers have been found to exert negative influence on their children in that maternal anxiety was found to be related to the child's behavioral problems.[57,124,125]

The parent's behavior before, during, and after dental treatment has a profound conscious and subconscious impact on the child. Parental behavior varies from family to family. Passive noninvolvement, attempting to obtain cooperation through threats and physical intervention, or attempting to reduce upset through verbal reassurance and physical contact are some of the possible behavioral patterns. Each, of course, may have a different effect according to the basic parent-child relationship of the family.

4. The Public View of Dentistry

As part of a community, the patient's attitudes toward dentistry and dental treatment are indirectly affected by the media and through social encounters. More than 25 years ago, Boissonneault[126] expressed the opinion that in the public's view, dentists have become known as a group who do nothing but practice dentistry; they do not provide community leadership or support community activities with either time or money.

This view may reflect only the personal opinion of the writer, now even outdated. Still, many dentists feel that they practice a profession which has a materialistic, and somewhat negative, image. In some studies, dental students thought of their chosen profession as a highly prestigious occupation.[92] However, many others perceived themselves as entering a profession which the public views somewhat unfavorably.[63] A high percentage of dental students feel people view dentists negatively because they have only mechanical skills (60% of the respondents), because of the pain they cause (44%), or because they charge high fees (32%).[63]

This unfavorable professional image is not necessarily true. However, since the interaction of people in social settings is influenced by the image one person believes is attributed to him by the other,[127] it can have a direct effect on the patient-dentist relationship.

Reports concerning the public view of the dental profession often conclude that there is no one image of dentistry but a variety of attitudes.[128] Generally, dentists are highly prestigious in the eyes of the public.[129-132] This prestige, however, is usually related to extrinsic, rather than intrinsic, aspects of the profession (the financial rewards involved with practicing dentistry).[123,131,132] In a study conducted in the Netherlands, respondents generally did not perceive dentists as caring, helping people; rather they found them to be remote and interested primarily in money.[123]

One of the charges most readily made against dentists by the American public is their apparent interest in "making money."[133] This is also the most frequently mentioned advantage of being a dentist by both adults and teenagers.[132] The dentist is often seen as one who is responsible for his own working hours and situation, but is less likely to have an interesting or satisfying job when compared to a physician or a high school teacher.[82]

The dental care system and dental education, as presently structured, does not serve the best interests of the public.[131] Dental science is generally isolated from the various branches of medicine, and active concern for dental health tends to be restricted to a small percentage of the affluent and educated. In 1987, about 71% of the dentists in the U.S. were solo practitioners.[61] This may be due, in part, to the general public view of the profession which causes large segments of the population to regard the dental professional as narrow minded and noninterested in the overall well-being of the person.

5. The Clinical Set-Up

The dental surgery itself, with its unfamiliar materials and instruments, serves as a stimulus which increases threat appraisal and causes a stress response. Smells of dental materials, the sight of sharp, unfamiliar instruments, and/or hearing threatening sounds are environmental factors which increase apprehension.

Even the architectural features of the dentist's office can convey many messages.[74] Decor, color design, illumination, wall pictures, and background music all contribute to create the general atmosphere.

Recently more attention is given to the organization of the dental clinic. Still, in many operatories, the display of the various instruments in front of the patient is quite threatening. Clinics especially designed for pedodontic practice and a modern approach to clinic design address some of these variables.

IX. THE DENTIST'S VIEW

Dentistry is commonly perceived as a stressful profession. The dental practitioner faces many physical environmental stressors — equipment noise, potential hazards from noxious gases, vapors, viruses, and bacteria, and the effects of working for extended periods of time.[134]

Christen[135] listed the stressors that dentists are subjected to during their professional work. These include operational stressors (working in a relatively restricted surrounding; compulsive cleanliness; working in confined, dark areas; time pressure; little peer support; high cost of equipment; etc.); interpersonal stressors (pressure of decision making, fear, anxiety, and pain associated with the dental treatment, rejection from patients, personnel management, etc.); and office environmental stressors (physical fatigue, inadequate lighting, noise, air pollution, eye and facial injuries, etc.).

Although most dentists are generally satisfied with their profession, some aspects of their work are often cited as more stressful than others. Trying to maintain a schedule and to cope with difficult patients are two important sources of stress.[97,99-101,136] Difficult, uncooperative patients, running behind schedule, constant time pressures, and nervous and dissatisfied patients rank high in the list of the most common sources of stress reported by British dentists.[99] Aspects of professional isolation, physical confinement, high caseloads, economic pressures, anxious patients, lack of recognition and appreciation by patients, and the stress of constantly striving for perfection were quoted by Forrest[137] as the most damaging stressors associated with the dental profession. Similarly, falling behind schedule, striving for technical perfection, causing pain and anxiety in patients, cancelled or late appointments, and lack of cooperation from patients in the chair are the most particularly noted stressors by American dentists.[100]

Dentistry is an almost "impossible" profession. To run a private dental practice, the competent dentist is required to[138]

- be a high level technician — work with utmost precision in a wet, contaminated environment with limited illumination and complicated access
- be a good "salesman" — persuade and "sell" the care and service needed which is not always understood or desired
- be a psychologist — refer to the stress and fear of the patients, be able to establish good interpersonal relationships, be trained in the various aspects of behavioral treatment
- be a businessman — hire and manage personnel, keep financial records, manage inventory, order supplies
- be a scientist — read scientific literature, understand relevant scientific issues, stay abreast of the field, attend meetings

To combine all these qualities in one person is almost impossible. To perform each one of the involved tasks well and find it pleasant or even bearable is extremely difficult. Herein lies the major stress of the profession: for most dentists some of their professional life is spent in work that, to them, is unpleasant or frustrating.[138]

Some authors have suggested that personality traits which characterize a good dentist are traits which predispose to depression, and that dental schools frequently select candidates with an obsessive-compulsive character.[137] In various studies, the average dental student was found to be "conventional, conforming, conservative, preferring the status quo, concerned about seeming proper or right, concerned about what others think of him, deferential to authority, unconsciously aggressive, persistent, conscientious, methodical, somewhat rigid and inflexible, neat and orderly, nonintraceptive, ..."[139] — all traits with some predisposition to stress.

Some of the data which reported an extraordinary high suicide rate among dentists[140,141] are considered unreliable today.[142,143] However, there is no dispute that dentistry is a difficult profession that causes considerable stress not only to the patient but also to the dental practitioner. When under stress, the dentist unwillingly conveys these feelings to the surroundings, including patients. Sensing an atmosphere of tension, patients react with stress of their own, thus creating a vicious cycle of mutual stress and tension.

X. SUMMARY

Stress is a common feature among both patients and dentists. The complex role of the oral cavity during the early stages of human development and throughout our life, makes this area in our body especially stress-prone. Furthermore, the dental situation itself bears numerous factors which act as potential "stressors," such as an imminence of physical harm, anticipation of harm, feeling of loss of control, etc.

Stress during dental treatment may originate in learned responses (such as former aversive encounters with a dentist), environmental factors (such as a public negative view of dentistry), or an impaired communication with the dentist. It is also affected by the dentist's own stress when facing the anxious, uncooperative patient.

Dental treatment is perceived as stress-inflicting in many patients. This leads to the development of various oro-related behavioral dysfunctions which pose a severe obstacle in administering proper dental care (see Chapters 4 to 9).

REFERENCES

1. **Lazarus, R. S.,** Some principles of psychological stress and their relation to dentistry, *J. Dent. Res.,* 45, 1620, 1966.
2. **Agras, S., Sylvester, D., and Oliveau, D.,** The epidemiology of common fears and phobias, *Compr. Psychiatry*, 10, 151, 1969.
3. **Fiset, L., Milgrom, P., and Melnick, S.,** Identification of the relationship between dental and non-dental fears, *J. Dent. Res.*, 67, 169, Abstr. No. 453, 1988.
4. **Morgan, C. T. and King, R. A.,** *Introduction to Psychology*, McGraw-Hill, New York, 1966.
5. **Lautch, H.,** Dental phobia, *Br. J. Psychiatry*, 119, 151, 1971.
6. **Duivenvoorden H. J., Schuurs, A. H. B., Thoden, van Velzen, S. K., Verhage, F., Makkes, P. C., and Eijkman, M. A. J.,** Influence of repression upon the measurement of dental anxiety, *Community Dent. and Oral Epidemiology*, 13, 315, 1985.
7. **Schuurs, A. H. B., Duivenvoorden, H. J., Thoden van Velzen, S. K., and Verhage, F.,** Three factors predicting irregular versus regular dental attendance: A model fitting to empirical data, *Community Dentistry Oral Epidemiol.*, 8, 413, 1980.
8. **Lazarus, R. S.,** *Psychological Stress and the Coping System*, McGraw-Hill, New York, 1966, 465.
9. **Freud, S.,** *The Standard Edition of the Complete Psychological Works of Sigmund Freud*, translated by Strachey, J. in collaboration with Freud, A., Hogarth, London, 1961.
10. **Erikson, E.,** *Childhood and Society,* W. W. Norton, New York, 1950.
11. **Piaget, J.,** *The Origins of Intelligence in Children*, International University Press, New York, 1952.
12. **Inhelder, B. and Piaget, J.,** *The Growth of Logical Thinking from Childhood to Adolescence*, Basic Books, New York, 1958.

13. **Levinson, N. A.,** Psychologic facets of esthetic dental health care: A developmental perspective, *J. Prosthet. Dent.*, 64, 486, 1990.
14. **Penfield, W. and Rasmussen, T.,** *The Cerebral Cortex of Man, A Clinical Study of Localization and Function*, MacMillan, New York, 1957.
15. **Maslow, A. H.,** *Motivation and Personality*, Harper & Row, New York, 1954, 411.
16. **Dworkin, S. F., Ference, T. P., and Giddon, D. B.,** *Behavioral Science and Dental Practice*, C. V. Mosby, St. Louis, 1978.
17. **Every, R. G.,** The teeth as weapons: their influence on behaviour (hypothesis), *Lancet*, March, 685, 1965.
18. **Every, R. G.,** The significance of extreme mandibular movements, *Lancet*, 2, 37, 1960.
19. **Kent, G.,** Anxiety, pain and type of dental procedure, *Behav. Res. and Ther.*, 22, 465, 1984.
20. **Stouthard, M. E. A. and Hoogstraten, J.,** Ratings of fears associated with twelve dental situations, *J. Dent. Res.*, 66, 1175, 1987.
21. **McNeil, D. W. and Berryman, M. L.,** Components of dental fear in adults?, *Behav. Res. and Ther.*, 27, 233, 1989.
22. **Corah, N. L. and Salmonson, R. J,** Psychologic response to a simulated dental procedure as a function of proximity to an actual dental appointment, *J. Dent. Res.*, 49, 438, 1970.
23. **Hall, E. T.,** *The Hidden Dimension*, Doubleday, New York, 1966.
24. **Abercrombie, M. L. J.,** Face to face — proximity and distance, *J. of Psychosom. Res.*, 15, 395, 1971.
25. **Argyle, M. and Ingham, R., Gaze,** mutual gaze, and proximity, *Semiotica*, 6, 32, 1972.
26. **Singer, J. E. and Davidson, L. M.,** Specifity and stress research, in *Dynamics of Stress*, Appley, M. H. and Trumbull, R., Eds., Plenum Press, New York, 1986.
27. **Lazarus, R. S. and Cohen, J. B.,** Environmental stress, in *Human Behaviour and the Environment: Current Theory and Research,* Vol. 2, Altman, I. and Wohlwill, J. F., Eds., Plenum Press, New York, 1977, 89.
28. **Mittwoch, T., Weisenberg, M., and Mikulincer, M.,** The influence of warning signal timing and cognitive preparation on the aversiveness of electric shock, *Pain*, 42, 373, 1990.
29. **Lindsay, S. J. E., Wege, P., and Yates, J.,** Expectations of sensations, discomfort and fear in dental treatment, *Behav. Res. Ther.*, 22, 99, 1984.
30. **Averill, J. R.,** Personal control over aversive stimuli and its relationship to stress, *Psychol. Bull.*, 80, 286, 1973.
31. **Logan, H. L. and Stein, S.,** Perceived control and dental fear revisited, *J. Dent. Res.*, 67, 170, Abstract 457, 1988.
32. **Tullman, G. M., Tullman, M. J., Rogers, B. J., and Rosen, J. B.,** Anxiety in dental patients: a study of three phases of state anxiety in three treatment groups, *Psychol. Rep.*, 45, 407, 1979.
33. **Morris, D.,** *The Naked Ape*, Jonathan Cape, London, 1967.
34. **Wolpe, J.,** *The Practice of Behavior Therapy*, Pergamon Press, Elmsford, N.Y., 1982.
35. **Pavlov, I. P.,** *Conditioned Reflexes*, translated by Anrep, G. V., Liveright, New York, 1927.
36. **Melamed, B. G. and Siegal, L. J.,** *Behavioral Medicine*, Springer-Verlag, New York, 1980.
37. **Watson, J. B. and Raynor, R.,** Conditioned emotional reactions *Exp. Psychol.*, 3, 1, 1920.
38. **Lautch, H.,** Dental phobia, *Br. J. Psychiatry*, 119, 151, 1971.
39. **Kleinknecht, R. A., Klepac, R. K., and Alexander, L. D.,** Origins and characteristics of fear of dentistry, *J. Amer. Dent. Assoc.*, 86, 842, 1973.
40. **Bernstein, D. A., Kleinknecht, R. A., and Alexander, L. D.,** Antecedents of dental fear, *J. Public Health Dent.*, 39, 113, 1979.
41. **Cohen, L. A., Snyder, T. L., and LaBelle, A. D.,** Correlates of dental anxiety in a university population, *J. Public Health Dent.*, 42, 228, 1982.
42. **Berggren, U. and Meynert, G.,** Dental fear and avoidance: causes, symptoms, and consequences, *J. Am. Dent. Assoc.*, 109, 247, 1984.

43. **Forgione, A. G. and Clark, R. E.,** Comments on an empirical study of the causes of dental fear, *J. Dent. Res.*, 53, 496, 1974.
44. **Lazarus, R. S.,** *Patterns of Adjustment and Human Effectiveness*, McGraw-Hill, New York, 1969.
45. **Bandura, A. L.,** *Principles of Behavior Modification*, Holt, Rinehart & Winston, New York, 1969.
46. **Bandura, A. L. and McDonald, F. J.,** The influence of social reinforcement and the behavior of models in shaping children's moral judgments, *J. Abnorm. Soc. Psychol.*, 67, 274, 1963.
47. **Whiting, J. W. M.,** Resource mediation and learning by identification, in *Personality Development in Children*, Iscoe, I. and Stevenson, H., Eds., University of Texas Press, Austin, 1960.
48. **Shoben, E. J., Jr. and Borland, L.,** An empirical study of the etiology of dental fear, *J. of Clin. Psychol.*, 10, 171, 1954.
49. **Shaw, O.,** Dental anxiety in children, *Br. Dent. J.*, 139, 134, 1975.
50. **Johnson, R. and Baldwin, D. C.,** Relationship of maternal anxiety to the behavior of young children undergoing dental extraction, *J. Dent. Res.*, 47, 801, 1968.
51. **Koenigsberg, S. R. and Johnson, R. J.,** Child behavior during sequential dental visits, *J. Am. Dent. Assoc.*, 85, 128, 1972.
52. **Holst, A., Schroder, U., Ek., L., Hallonsten, A.-L., and Crossner, C.-G.,** Prediction of behavior management problems in children, *Scand. J. Dent. Res.*, 96, 457, 1988.
53. **Johnson, R.,** Maternal influence on child behavior in the dental setting, *Psychiatry Med.*, 2, 221, 1971.
54. **Ellis, A.,** *Reason and Emotion in Psychotherapy*, Lyle Stuart, Secaucus, NJ, 1975.
55. **Lazarus, A.,** *Multi-Modal Behavioral Therapy*, Springer-Verlag, New York, 1976.
56. **Mahoney, M. J.,** *Cognition and Behavior Modification*, Ballinger, Cambridge, MA, 1974.
57. **Meichenbaum, D.,** *Cognitive Behavior Modification*, General Learning Press, Morristown, NJ, 1974.
58. **Anderson, D. B. and Pennebaker, J. W.,** Pain and pleasure: alternative interpretations for identical stimulation, *Eur. J. Soc. Psychol.*, 10, 207, 1980.
59. **Wardle, J.,** Fear of dentistry, *Br. J. Med. Psychol.*, 55, 119, 1982.
60. **Szasz, T. S. and Hollender, M. H.,** A contribution to the philosophy of medicine — the basic models of the doctor-patient relationship, *Arch. Intern. Med.*, 97, 585, 1956.
61. The American Dental Association, Dentists in Nonsolo and Solo Practice, The 1987 Survey of Dental Practice, Bureau of Economic and Behavioral Res.
62. **Hall, O.,** The stages of a medical career, *Am. J. Sociol.*, 53, 327, 1948.
63. **Quarantelli, E. L.,** The dental student image of the dentist-patient relationship, *J. Public Health*, 51, 1312, 1961.
64. **DiMatteo, M. R. and DiNicola, D. A.,** *Achieving Patient Compliance*, Pergamon Press, Oxford, 1982.
65. **Kent, G.,** Satisfaction with dental care: its relationship to utilization and allegiance, *Med. Care*, 22, 583, 1984.
66. **Bernstein, D. A., Kleinknecht, R. A., and Alexander, L. D.,** Antecedents of dental fear, *J. Public Health Dent.*, 39, 113, 1979.
67. **Craft, M. and Croucher, R.,** *The 16-20 Study*, Health Education Council, London, 1980.
68. **Bulman, J. S., Richard, N. D., Slack, G. C., and Willcocks A. J.,** *Demand and Need for Dental Care: A Socio-Dental Study*, Oxford University Press, London, 1968.
69. **Corah, N. L., O'Shea, R. M., and Bissell, G. D.,** The dentist-patient relationship: perceptions by patients of dentist behavior in relation to satisfaction and anxiety, *J. Am. Dent. Assoc.*, 111, 443, 1985.
70. **Corah, N. L., O'Shea, R. M., Bissell, G. D., Thines, T. J., and Mendola, P.,** The dentist-patient relationship: perceived dentist behaviors that reduce patient anxiety and increase satisfaction, *J. Am. Dent. Assoc.*, 116, 73, 1988.

71. **Gale, E. N., Carlsson, S. G., Eriksson, A., and Jontell, M.,** Effects of dentists' behavior on patients' attitudes, *J. Am. Dent. Assoc.*, 109, 444, 1984.
72. **Rouse, R. A. and Hamilton, M. A.,** Dentists' technical competence, communication, and personality as predictors of dental patient anxiety, *J. Behav. Med.*, 13, 307, 1990.
73. **McKeithan, E. J.,** The patients' image of the dentist, *J. Am. Coll. Dent.*, 33, 171, 1966.
74. **Kent, G. G.,** *The Psychology of Dental Care*, Wright and Sons, Bristol, England, 1984.
75. **Van Groenestijn, M. A. J., Maas-de Waal, C. J., Mileman, P. A., and Swallow, J. N.,** The ideal dentist, *Soc. Sci. Med.*, 14A, 533, 1980.
76. **Wurster, C. A., Weinstein, P., and Cohen, A. J.,** Communication patterns in pedodontics, *Percept. Mot. Skills*, 48, 159, 1979.
77. **Ayer, W. A.,** The dentist-patient relationship, *Int. Dent. J.*, 32, 56, 1982.
78. **Berkanovic, E. and Reeder, L. G.,** Can money buy the appropriate use of services? Some notes on the meaning of utilization data, *J. Health Soc. Behav.*, 15, 93, 1974.
79. **Wills, T. A.,** Perceptions of clients by professional helpers, *Psychol. Bull.*, 85, 968, 1978.
80. **Frazier, P. J., Jenny, J., Bagramian, R. A., Robinson E., and Proshek, J. M.,** Provider expectations and consumer perceptions of the importance and value of dental care, *Am. J. Public Health*, 67, 37, 1977.
81. **Weinstein, P., Milgrom, P., Ratener, P., and Morrison, K.,** Patient dental values and their relationship to oral health status, dentist perceptions and quality of care, *Community Dent. Oral Epidemiol.*, 7, 121, 1979.
82. **Fusillo, A. E. and Metz A. S.,** Social science research on the dental student, in *Social Sciences and Dentistry*, Richards, N. D. and Cohen, L. K., Eds., Federation Dentaire Internationale, The Hague, 1971, 15.
83. **Morris, R. T. and Sherlock, B. J,** Decline of ethics and the rise of cynicism in dental schools, *J. Health Soc. Biol.*, 12, 290, 1971.
84. **Sherlock, B. J. and Morris, R. T.,** *Becoming a Dentist*, Charles C. Thomas, Springfield, IL, 1972.
85. **Vinton, J. C.,** A four year longitudinal study of the impact on learning structure on dental student lifestyle values, *J. Dent. Educ.*, 42, 251, 1978.
86. **Moody, P. M., Van Tassel, C., and Cash, D. M.,** Cynicism, humanitarianism and dental career development, *J. Dent. Educ.*, 38, 645, 1974.
87. **Eli, I. and Shuval, J. T.,** Professional socialization in dentistry: a longitudinal study of attitude changes among dental students toward the dental profession, *Soc. Sci. Med.*, 16, 951, 1982.
88. **Eli, I.,** Professional socialization in dentistry: a longitudinal analysis of changes in students' expected professional rewards, *Soc. Sci. Med.*, 18, 297, 1984.
89. **Eli, I.,** The dental student and his teacher — Model or anti-model, *Isr. J. Dent. Sci.*, 2, 71, 1988.
90. **More, D. M.,** The dental student approaching graduation, *J. Am. Coll. Dent.*, 29, 115, 1962.
91. **Richardson, J. E.,** Expression of Satisfaction in Dental School, Dissertation, University of Iowa, Microfilm No. 680969, 1967.
92. **O'Shea, R. M., Lefkowitz, M. L., and Gray, S. B.,** Sociological perspective on the dental student, *J. Dent. Educ.*, 30, 311, 1966.
93. **Shuval, J. T.,** The roles of models in professional socialization, in *Entering Medicine: The Dynamics of Transition*, Pergamon Press, Oxford, 1980, 143.
94. **MacKenzie, R. S.,** Social science techniques in dental education, in *Social Science and Dentistry — A Critical Bibliography*, Richards, N. D. and Cohen, L. K., Eds., Federation Dentaire Internationale, The Hague, 1971.
95. **Eli, I., Judes, H., and Allerhand-Alexander, Y.,** Dentists and dentistry: attitude changes toward the chosen profession, *Hum. Relat.*, 41, 929, 1989.
96. **Weinstein, P., Smith, T. A., and Bartlett, R. C.,** A study of the dental student-patient relationship, *J. Dent. Res.*, 52, 1287, 1973.
97. **Cooper, C. L.,** Dentists under pressure: a social psychological study, in *White Collar and Professional Stress*, Cooper, C. L. and Marshall, J., Eds., John Wiley & Sons, London, 1980.

98. **Cooper, C. L., Mallinger, M., and Kahn, R.,** Identifying sources of occupational stress among dentists, *J. Occup. Psychol.*, 51, 227, 1978.
99. **Cooper, C. L., Watts, J., and Kelly, M.,** Job satisfaction, mental health, and job stressors among general dental practitioners in the UK, *Br. Dent. J.*, 162, 77, 1987.
100. **O'Shea, R. M., Corah, N. L., and Ayer, W. A.,** Sources of dentists' stress, *J. Am. Dent. Assoc.,* 109, 48, 1984.
101. **Corah, N. L., O'Shea, R. M., and Ayer, W. A.,** Dentists' management of patients' fear and anxiety, *J. Am. Dent. Assoc.*, 110, 734, 1985.
102. **Cheney, H. G.,** Effect of patient behavior and personality on treatment planning, *Dent. Clin. North Am.*, 21, 531, 1977.
103. **Duke, M. P. and Cohen, B.,** Locus of control as an indicator of patient cooperation, *J. Am. Coll. Dent.*, 42, 174, 1975.
104. **Ayer, W. A., Barnes, G. P., and Macy, P. G.,** Personality correlates and plaque scores, *Va. Dent. J.*, 50, 19, 1973.
105. **Froelich, R. E., Bishop, F. M., and Dworkin, S. F.,** *Communication in the Dental Office: A Programmed Manual for the Dental Professional*, C. V. Mosby, St. Louis, 1976.
106. **Liddell, A., Ackerman, C., and Locker, D.,** What dental phobics say about their dental experiences, *J. Can. Dent. Assoc.*, 56, 863, 1990.
107. **Hansen, R. G.,** The need for effective communication in dentistry, in *Communication in the Dental Office*, Froelich, R. E., Bishop, F. M., and Dworkin, S. F., Eds., C. V. Mosby, St. Louis, 1976.
108. **Argyle, M.,** *Social Interaction*, Methuen, London, 1969.
109. **Argyle, M., Alkema, F., and Gilmour, R.,** The communication of friendly and hostile attitudes by verbal and non-verbal signals, *Eur. J. Soc. Psychol.*, 1, 385, 1971.
110. **DiMatteo, M. R., Friedman, H. S., and Taranta, A.,** Sensitivity to bodily nonverbal communication as a factor in practitioner-patient rapport, *J. Nonverbal Behav.*, 4, 18, 1979.
111. **DiMatteo, M. R., Taranta, A., Friedman, H. S., and Prince, L. M.,** Predicting patient satisfaction from physicians' nonverbal communication skills, *Med. Care*, 18, 376, 1980.
112. **Dittmann, A. T.,** *Interpersonal Messages of Emotion*, Springer-Verlag, New York, 1972.
113. **LeResche, L.,** Facial expression in pain: a study of candid photographs, *J. Nonverbal Behav.*, 7, 46, 1982.
114. **LeResche, L. and Dworkin, S. F.,** Facial expression accompanying pain, *Soc. Sci. Med.*, 19, 1325, 1984.
115. **Friedman, N., Sugiyama, J., and Slavin, W.,** Clinical manual for pre-data publication, Publication of the Section of Behavioral Dentistry, University of Southern California.
116. **Kiyak, H. A.,** Dental beliefs, behaviors and health status among Pacific Asians and Caucasians, *Community Dent. Oral Epidemiol.*, 9, 10, 1981.
117. **Kiyak, H. A.,** Comparison of esthetic values among Caucasians and Pacific Asians, *Community Dent. Oral Epidemiol.*, 9, 219, 1981.
118. **Price, S. C. and Kiyak, H. A.,** A behavioral approach to improving oral health among the elderly, *Spec. Care Dent.*, 1, 267, 1981.
119. **Domoto, P. K., Weinstein, P., Melnick, S., Ohmura, M., Uchida, H., Ohmachi, K., Hori, M., Okazaki, Y., Shimamoto, T., Matsumura, S., and Shimono, T.,** Results of a dental fear survey in Japan: implications for dental public health in Asia, *Community Dent. Oral Epidemiol.*, 16, 199, 1988.
120. **Davis, P.,** Culture, inequality and the pattern of dental care in New Zealand, *Soc. Sci. Med.*, 15A, 801, 1981.
121. **Zborowski, M.,** Cultural components in responses to pain, *J. Soc. Issues*, 8, 16, 1952.
122. **Jenny, J., Frazier, P. J., Bagramian, R. A., and Proshek J. M.,** Parents' satisfaction and dissatisfaction with their children's dentist, *J. Public Health Dent.*, 33, 211, 1973.
123. **Van Groenestijn, M. A. J., Maas-de Waal, C. J., Mileman, P. A., and Swallow, J. N.,** The image of the dentist, *Soc. Sci. Med.*, 14A, 541, 1980.
124. **Johnson, R. and Baldwin, D. C.,** Maternal anxiety and child behavior, *J. Dent. Child.*, 36, 87, 1969.

125. **Bailey, P. M., Talbot, A., and Taylor, P. P.,** A comparison of maternal anxiety levels with anxiety levels manifested in the child dental patient, *J. Dent. Child.*, 40, 284, 1973.
126. **Boissonneault, G. A.,** A newspaperman looks at the dentist's image, *J. Am. Dent. Assoc.*, 66, 303, 1963.
127. **Strauss, A.,** *Mirrors and Masks: A Search for Identity*, Free Press, Glencoe, 1959.
128. **Willcocks, A. J. and Richards, N. D.,** Dental manpower and dentistry as an institution, in *Social Sciences and Dentistry*, Richards, N. D. and Cohen, L. K., Eds., Federation Dentaire Internationale, The Hague, 1971.
129. **Hodge, R., Treeman, P. H., and Russi, A.,** A comparative study of occupational prestige, in *Class, Status and Power*, Bendix, R. and Lipsit, S. M., Eds., Free Press, New York, 1966.
130. **O'Shea, R. M. and Cohen, L. K.,** The social sciences and dentistry, *J. Public Health Dent.*, 27, 45, 1967.
131. **Cohen, R.,** The quality of life of the dentist as perceived by society, *Int. Dent. J.*, 28, 332, 1978.
132. **Kreisberg, L. and Treiman, B. R.,** The public's view on dentistry as a profession, *J. Dent. Educ.*, 24, 247, 1961.
133. **Kreisberg, L. and Treiman, B. R.,** Dentists and the practice of dentistry as viewed by the public, *J. Am. Dent. Assoc.*, 64, 806, 1962.
134. **Katz, C. A.,** Stress factors operating in the dental office environment, *Dent. Clin. North Am.*, 30, S29, 1986.
135. **Christen, A.,** Stress and distress in dental practice, in *Occupational Hazards in Dentistry*, Goldman, H., Hartman, S., and Messite, J., Eds., Yearbook Medical Publishers, Chicago, 1984.
136. **Cooper, C. L.,** Dentists under pressure: a social psychological study, in *White Collar and Professional Stress*, Cooper, C. L. and Marshall, J., Eds., John Wiley & Sons, New York, 1980, 3.
137. **Forrest, W.,** Stresses and self destructive behaviors of dentists, *Dent. Clin. North Am.*, 22, 361, 1978.
138. **Jackson, E. and Mealiea, W. L.,** Stress management and personal satisfaction in dental practice, *Dent. Clin. North Am.*, 21, 559, 1977.
139. **Kirk, B. A., Cummings, R. W., and Hackett, H. T.,** Personal and vocational characteristics of dental students, *Personnel Guidance J.*, 41, 522, 1963.
140. **Blachly, P. H., Osterud, H. T., and Josslin R.,** Suicide in professional groups, *N. Engl. J. Med.*, 268, 1278, 1963.
141. **Glass, R.,** Mortality of New England Dentists 1921-1960, U. S. Department of Health, Education and Welfare, Washington, D. C., 1966.
142. **Rose, K. D. and Rosow, I.,** Physicians who kill themselves, *Arch. Gen. Psychiatry*, 29, 800, 1973.
143. **Orner, G.,** Mortality study of dentists: final report, *International Institute of Safety and Health*, Temple University, Philadelphia, 1976.

Chapter 3

THE EXPERIENCE OF PAIN — PSYCHOLOGICAL ASPECTS

Pain is a common and powerful "stressor" which causes threat appraisal. It is impossible to look at pain as a unique sensory reaction. Pain has a sensory component; however, it also is a psychological experience involving variables of behavioral, cognitive, and emotional origins. Like other "stressors," pain is influenced by variables dependent on culture, attention, anxiety, and cognition.

Pain is frequently associated with the dental situation. Fear of pain is the most significant predictor of dental fear in man.[1] Subjects who reported never having had anxieties concerning dental treatment were found less likely to have had a painful dental treatment than subjects who did report an anxiety.[2] Although many dentists deny that their patients experience pain during treatment,[3] up to 77% of patients report some degree of pain during their visits.[4] Furthermore, 46% of fearless and 70% of fearful patients expect treatment to be painful.[5]

Most of these patients refer to incidents of acute pain caused by the dental procedures. However, symptoms of chronic pain can also lead to severe oro-related behavioral dysfunctions (see Chapter 6). To better understand the complex nature of pain, some of the biological and psychological aspects will be explained, as related to the dental situation.

I. DEFINITION OF PAIN

Similar to the term "stress," the definition of "pain" has undergone basic changes in recent years, placing an increasing emphasis on the psychological, social, and cognitive aspects of the experience.

Initially, pain was defined merely with aspects of physical injury — "an unpleasant experience which we primarily associate with tissue damage or describe it in terms of tissue damage or both".[6] In 1979, the definition was changed to include aspects of the emotional experience involved — "an unpleasant *sensory and emotional* experience associated with *actual or potential* tissue damage, or described in terms of such damage"[7] (author's emphasis).

The latter definition recognizes and accepts that pain is also a psychological phenomenon. It is always subjective and unpleasant, therefore, an emotional experience. It is not necessarily connected to a stimulus and can sometimes be reported without direct tissue damage. Usually this happens for psychological reasons. There is no way to distinguish between pain reported due to psychological reasons and pain originating from actual tissue damage. In both cases, it is regarded and reported by the patient as pain and has to be accepted as such.[7]

It is generally accepted that pain serves as a "warning signal" — it enables the organism to sense impending tissue damage and thus avoid harm and prolong survival.[8] Inability to feel pain because of congenital factors considerably shortens life expectancy[9,10] and is often a direct cause of death.[11] On the other hand, chronic, uncontrolled pain can be detrimental to the patient's physical, psychological, and social well being.[12]

Wall[13] claimed that pain is a poor protector against injury for it occurs far too late to provide useful preventive measures. Its main role is to force the damaged organ to rest, or to still behavior of the injured organism, in order to promote healing and recuperation. Wall suggested the classification of pain together with other bodily sensations, such as hunger or thirst ("need states"), evoked by internal events, rather than classifying it with sensations such as seeing and hearing that are evoked by external events. Much like other "need states," pain is strongly affected by distraction, suggestion, culture, learning, and closely associated with predictable behavior (eating when hungry, drinking when thirsty, or resting when in pain). Thus, pain serves not only as a signal of occurring damage, but also as a signal which impedes the onset of a form of behavior.

II. GATE CONTROL THEORY OF PAIN

In 1965, Melzack and Wall[14] proposed a new theory, which provided explanations for many of the phenomena associated with the experience of pain — the gate control theory. The conceptual model of this theory is presented in Figure 3, and includes the following points.

1. Spinal cord cells (T), located in the dorsal horn, receive impulses from the peripheral nerves. Their action is modulated (inhibited) by a spinal gating mechanism located in the substantia gelatinosa (SG) cells in the dorsal horn.
2. The SG and T cells receive information from the periphery through large (L) and small (S) diameter fibers. While both the L and S fibers excite (+) the T cells, they have a different activity on the spinal gate (SG) mechanism. Activity in the L fibers tends to inhibit (–) transmission (close the gate), and activity in the S fibers tends to facilitate (+) transmission (open the gate).

   The spinal cord is continually bombarded by incoming nerve impulses carried predominantly by the S fibers that are tonically active and adapt slowly. This holds the gate in a relatively open position. Most of the L fibers are inactive in the absence of stimulus. L fiber stimulation and activity begin when a stimulus is applied. The increased proportion of L fiber activity, compared to the continuous S fiber activity, causes partial closure of the gate. As the intensity of the stimulus increases, receptor fibers are activated and the positive and negative effects of the L and S fibers tend to counteract each other.

   The effect of both types of fibers on the T cells causes a slow increase in output. If stimulation is prolonged, the L fibers begin to adapt, while the S fibers remain active. The balance between the activity of the L and S

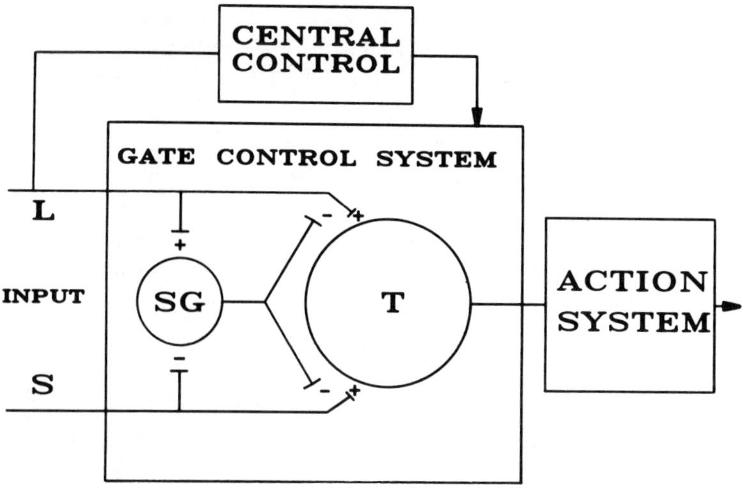

FIGURE 3. Schematic diagram of the gate control theory of pain mechanisms: L, the large-diameter fibers; S, the small-diameter fibers. The fibers project to the substantia gelatinosa (SG) and first central transmission (T) cells. The inhibitory effect exerted by SG on the afferent fiber terminals is increased by activity in L fibers and decreased by activity in S fibers. The central control trigger is represented by a line running from the large-fiber system to the central control mechanisms; these mechanisms, in turn, project back to the gate control system. The T cells project to the entry cells of the action system. Excitation (+); inhibition (–). (From Melzack, R. and Wall, P. D., *Science*, 150, 975, 1965.)

fibers shifts to the latter and a relative increase in S fiber activity occurs, causing the gate to open and increasing T cell output. When the T cell output exceeds a critical level, it activates the action system — the patterns of behavior and experience, characteristic of pain.
The inhibitory effect of the L fibers explains some of our subconscious reactions when feeling pain. Rubbing an aching area overcomes the tendency of the large fibers to adapt and artificially raises their activity. This tends to close the gate and reduce the sensation of pain.

3. The whole complex of the gate control system is influenced by nerve impulses that descend from the brain. Stimulation of the brain activates descending afferent fibers (central control) and makes it possible for the brain to activate selective cognitive processes. Attention, emotion, and memories of prior experiences can mediate the perception of pain through the gate control system. While some central activities, such as anxiety or excitement, may open or close the gate for all inputs from any part of the body, others involve selective, localized gate activity. One mechanism — the central control trigger — activates particular, selective brain processes that are specific to each stimulus. These brain activities act, by way of central control afferent fibers, on the gate control system. Part of their function may be to activate selective brain processes (memories of prior experiences) and pre-set response strategies that influence the arriving information.[14,15]

The gate control theory explains many phenomena associated with pain — hyperalgesia, spontaneous pain, referred pain, prolonged pain, and the effect of cultural cognitive and emotional parameters.[16] Since its initial presentation, the gate control theory has undergone further elaboration and modifications [16-19] and has been subjected to some criticism.[20-23] However, it is still the most relevant theory for understanding the various cognitive and psychological aspects of pain.[15,18,19,24,25]

Recently, Wall[18] referred to the term "gate control," restricting it to the rapidly acting mechanisms that receive and control the transfer of impulses from the input afferent fibers to cells which, in turn, trigger the various effector systems and evoke sensations. However, ongoing pain is a continuing process that cannot be explained simply as a series of repetitive responses to a series of abrupt stimuli. Tissue damaged in the periphery receives an afferent barrage in nociceptors from the central nervous system which produces rapid central inhibitors and excitations as determined by the gate control mechanism. This process is accompanied by further central and peripheral changes which may explain the widespread effects of peripheral damage. While cutaneous injuries (i.e., skin lesions) are associated with pain and tenderness in the immediate area of the damage, deep lesions are associated with distant referred areas of pain and tenderness. This may be explained by slow-onset, long-duration changes that are triggered by impulses in unmyelinated afferents, particularly those originating from deep tissue. These central changes consist of widespread increases of excitability of nerve cells projecting to the brain and to reflex circuits. This causes some of the cells, previously excited only by nociceptors, to also respond to low-threshold inputs. Wall suggested that this provides a basis for the widespread secondary tenderness and allodynia which characterize many pains.

Rugh[26] presented the various psychological factors involved in the perception and behavior of pain in the form of a multidimensional model. The model, based on the gate control theory, consists of seven basic components that modify the different aspects of the pain experience: the pain stimulus, the receptor system, the perceptual sensory system, the cognitive processes, the motivational-affective component, the behavioral response system, and the environment. All seven components interact and affect the experiences of pain and pain behavior.

III. ACUTE VS. CHRONIC PAIN

Chronic and acute pain differ. It is not an artificial distinction created by imposing a concept of time on a biological event, but an observable and measurable process.[8,15,27,28]

A. FORMS OF PAIN AND ITS FUNCTIONS

Melzack and Dennis[28] defined a short-duration, acute pain, occurring at the onset of injury, as "phasic pain". Its immediate behavioral manifestations are characterized by an attempt to relieve pain and by efforts to withdraw from the source of injury. At that point, pain serves as a protection mechanism, signaling the presence of an immediate danger which must be avoided to prevent further harm.

Phasic pain is often encountered in the dental situation. Pain during administration of local analgesia; pain caused by drilling in vital, insufficiently anesthesized dentinal tissue; pain due to exposure of a vital pulp are some of the phasic acute pains possible during dental treatment.

Although such pain is rather easily controlled (it usually ceases with the discontinuation of the inflicting stimulus) it nevertheless can have long-term, behavioral effects. Fear, anxiety, and apprehension caused by the painful stimulus often result in an initial overt avoidance reaction which influences the future attitude of the patient to dental care (see Chapter 4).

In many instances, the pain-inflicting stimulus causes damage to the affected tissues. In these cases, the phasic component is replaced by a tonic component which persists for variable time periods until healing takes place.[15,28] The two components (phasic and tonic) are referred to as acute pain.

Acute pain is usually associated with a well-defined cause (acute pulpitis, pain from a carious tooth, pain caused by a dento-alveolar abscess) and has a characteristic time course (it vanishes after healing). Aside from its role in signaling the site of injury, it also has a role in promoting actions directed at healing (rest of the injured organ) rather than resulting in avoidance behavior.[13] While at the moment of injury, passivity and rest would be maladaptive; after the danger has passed, resting and immobilization are appropriate to enhance recuperation.

Chapman[29] defined two functions of nociception. The first acts as a warning system, providing immediate information about the presence, extent, and location of the injury. The second acts as a reminding system. By generating slow, diffuse, nagging pain, it repeatedly reminds the brain that injury has occurred and should be given proper attention. In the case of acute dental pain, the initiated attention and behavior include actions oriented towards pain elimination, namely the start of dental treatment. "Rest behavior," typical to the recuperation period of other wounds, is not always effective where pain is from a dental origin. Other modes of action are initiated, including possible attempts for self-care (e.g., administration of chemical agents at the affected site) or seeking professional help.

Unlike acute pain, chronic pain usually persists beyond the time required for healing[15,30] and can occur due to organic and/or psychogenic causes. The role of chronic pain in man is puzzling. It does not allow one to escape from harm and avoid further trauma, nor does it result in rest which is essential for recuperation. On the contrary, it is often destructive physically, psychologically, and socially.[12]

In the oro-facial area, there are several potential sources of chronic pain which pose severe problems to the patient and dentist. Their behavioral aspects are discussed in Chapter 6.

B. EFFECT OF ACUTE AND CHRONIC PAIN ON BEHAVIOR

Both acute and chronic pain are associated with specific modes of behavior. Phasic pain is typically accompanied by fear and concerted defensive, self-preservative efforts.[31] It usually provokes characteristic withdrawal behavior aimed at relieving the pain and is associated with verbal and nonverbal behavior typical to pain,[32,33] including distinct facial expressions.[34,35]

In prolonged acute, tonic pain, three main phases of behavior have been suggested.[19] The immediate phase (occurring immediately after acute injury) is characterized by a variety of reactions, from absolute lack of pain to differing degrees. The effect of the same injury can vary immensely among individuals, as well as in cases of different injuries in the same individual. The secondary phase (occurring sometime after injury) is characterized by agitation and aggressive behavior. The tertiary phase (beginning of recovery) is characterized by minimal movement, minimal eating, minimal noise, and prolonged sleep.[13,19]

Unlike prolonged acute pain, which imposes the behavior of rest and recuperation, chronic pain is frequently associated with sleep disturbances, irritability, and depression.[8,36] In prolonged chronic pain, the patient is depressed, withdrawn, irritable, and has a somatic preoccupation directly related to the duration of pain. Some patients become angry, demanding, and manipulative with high probability for psychological and social dysfunctions.[12,36]

C. EMOTIONAL ASPECTS OF ACUTE AND CHRONIC PAIN

Pain is an emotional and usually unpleasant experience.[7] The recognition and tolerance of noxious stimuli are modified by the emotional-affective system and by cognitive processes.[26] There is evidence that pain and mood are related and that there may be a chemical basis for this reciprocal relationship. Mood changes can precede or follow pain, suggesting an interactive system: changes in mood can result in pain, and conversely, changes in pain can cause alterations in mood.[37]

The most common emotional concomitants of pain are anxiety, fear, and depression, but other emotional states may be present including anger, aggression, guilt, subservience, and sexual arousal.[36]

1. Fear and Anxiety

Fear and anxiety are emotions most often associated with situations of acute pain. In their perceptual-defensive-recuperative model of fear and pain, Bolles and Fanselow[31] suggested that fear, produced by the stimulus associated with the painful event, results in the inhibition of pain and pain-related behavior during the defensive phase of the traumatic situation. Only later, when immediate danger no longer exists, does a phase of recuperation begin, during which, behavior is motivated by pain and oriented towards recuperation.

Whichever of the two components comes first, acute pain and fear usually come together, with mutual effect on one another. Both components bear high relevancy to the dental situation. Unexpected acute pain, experienced during treatment, is a common cause for developing dental anxieties and phobia.[2] In many cases, pain triggers the development of dental anxiety which, in turn, contributes to the development of the vicious cycle of pain-fear-anxiety-avoidance-more pain, etc. (see Chapter 4).

Generally, when anxiety exists, it increases the perception of noxious events as painful.[38-41] In the dental setting, the amount of pain expected and experienced by patients is directly related to the patient's anxiety.[42-46] Highly fearful dental patients were found not to be different from nonfearful patients with regard to their pain threshold or pain tolerance of nondental stimuli (electric stimulation of the forearm). They did, however, rate dental stimuli (tooth pulp stimulation) as more painful than did the non-fearful patients.[43,47]

Anxiety poses a severe obstacle in the administration of dental treatment. It can lead the patient to report pain during treatment even after local anesthetic has been given. In a survey concerning the difficulties in achieving local anesthesia, dentists indicated that a high percentage of patients who do not experience numbness after injection are fearful or anxious.[48] Similarly, fear of dental treatment has been found to be positively associated with the likelihood of failure to achieve optimal local anesthesia.[49]

Anxiety is also associated with conditions of chronic pain. When the cause of pain is not sufficiently understood and no effective cure can be immediately suggested, patients may experience anxiety arising from the helplessness and hopelessness of the situation. The inability to control pain and the anticipation of unavoidable, uncontrollable, and unpredicted pain can cause a high degree of apprehension.

2. Depression

Whereas acute pain and fear share many autonomic signs, chronic pain is more closely associated with the state of depression.[12] A high prevalence of depressive symptoms has been found, not only among selected groups of chronic pain patients treated in hospitals or pain clinics, but also in chronic pain subjects from a general population in the U.S.[50]

Although some theoretical models have been suggested to explain the relationship between chronic pain and depression, no evidence has been found to support any approach.[51] Some hypothesize that chronic pain and depression are closely related, due to similar neurochemical mechanisms involved in both disorders,[52,53] and that chronic pain should be viewed as a variant of depressive disease.[54,55] Other explanations tie the depression associated with chronic pain to reasons such as the decline in social activities and social rewards associated with prolonged pain.[56]

Rudy et al.[57] suggested a cognitive-behavioral mediation model in which the depressed mood among chronic pain patients is explained by their appraisals of the degree to which pain interferes with important areas of functioning and perceptions of self-control. It has also been suggested[58] that the patient's locus of control is significantly related to pain-coping strategies and psychological distress. Patients who perceive outcomes as controlled by chance factors (fate or luck) are more likely to report depression, anxiety, and obsessive-compulsive symptoms.

Depression is often associated with chronic pain conditions in the oro-facial region (see Chapter 6). Understanding the various emotional factors associated with these conditions is essential to undertake a proper treatment approach.

D. COGNITIVE ASPECTS OF PAIN

The experience of pain includes a confrontation with harm and can therefore be perceived as a threatening stimulus. As in other situations of actual confrontation with harm, threat appraisal is affected not only by the potency of the stimulus but also by counter-harm resources of the individual.[59] The individual's cognitive view of the stressful situation influences the coping process; variables such as a perception of the consequences, the importance of the event to well-being, and the resources with which to cope all affect the process.[60] Furthermore, various cognitive strategies have a positive effect in enhancing pain tolerance/threshold or attenuating pain ratings.[61]

1. Control

The cognition of control vs. helplessness is a major factor in threat appraisal. It is the individual's conception of self-power rather than actual power that is important, and it affects reaction to the pain stimulus. Research has shown that providing patients with control over pain stimulation reduces pain and increases tolerance.[62,63]

In the dental setting, children who were provided with a method to signal the dentist to stop treatment showed less response to high arousal procedures.[64] This, however, has not been confirmed with regard to adults, probably due to the fact that adults have learned control responses for the dental context (movements, grunts, groans) which make the external control devices redundant.[65]

As people in pain usually search for information to give meaning to the experience,[66] a sense of control can be achieved not only by direct control of the actions of the dentist (or physician),[63] but also by the means of information concerning the anticipated and ongoing treatment. Dworkin et al.[67] have shown that subjects who were provided with high levels of information on N_2O analgesia had higher sensation and pain tolerance thresholds to tooth pulp stimulation than low information controls.

Although the effect of preoperative information on postoperative pain is not always consistent,[68,69] it seems to have a generally beneficiary effect in the dental situation as far as acute pain is concerned. The fear of uncontrolled, sudden, acute pain is a primary concern of the majority of patients.[70] Therefore, continuous information about the ongoing procedures is one way of providing the patient with some sense of control or involvement.

The issue of control loss is especially important with patients suffering from prolonged chronic pain. The inability to find relief from the pain contributes to feelings of hopelessness, helplessness, despair, and pessimism.[36] The degree to which these patients feel control over their pain affects their ability to cope with it.

2. Beliefs

Reaction to a stimulus, whether acute or chronic, is always affected by its meaning to the individual. For example, in the dental situation, unexpected, acute pain can be interpreted as a sign of insufficient control by the dentist and lead to mistrust in the dentist's skills. In such cases, any minor stimulus is interpreted as a threat and evokes a pain reaction. Conversely, when mutual trust exists, the patient's belief in the necessity of treatment and in the skills of the dentist makes such incidences bearable and less traumatic.

In cases of chronic pain, the patient's beliefs play a major role in attitude and reaction to the stimulus. Those who express belief that pain will be enduring, usually report an increase in pain intensity.[71] Furthermore, if the pain is believed (rightfully or not) to be a signal of a life-threatening illness (e.g., malignant tumor), the ability to tolerate it is affected. Pain is better tolerated when its origin is known not to be a sign of a life threatening disease.[26]

In stressful situations, behavior, thoughts, and emotional reactions are influenced by the patient's perception of "self-efficacy," namely the belief in possession of relevant, necessary coping skills.[72] In pain situations, perceived self-efficacy has been shown to affect tolerance.[25] Generally, patients who avoid dental care due to fear and anxiety were found to have a lower tolerance level to pain than nonfearful patients, and they perceived themselves reliably less able to tolerate it (lower on measures of "efficacy"). No such differences were found between the groups with regard to nondental pain.[48,73,74]

3. Expectations

A person's expectations of a given situation influence the final interpretation of the stimulus as painful or nonpainful. An ambiguous sensation can be perceived as either pleasurable or painful based on one's expectancy or schematic representation of the stimulus. In an experiment conducted by Anderson and Pennebaker,[75] subjects touched a vibrating surface for 1 s. Some believed the surface would cause pain, others expected it to produce pleasure, and a third group had no preestablished way of evaluating the vibrations. As predicted, pain subjects usually reported the vibrations to be painful, pleasure subjects as pleasurable, and the control subjects as neutral sensations. These results suggest that settings typically associated with pain or aversive sensations (e.g., the dental situation) increase the probability that pain is perceived.

Studies of tooth pulp shock (acute, phasic pain) delivered in laboratory and clinical settings produced evidence that responses to pain change according to the situational context in which the pain is experienced. In a study conducted by Dworkin and Chen,[76] subjects served as their own control when tooth pulp shock was delivered in laboratory and clinical situations. The responses of the subjects to the pain evoked by the pulp stimulations were recorded on two occasions for each subject: the first in a psychological laboratory, the second either in the laboratory setting (for half of the subjects) or in a clinical dental setting (for the other half). Results showed a substantial decrease in the subjects threshold for sensation and pain, and in pain tolerance, when tested in the clinical setting, indicating that the anticipation of threat in the dental setting and the associated anxiety are prepotent cognitive mediators of pain behavior.

4. Attention and Distraction

Perception depends on the constant monitoring of impulses from the many intero-, proprio-, and exteroceptors and the filtering of this input to select information which is relevant and useful. This selection process is called *attention* and involves the filtering of relevant signals and integrating of information to permit the organization of meaningful forms of experience.[29]

Melzack[17] summarized many classic examples of the effects of attention and distraction on the intensity of pain experience. Apparently, almost any situation that attracts a sufficient degree of intense, prolonged attention (e.g., sports, battle) can provide the conditions for other stimulation to go unnoticed, including wounds that would cause considerable suffering under normal circumstances.

In an extensive review, McCaul and Malott[77] summarized the effect of distraction on the pain experience. Numerous data were presented to support the major principles of the effect of distraction on pain:

1. Distraction reduces pain as compared to undistracted and placebo control conditions. Patients who were asked to perform an attention demanding task exhibited less distress to a painful stimulus than subjects provided with either no instructions or placebo instructions.
2. Distraction techniques that require more attention capacity are more effective in reducing pain-related distress.
3. Distraction has stronger effects in reducing distress in mild, as opposed to intense pain stimuli.
4. Distraction is more effective than sensation redefinition for mild pain stimuli.

Many dentists subconsciously use distracting methods while treating anxious children and adults. Background music and constant talking to the patient during treatment are common methods.

E. MEMORY OF PAIN

The cognitive aspects of the pain experience (beliefs, expectations) are affected by the extent to which the individual recalls a former painful experience. Although research on the memory of pain is a relatively new area, an increasing amount of information suggests that the accuracy of such memory is dependent on a number of variables.

In a recent literature review, Erskine et al.[78] presented the data accumulated in this field with regard to chronic vs. acute pain and whether the pain was naturally occurring or part of a clinical or experimental procedure. Although somewhat reserved as to drawing definite conclusions from the reviewed data, three possible emerging patterns are shown:

1. Overall correlations between actual pain experience and pain recall are positive but rather weak.
2. Recall of pain intensity is more accurate for acute than for chronic pain or repeated episodic experience of the pain.
3. Mood and affective states influence the memory of pain.

The last two points are especially relevant to the dental setting. When patients experience recurrent acute pain during dental treatment, their recall of the experience may increase in magnitude. This indirectly supports the notion that when dental anxiety is anteceded by former aversive encounters in the dental office, usually more than one such encounter is involved[79,80] (see also Chapter 4). It is possible that part of the aversive learning process lies in the increasing memory of the pain experienced during treatment which concomitantly leads to increased anxiety, increased pain perception, increased memory of the involved pain, etc.

A patient's memory of acute pain during dental treatment is often affected by the level of dental anxiety.[46] Anxious patients reported more pain 3 months after a dental appointment than immediately after treatment. The level of pain remembered by the patients was more closely associated with their expectations of pain than to their real previous experience.

In another study designed to explore the relevance of anxious mood on recall of previous dental experiences, Kent[81] found that incidents recalled by patients with high anxiety were significantly more unpleasant than those with moderate and low anxiety, indicating that anxiety affects the description of previous experiences.

The correlation between patient anxiety and memory of pain was not confirmed in patients suffering from recurrent episodes of pain (menstrual and headache). In a study by Rachman and Eyrl,[82] all patients recalled their pain as being higher than it actually was, but the correlations between pain reports and pain recall were positive. This study did not confirm the relationship between accuracy of recall and anxiety reported by Kent,[46,81] presumably because the pain experienced during dentistry is more anxiety-evoking than the naturally occurring, regular episodes of menstrual pain or headaches.

In situations of chronic pain, memory of past pain experience depends significantly on the intensity of present pain and the patient's emotional state. When chronic pain patients (headache of myofacial origin) were asked to rate former pain experiences, they were significantly affected by the intensity of their present pain. Namely, when present pain intensity was high, patients rated the levels of their prior pain as being more severe than originally recorded. When present pain intensity was low, the same patients remembered prior pain as being less severe.[83] Furthermore, chronic pain patients who reported more emotional distress, who had conflicts at home, and who were less active were less accurate in remembering their pain.[84]

F. LEARNED ASPECTS OF PAIN

As in any other "stressor", the experience of pain is also influenced by individual learned responses. Respondent and operant conditioning, vicarious learning through modeling and suggestions, and social learning have a significant impact on the pain experience.[85]

1. Direct Learning and Pain

Direct, operant conditioning plays a significant role, especially in situations where chronic pain is involved. Chronic pain is a prolonged phenomenon which presents a new reality to the suffering person. In this generally unpleasant reality, several reinforcing events exist which can be pain contingent.[86,87] Sympathy and attention from the environment, and avoidance of unpleasant work or duties, are some secondary gains which are not easily abandoned. Fordyce[87] paraphrased this reinforcement as "good things happen when I hurt, that otherwise would not."

Reinforcement of pain behavior can also take place with pain medications. For some, the effects of pain medications reinforce pain behavior due to the development of physiological and psychological addiction. These individuals hang on to the pain behaviors necessary and sufficient to lead to delivery of medications even after the original nociceptive stimulus has resolved.[87]

2. Indirect Learning and Pain

Pain behavior may sometimes lead to effective avoidance of aversive or unpleasant consequences. Such reinforcement is especially effective in the development of chronic pain. Indirect reinforcement of pain behavior was paraphrased by Fordyce[87] as "when I hurt, bad things do not happen to me which otherwise would." A relevant example cited by Fordyce is that of an elderly woman who, due to insult to her memory, found participation in a bridge club increasingly stressful. Episodes of pain enabled her to stay home and avoid the unpleasant encounter. The secondary gain achieved this way served as an indirect factor reinforcing the pain behavior and preventing a possible cure.

Similar relevant examples exist in the dental situation. Avoidance of dental treatment due to temporomandibular joint (TMJ) pain which prevents prolonged opening of the mouth, is one possible example.

Other processes of indirect learning (i.e., modeling) also affect situations of acute pain. Observation of others responding to painful stimulation may provoke or reduce the pain response of the observer. Observing another person experiencing noxious stimuli without apparent distress was shown to reduce pain reactions in experimental settings.[88,89]

G. SOCIAL AND CULTURAL ASPECTS OF PAIN

The suffering patient is part of a sociocultural environment and, as such, influences his/her surroundings and is influenced by them. Both acute and chronic pain are profoundly affected by social and cultural factors.

The effect of social modeling of pain has been studied in laboratory settings, especially with regard to stimuli resulting from acute-phasic pain (it is practically impossible to imitate chronic pain under controlled conditions in the laboratory). Craig et al.[89-92] demonstrated the influence of models on patient pain tolerance in a laboratory setting. In all studies the subject's assessment of the inflicted noxious stimuli was significantly affected by the response of a confederate model.

The reinforcing influence of social environmental factors on an individual's chronic pain behavior has frequently been discussed. Several studies suggest that the level of approval given by different societies for the public expression of pain has a significant impact on the individual's behavior. Differences in the response to pain of patients from different origins have been shown by Zola,[93] Zborowski,[94,95] and others.[96,97]

Zborowski[95] suggested the arrangement of behavioral responses to pain in five groups: (1) motor responses (twisting, bodily movement), (2) vocal responses (groaning, crying, screaming), (3) verbal responses (complaining, cursing, talking about pain, asking for help), (4) social responses (withdrawal from people, changes in communication patterns); and (5) the absence of manifest behavior (hiding or suppressing external signs of pain).

The individual's behavior in pain is a combination of these responses, each of which is subjected to cultural and social influences. For example, while Irish patients tend to deny their problems and complain less, Italians are more dramatizing, with more symptoms and bodily dysfunctions.[93] American patients of Jewish and Italian origin prefer company while in pain, whereas patients from "Old American" and Irish origin tend to withdraw socially. "Old American" and Irish patients are usually nonexpressive, whereas Jews and Italians usually make no effort to control their emotional reactions to pain.[94,95]

The cultural significance attributed to pain, symbols of pain, and situations associated with pain make them acceptable or avoidable regardless of the actual intensity of the sensation (e.g., acceptance of pain inflicted during the administration of local anesthesia as good and serving a positive purpose, rejection of pain caused by a needle puncture in the finger as bad and symbolizing injury). Zborowski[95] pointed out that the acceptance of pain does not mean that the feeling quality of the sensation has changed. The sensation is always unpleasant, but the unpleasantness is tolerated when cultural traditions call for its acceptance.

Although pain expressions are highly divergent among different cultural groups, there is no evidence to indicate that any group is deficient in aspects of the pain experience.[37] Recent studies suggest that while ethnic groups differ with regard to factors which influence responses to pain, similarities exist in their reporting of the responses. For example, responses, attitudes, and descriptions were found to be relatively similar in Black, Irish, Italian, Jewish, and Puerto Rican facial pain patients. The majority of items for which interethnic differences were found concern the patient's emotions (stoicism vs. expressiveness) in response to pain, and interference in daily functioning attributed to pain.[98]

Further evidence exists that some dimensions of pain (time, intensity, location, quality, cause, and curability) are universal, while others are culture-specific ("suantong" in Chinese dentists and dental patients, "real" and "imagined" pains in Western subjects).[99,100]

IV. SUMMARY

Rightfully or not, the experience of pain is closely associated with dental care, and is a common cause for stress in the dental situation.

Pain is a sensory as well as an emotional experience. The experience of pain involves, and is influenced by, variables such as fear, anxiety, depression, perception of control, beliefs, expectations, attention, distraction, and learning.

While acute pain may directly lead to the development of fear, anxiety, and phobia towards dental care, prolonged chronic pain in the oro-facial region is often a source of depression and social impairment. Both acute and chronic pain have an intense impact on human behavior, emotions, and cognitions, and as such affect the development of various oro-related behavioral dysfunctions.

REFERENCES

1. **McNeil, D. W. and Berryman, M. L.,** Components of dental fear in adults?, *Behav. Res. Ther.*, 27, 233, 1989.
2. **Davey, G. C. L.,** Dental phobias and anxieties: evidence for conditioning processes in the acquisition and modulation of a learned fear, *Behav. Res. Ther.*, 27, 51, 1989.
3. **Dangott, L., Thornton, B. C., and Page, P.,** Communication and pain, *J. Commun.*, 28, 30, 1978.
4. **Klepac, R. K., Dowling, J., Hauge, G., and McDonald, M.,** Reports of pain after dental treatment, electrical tooth pulp stimulation and cutaneous shock, *J. Am. Dent. Assoc.*, 100, 692, 1980.

5. **Wardle, J.,** Fear of dentistry, *Br. J. Med. Psychol.*, 55, 119, 1982.
6. **Merskey, H. and Spear, F. G.,** *Pain: Psychological and Psychiatric Aspects*, Williams and Wilkins, Baltimore 1967.
7. IASP Subcommittee on Taxonomy, Pain terms; a list with definitions and notes on usage, *Pain*, 6, 249, 1979.
8. **Sternbach, R. A.,** Acute versus chronic pain, in *Textbook of Pain*, 2nd ed., Wall, P. A. and Melzack, R., Eds., Churchill Livingstone, London, 1989.
9. **Sternbach, R. A.,** Congenital insensitivity to the pain: A critique, *Psychol. Bull.*, 60, 252, 1963.
10. **Sternbach, R. A.,** *Pain: A Psychophysiological Analysis*, Academic Press, New York, 1968.
11. **Baxter, D. W. and Olszewski, J.,** Congenital insensitivity to pain, *Brain*, 83, 381, 1960.
12. **Sternbach, R. A.,** *Pain Patients: Traits and Treatment*, Academic Press, New York, 1974.
13. **Wall, P. D.,** On the relation of injury to pain, *Pain*, 6, 253, 1979.
14. **Melzack, R. and Wall, P. D.,** Pain mechanisms: a new theory, *Science*, 150, 971, 1965.
15. **Melzack, P. and Dennis, S. G.,** Neurophysiological foundations of pain, in *The Psychology of Pain*, Sternbach, R. A., Ed., Raven Press, New York, 1978, 1.
16. **Casey, K. L. and Melzack, R.,** Neural mechanisms of pain: a conceptual model, in *New Concepts in Pain and its Management*, Way, E. L., Ed., F. A. Davis, Philadelphia, 1967, 13.
17. **Melzack, R.,** *The Puzzle of Pain*, Basic Books, New York, 1973.
18. **Wall, P. D.,** Modulation of pain by nonpainful events, in *Advances in Pain Research and Therapy*, Vol. 1, Bonica, J. J. and Albe-Fessard, D. G., Eds., Raven Press, New York, 1976, 1.
19. **Wall, P. D.,** Introduction, in *Textbook of Pain*, 2nd ed., Wall, P. D. and Melzack, R., Eds., Churchill Livingston, London, 1989.
20. **Perl, E. R.,** Is pain a specific sensation?, *J. Psychiatric Res.*, 8, 273, 1971.
21. **Nathan, P. W. and Rudge, P.,** Testing the gate-control theory of pain in man, *J. Neurol., Neurosurg. Psychiatry*, 37, 1366, 1974.
22. **Kerr, F. W. L.,** Neuroanatomical substrates of nociception in the spinal cord, *Pain*, 1, 325, 1975.
23. **Nathan, P. W.,** The gate-control theory of pain: a critical review, *Brain*, 99, 123, 1976.
24. **Liebeskind, J. C. and Paul, L. A.,** Psychological and physio-logical mechanisms of pain, *Ann. Rev. Psychol.*, 28, 41, 1977.
25. **Weisenberg, M.,** Cognitive aspects of pain, in *Textbook of Pain*, 2nd ed., Wall, P. D. and Melzack, R., Eds., Churchill Livingston, London, 1989.
26. **Rugh, J. D.,** Psychological components of pain, *Dent. Clin. North Am.*, 31, 579, 1987.
27. **Melzack, P.,** Neurophysiological foundations of pain, in *The Psychology of Pain*, Sternbach, R. A., Ed., Raven Press, New York, 1978, 1.
28. **Melzack, R. and Dennis, S. G.,** Phylogenetic evolution of pain expression in animals, in *Pain and Society*, Kosterlitz, H. W. and Terenius, L. Y., Eds., Verlag Chemie, Weinheim, West Germany, 1980, 13.
29. **Chapman, C. R.,** Pain: the perception of noxious events, in *The Psychology of Pain*, Sternbach, R. A., Ed., Raven Press, New York, 1978, 169.
30. **Merskey, H., Ed.,** Classification of chronic pain: descriptions of chronic pain syndromes and definitions of pain terms, *Pain* (Suppl.) 3, 1, 1986.
31. **Bolles, R. C. and Fanselow, M. S.,** A perceptual-defensive-recuperative model of fear and pain, *Behav. Brain Sci.*, 3, 291, 1980.
32. **Craig, K. D. and Prkachin, K. M.,** Non-verbal measures of pain, in *Pain Measurement and Assessment*, Melzack, R., Ed., Raven Press, New York, 1982, 173.
33. **Patrick, C. J., Craig, K. D., and Prkachin, K. M.,** Observer judgments of acute pain: Facial action determinants, *J. Pers. Soc. Psychol.*, 50, 1291, 1986.
34. **LeResche, L.,** Facial expression in pain: a study of candid photographs, *J. Nonverbal Behav.*, 7, 46, 1982.

35. **LeResche, L. and Dworkin, S. F.,** Facial expression accompanying pain, *Soc. Sci. Med.*, 19, 1325, 1984.
36. **Craig, K. D.,** Emotional aspects of pain, in *Textbook of Pain*, 2nd ed., Wall, P. D. and Melzack, R., Eds., Churchill Livingston, London, 1989.
37. **Wolff, B. B., Bond, M. R., Brinkhus, H., Carli, G., Craig, K. D., Dum, J. E., Kosterlitz, H. W., Melzack, R., and Tu, W.,** Evolution of expression of pain (acute and chronic) group report, in *Pain and Society*, Kosterlitz, H. W. and Terenius, L. Y., Verlag Chemie, Weinheim, West Germany, 1980, 81.
38. **Weisenberg, M.,** Pain and pain control, *Psychol. Bull.*, 84, 1008, 1977.
39. **Von Graffenried, B., Adler, R., Abt, K., Nuesch, E., and Spiegel, R.,** The influence of anxiety and pain sensitivity on experimental pain in man, *Pain*, 4, 253, 1978.
40. **Sternbach, R. A.,** Clinical aspects of pain, in *The Psychology of Pain*, 2nd ed., Sternbach, R. A., Ed., Raven Press, New York, 1986, 223.
41. **Robin, O., Vinard, H., Vernet-Maury, E., and Saumet, J. T.,** Influence of sex and anxiety on pain treshold and tolerance, *Functional Neurol.*, 2, 173, 1987.
42. **Bowers, K. S.,** Pain, anxiety, and perceived control, *J. Consult. Clin. Psychol.*, 32, 596, 1968.
43. **Klepac, R. K., McDonald, M., Hauge, G., and Dowling, J.,** Reactions to pain among subjects high and low in dental fear, *J. Behav. Med.*, 3, 373, 1980.
44. **Kent, G.,** Anxiety, pain and type of dental procedure, *Behav. Res. Ther.*, 22, 465, 1984.
45. **Green, R. M. and Green, A.,** Adult attitudes to dentistry among dental attenders in South Wales, *Br. Dent. J.*, 159, 157, 1985.
46. **Kent, G.,** Memory of dental pain, *Pain*, 21, 187, 1985.
47. **Klepac, R. K., Dowling, J., and Hauge, G.,** Characteristics of clients seeking therapy for the reduction of dental avoidance: reactions to pain, *J. Behav. Ther. Exp. Psychiatry*, 13, 293, 1982.
48. **Kaufman, E., Weinstein, P., and Milgrom, P.,** Difficulties in achieving local anesthesia, *J. Am. Dent. Assoc.*, 108, 205, 1984.
49. **Weinstein, P., Milgrom, P., Kaufman, E., Fiset, L., and Ramsay, D.,** Patient perceptions of failure to achieve optimal local anesthesia, *Gen. Dent.*, 33, 218, 1985.
50. **Magni, G., Caldieron, C., Rigatti-Luchini, S., and Merskey, H.,** Chronic musculoskeletal pain and depressive symptoms in the general population. An analysis of the 1st National Health and Nutrition Examination Survey data, *Pain*, 43, 299, 1990.
51. **Romano, J. M. and Turner, J. A.,** Chronic pain and depression: does the evidence support a relationship, *Psychol. Bull.*, 97, 18, 1985.
52. **Hendler, N.,** Depression caused by chronic pain, *J. Clin. Psychiatry*, 45, 30, 1984.
53. **Ward, N. G., Bloom, V. L., Dworkin, S., Fawcett, J., Nara-Simhachari, N., and Friedel, R. O.,** Psychobiological markers in coexisting pain and depression: Towards a unified theory, *J. Clin. Psychiatry*, 43, 32, 1982.
54. **Engel, G. L.,** "Psychogenic" pain and the pain-prone patient, *Am. J. Med.*, 26, 899, 1959.
55. **Blumer, D. and Heilbronn, M.,** Chronic pain as a variant of depressive disease: the pain-prone disorder, *J. Nerv. Ment. Dis.*, 170, 381, 1982.
56. **Turk, D. C., Meichenbaum, D., and Genest, M.,** *Pain and Behavioral Medicine: A Cognitive-Behavioral Perspective*, Guilford Press, New York, 1983.
57. **Rudy, T. E., Kerns, R. D., and Turk, D. C.,** Chronic pain and depression: Toward a cognitive-behavioral mediation model, *Pain*, 35, 129, 1988.
58. **Crisson, J. E. and Keefe, F. J.,** The relationship of locus of control to pain coping strategies and psychological distress in chronic pain patients, *Pain*, 35, 147, 1988.
59. **Lazarus, R. S.,** *Psychological Stress and the Coping System*, McGraw-Hill, New York, 1966, 465.
60. **Roskies, E. and Lazarus, R. S.,** Coping theory and the teaching of coping skills, in *Behavioral Medicine: Changing Health Lifestyles*, Davidson, P. O. and Davidson, S. M., Eds., Brunner/Mazel, New York, 1980, 38.

61. **Fernandez, E. and Turk, D. C.,** The utility of cognitive coping strategies for altering pain perception: a meta-analysis, *Pain*, 38, 123, 1989.
62. **Staub, E., Tursky, B., and Schwartz, G. E.,** Self-control and predictability: Their effects on reactions to aversive stimulation, *J. Pers. Soc. Psychol.*, 18, 157, 1971.
63. **Bowers, K. S.,** Pain, anxiety and perceived control, *J. Consult. Clin. Psychol.*, 32, 596, 1968.
64. **Corah, N. L.,** Effect of perceived control on stress reduction in pedodontic patients, *J. Dent. Res.*, 52, 1261, 1973.
65. **Corah, N. L., Bissell, G. D., and Illig, S. J.,** Effect of perceived control on stress reduction in adult dental patients, *J. Dent. Res.*, 57, 74, 1978.
66. **Craig, K. D.,** Social modeling influences: pain in context, in *The Psychology of Pain*, 2nd ed., Sternbach, R. A., Ed., Raven Press, New York, 1986, 67.
67. **Dworkin, S. F., Chen, A. C. N., Schubert, M. M., and Clark, D. W.,** Cognitive modification of pain: information in combination with N_2O, *Pain*, 19, 339, 1984.
68. **Scott, L. E., Clum, G. A., and Peoples, J. B.,** Preoperative predictors of postoperative pain, *Pain*, 15, 283, 1983.
69. **Bradlyn, A. S., Christoff, K., Sikora, T., O'Dell, S., and Harris, C. V.,** The effects of a videotape preparation package in reducing children's arousal and increasing cooperation during cardiac catheterization, *Behav. Res. Ther.*, 24, 453, 1986.
70. **Lindsay, S. J. E., Humphris, G., and Barnby, G. J.,** Expectations and preferences for routine dentistry in anxious adult patients, *Br. Dent. J.*, 163, 120, 1987.
71. **Williams, D. A. and Thorn, B. E.,** An empirical assessment of pain beliefs, *Pain*, 36, 351, 1989.
72. **Bandura, A.,** Self-efficacy: toward a unifying theory of behavioural change, *Psychol. Rev.*, 84, 191, 1977.
73. **Kent, G.,** Self-efficacious control over reported physiological, cognitive and behavioural symptoms of dental anxiety, *Behav. Res. Ther.*, 25, 341, 1987.
74. **Kent, G. and Gibbons, R.,** Self-efficacy and the control of anxious cognitions, *J. Behav. Ther. Exp. Psychiatry*, 18, 33, 1987.
75. **Anderson, D. B. and Pennebaker, J. W.,** Pain and pleasure: alternative interpretations for identical stimulation, *Eur. J. Soc. Psychol.*, 10, 207, 1980.
76. **Dworkin, S. F. and Chen, A. C.,** Pain in clinical and laboratory contexts, *J. Dent. Res.*, 61, 772, 1982.
77. **McCaul, K. D. and Malott, J. M.,** Distraction and coping with pain, *Psychol. Bull.*, 95, 516, 1984.
78. **Erskine, A., Morley, S., and Pearce, S.,** Memory for pain: a review, *Pain*, 41, 255, 1990.
79. **Lautch, H.,** Dental phobia, *Br. J. Psychiatry*, 119, 151, 1971.
80. **Bernstein, D. A., Kleinknecht, R. A., and Alexander, L. D.,** Antecedents of dental fear, *J. Public Health Dent.*, 39, 113, 1979.
81. **Kent, G.,** Memory of dental experiences as related to naturally occurring changes in state anxiety, *Cognit. Emotion*, 3, 45, 1989.
82. **Rachman, S. and Eyrl, K.,** Predicting and remembering recurrent pain, *Behav. Res. Ther.*, 27, 621, 1989.
83. **Eich, E., Reeves, J., Jaeger, B., and Graf-Radford, S. B.,** Memory for pain: relation between past and present pain intensity, *Pain*, 23, 375, 1985.
84. **Jamison, R. N., Sbrocco, T., and Parris, W. C. V.,** The influence of physical and psychosocial factors on accuracy of memory for pain in chronic pain patients, *Pain*, 37, 289, 1989.
85. **Burdette, B. H. and Gale, E. N.,** Pain as a learned response: a review of behavioral factors in chronic pain, *J. Am. Dent. Assoc.*, 116, 881, 1988.
86. **Fordyce, W. E.,** *Behavioral Methods in Chronic Pain and Illness*, C. V. Mosby, St. Louis, 1976.

87. **Fordyce, W. E.,** Learning processes in pain, in *The Psychology of Pain*, Sternbach, R. A., Ed., Raven Press, New York, 1978, 49.
88. **Neufeld, R. W. J. and Davidson, P. O.,** The effects of vicarious and cognitive rehearsal on pain tolerance, *J. Psychosom. Res.*, 15, 329, 1971.
89. **Craig, K. D. and Weiss, S. M.,** Vicarious influences on pain threshold determinations, *J. Pers. Soc. Psychol.*, 19, 53, 1971.
90. **Craig, K. D. and Neidermayer, H.,** Autonomic correlates of pain thresholds influenced by social modelling, *J. Pers. Soc. Psychol.*, 29, 246, 1974.
91. **Craig, K. D. and Weiss, S. M.,** Verbal reports of pain without noxious stimulation, *Percept. Mot. Skills*, 34, 943, 1972.
92. **Craig, K. D. and Best, J. A.,** Perceived control over pain: individual differences and situational determinants, *Pain*, 3, 127, 1977.
93. **Zola, K.,** Culture and symptoms: an analysis of patient presenting complaints, *Am. Soc. Rev.*, 66, 615, 1966.
94. **Zborowski, M.,** Cultural components in responses to pain, *J. Soc. Issues*, 8, 16, 1952.
95. **Zborowski, M.,** *People in Pain*, Jossey-Bass, San Francisco, 1969.
96. **Sternbach, R. A. and Tursky, B.,** Ethnic differences among housewives in psychophysical and skin potential responses to electric shock, *Psychophysiology*, 1, 241, 1965.
97. **Lambert, W. E., Libman, E., and Poser, E. G.,** The effect of increased salience of a membership group on pain tolerance, *J. Pers.*, 28, 350, 1960.
98. **Lipton, J. A. and Marbach, J. J.,** Ethnicity and the pain experience, *Soc. Sci. Med.*, 19, 1279, 1984.
99. **Moore, R., Miller, M. L., Weinstein, P., Dworkin, S. F., and Liou, H.-H.,** Cultural perceptions of pain and pain coping among patients and dentists, *Community Dent. Oral Epidemiol.*, 14, 327, 1986.
100. **Moore, R. A. and Dworkin, S. F.,** Ethnographic methodologic assessment of pain perceptions by verbal description, Pain, 34, 195, 1988.

SECTION II

BEHAVIORAL ASPECTS OF DENTAL TREATMENT

Chapter 4

DENTAL FEAR, ANXIETY, AND PHOBIA

The complex factors of stress in the orofacial region influence both the physiology, and the psychology of the dental experience, and lead to a large variety of behavioral dysfunctions related to dental treatment. The most quoted and investigated oro-related behavioral dysfunctions are those originating from fear and anxiety.

I. DEFINITIONS

Anxiety is the apprehension caused by a threat to values (physical, psychological, or social) that are held essential to one's existence (e.g., physical threat, threat to success, threat to the love of another person, etc.).[1]

Anxiety consists of both a somatic physiological aspect and a psychological one. It includes (1) physical and mental awareness of being powerless, (2) presence of an impending and almost inevitable danger, (3) alertness as if facing emergency, (4) apprehensive self-absorption which interferes with an effective and advantageous solution of reality problems, and (5) an irresoluble doubt concerning the nature of the threat, the probability of its actual appearance, the best means of reducing it, and one's subjective capacity to make effective use of those means.[2]

While anxiety is more typically a reaction to an unreal or imagined danger, fear is considered a reaction to a real or threatened danger, and usually lacks components 4 and 5 typical to anxiety. Phobia is a "morbid fear associated with morbid anxiety"[2] or, in other words, "persistent and irrational fear…that results in a compelling desire to avoid the dread object, activity, or situation".[3]

It is clear that in the dental situation fear and anxiety are practically indistinguishable. The patient is confronted with both "real" and "imagined" threats (see Chapter 2) and reacts with different degrees of apprehension. Usually, the term "dental fear" is used to describe moderate apprehension which causes tension before and during treatment, but enables the patient to receive dental care. Dental anxiety describes a more profound apprehension which actually interferes with routine treatment and requires special attention. The term "dental phobia" is typically used to refer to patients whose anxiety is so great that it leads to total avoidance of dental care, including practical oral neglect. In the present text the terms "dental fear" and "dental anxiety" will be used interchangeably.

Anxiety bears two distinct components: state and trait anxiety. State anxiety is the individual's response to the specific situation, varying in intensity and fluctuating over time (e.g., increasing when facing dental treatment, decreasing when the treatment is over). Trait anxiety is part of the personality, involving the individual's predisposition to become anxious under a variety of circumstances. It refers to relatively stable individual differences in anxiety proneness which results in the disposition to perceive a wide range of stimulus situations as dangerous, and in the tendency to respond to such threat with state anxiety reactions.[4]

II. PREVALENCE

There is general agreement as to the prominence of dental fear and anxiety, however, it is somewhat difficult to assess the exact prevalence of the problem. Various studies have used different means to survey different populations (telephone surveys vs. personal self-report, population of college students vs. general population of major cities, different kinds of questionnaires, etc.). Measures of dental anxiety range from reports on avoiding dental treatment due to fear, avoiding treatment except when symptomatic, or direct reports of high dental fear.

The prevalence of dental fear in the American population in the late 1950s and early 1960s was estimated at about 5 to 9%.[5,6] Crockett[6] reported that about 6% of his study group avoided dental care even when necessary; Friedson and Feldman[5] reported that 9% of the people who did not use dental services regularly indicated that their reluctance to do so was based on fear ("afraid of dentists, it hurts..."); and in Sweden up to 9% of the adult population was found to avoid dental care due to fear of treatment.[7]

Later studies, conducted in the 1970s and 1980s, reported even higher numbers for the prevalence of dental fear in different populations. In a survey conducted on the Swedish population (ages 12 to 75), 14% were found to regard dental visits as "so uncomfortable that they were unable to follow through treatment."[8] In England, out of 419 respondents surveyed, 15% reported being very or extremely anxious about conservation treatment, 30% were very or extremely anxious about drilling, and 28% were very or extremely anxious about oral injections. About 13% reported that they "always" or "very often" postponed visits to the dentist because of anxiety.[9]

Ayer and Corah[10] estimated that up to 25% of the American population avoids dental treatment except when symptomatic. In a Dental Fear Survey conducted in the states of Florida and Washington, about 5% reported that they postponed making dental appointments due to fear "nearly every time", while another 9% did it "often", and another 10% "a few times". When asked to rate how fearful they were of having dental work, about 7% ranked it "very much", 10% "much", and 20% "somewhat".[11]

High levels of dental fear were also found in the population of several major western cities.[12-14] In Dallas about 12% of respondents reported high dental fear and another 17% reported moderate dental fear. Results disclosed that 36% of those surveyed had not been to the dentist in over a year.[12] In a survey conducted on 1019 residents of Seattle, 50% reported some dental fear, with about 30% acknowledging being a little afraid, 13% being somewhat afraid, 4% being very afraid, and 3% being terrified of dental treatment.[13] In Toronto and North York, Ontario, approximately 13% of those surveyed (age 50 and over) were found to be anxious or highly anxious about dental care (total number of respondents: 2007).[14]

In a survey of dental fear in Japan, up to 80% of Japanese college students reported some fear, while 6 to 14% reported to be "very afraid" or "terrified" of the treatment. When the group of "somewhat afraid" was added to these two categories (similar to the calculations carried out in the survey in Seattle), the range was from 21 to 33%.[15] In Singapore, 68 out of 505 primary school children, age 10 to 14, were classified as having a high level of fear (prevalence of 177 fearful children per 1000 population).[16]

Although some surveys have not found significant correlations between gender and fear level of the respondents,[17-21] many others indicate higher levels of anxiety among women.[11-13,15,22-27] This may be due to a higher percentage of women respondents in some of the studies,[9,12,13,19,23] but may also originate from the generally accepted social norm which allows women to more freely express their anxieties.

Based on different social roles and expectations, it is possible that men and women differ in their willingness (or ability) to admit their anxiety feelings.[24] Duivenvoorden et al.[28] claimed that anxiety experienced by both genders is more readily reported by women. In their study, four times as many men as women showed patterns of repression and denial regarding their dental anxiety (probably due to learned behavior in which anxiety should not be expressed). Similarly, Kent[29] reported that men claim more control over dental anxiety than women.

Presumably, in many of the cases, dental anxiety in men is expressed in other, less direct, ways (e.g., excessive gagging reflex; see Chapter 5). Indirect support for this premise may be found in the fact that among patients suffering from severe dental fear, oral health is significantly more deteriorated in men than in women.[30] Furthermore, many clinics specializing in the treatment of dental fear and phobia report a higher number of female patients.[11,24,26,30,31] This indicates that women are probably more open to admitting anxiety and initiating treatment.

Taking the various data together, it is clear that dental fear and anxiety pose a major community health problem. If we consider that about 15% of the adult population suffer from partial avoidance of dental care (attending treatment only when symptomatology arises) and another 6% suffer from total avoidance (not attending dental treatment at all), we are facing a population of millions of patients all over the world. These patients need special attention and treatment (sedation, general anesthesia, behavioral modification, etc.) which will enable them to obtain proper dental care. Additionally, the emotional status of these individuals has an extreme adverse effect on their oral health, a fact which affects the financial costs (private, insurance, community) involved.

III. INFLUENCE ON ORAL HEALTH

Dental anxiety is detrimental to the oral health of the patient. Although this statement is almost self-explanatory, relatively few studies precisely assess the oral condition of patients who are afraid of dental treatment.

Dental anxiety plays a significant role in nonattendance for dental treatment.[17] One method used to assess anxiety in patients involves the tabulation of missed or cancelled dental appointments.[20,24] Damage and neglect are the obvious consequences of such avoidance behavior. This leads to pain, and further contributes to the existing stress, additional avoidance, more neglect and vice versa. The vicious cycle is reinforced by feelings of shame due to the oral condition and to the inability to cope with the situation. Other defensive adjustment mechanisms, such as suppression ("...I don't even want to think of it"), denial ("...there is nothing wrong with my teeth"), projection ("...it is the dentists who have ruined my teeth") further contribute to the inability (and often also the unwillingness) of the patient to cope with the situation (Figure 4).

As time elapses, past dental experiences tend to gain in negative impact. When asked retrospectively how they felt, many patients recall more anxiety than when actually seated in the dental chair.[32] Similarly, anxious patients report more pain 3 months after the appointment than they do immediately following treatment, probably due to the reconstruction of memories to make them consistent with their existing level of anxiety.[33]

Dental anxiety is usually associated with a range of variables describing behavioral and oral health outcomes. The dentally anxious individuals were found to be less likely to use dental services, less satisfied with dental care, and have poorer self-perceived oral health.[14]

Duivenvoorden et al.[28] pointed out that it is not anxiety itself but rather the way one deals with it which determines the behavioral consequences (regular or irregular attendance of dental treatment). A desire for a well cared for mouth may be a powerful incentive for some regular attenders even when it is occasionally concomitant with dental fear. On the other hand, repression and denial leads to neglect of dental care. It seems that irregular dental attendance depends on the level of the variables involved (dental anxiety, family dental pattern, and preference for preserving teeth).[33]

The consequences are often catastrophic. In the Netherlands,[35] about 80% of the patients who reached the state of full mouth extractions did not visit a dentist on a regular basis, with anxiety probably being the major factor in their poor attendance. In a study conducted on 160 patients referred to a specialist clinic because of severe dental fear and avoidance, the mean DMFS-rate (Decayed, Missing, Filled per Surface) was 76.6 (range 20 to 126). On the average, there were 37 carious tooth surfaces (range 3 to 75), 26 restored surfaces (range 0 to 25), and 5 missing teeth (range 0 to 25), 3 remaining teeth with a total destruction of the crown, and 4 periapical lesions. More than half

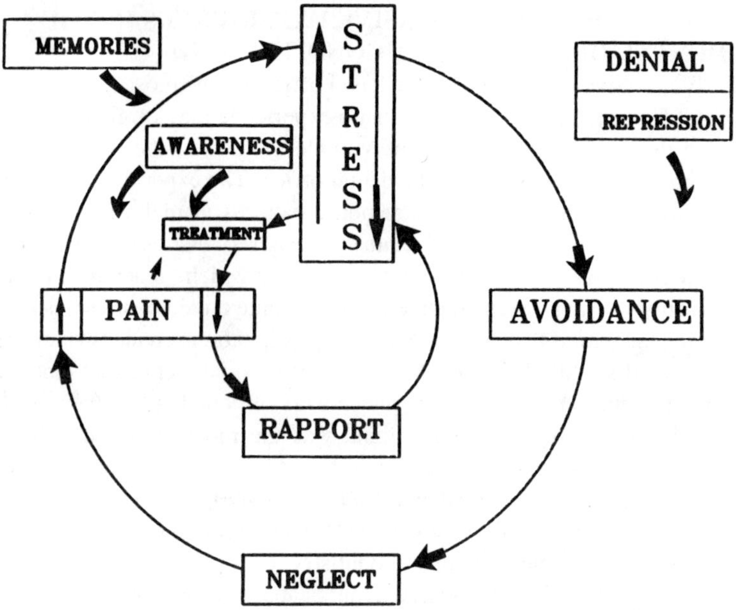

FIGURE 4. The vicious cycle of stress, avoidance, and pain in dentistry. The stress aroused by the dental situation leads to avoidance of treatment and neglect of oral health. This leads to increased pain, more stress, and further avoidance. The cycle is enhanced by memories of past traumatic experiences and by defensive adjustment mechanisms, such as denial and repression. Occasionally, when the experienced pain is higher than the stress aroused by the possibility of treatment, treatment is initiated. If, at this stage, a proper interpersonal relationship with the dentist is established, this will lead to a continuation of treatment, a decrease in experienced pain, an increase in rapport, a further decrease in stress, and vice versa. The positive cycle of treatment and rapport can be enhanced by the patient's awareness and desire for a well cared for mouth.

of the patients had visible dental plaque on all tooth surfaces, 13% had one or two crowns, and 9% wore dentures.[30] In another study of 11 patients treated for dental fear, the mean DMFS rate was 60.5 (ranging from 36 to 88) and an average of 8 years elapsed since their last dental treatment.[31]

IV. ANTECEDENTS OF DENTAL FEAR/ANXIETY/PHOBIA

The dental situation is complex and involves physical, psychodynamic, cognitive, and learned factors (see Chapter 2). Generally, a combination of several factors leads to the development of dental anxiety. We can investigate some of them and speculate about others, but the final result is the same: emotional arousal that does not allow routine dental care leads to severe impairment of oral health.

A. EFFECT OF EARLY AVERSIVE EXPERIENCES IN THE DENTAL OFFICE (DIRECT CONDITIONING)

Early, aversive encounters in the dental office are the most common causes of dental fear and anxiety. The traumatic experience may originate from pain inflicted during treatment, from unfavorable attitude of the dentist, or from other unpleasant experiences in the dental office. The experience serves as an initial stimulus triggering specific response patterns, namely, fear or anxiety. If the dentist fails to perceive and relate to the signs of distress at this point, that behavior serves as a negative reinforcing factor which "teaches" the patient that the only way to avoid punishment (in this context pain or stress) is to avoid the dental encounter. A new learned, unadaptive, habit is created which affects the individual's future behavior. Many studies found direct negative or painful dental experiences to be the main antecedents of dental fear.[18,22,23,25,30,36-38]

Lautch[37] claimed that dental trauma was the most important etiological factor in the development of dental fear, but at least two such experiences are generally necessary for severe dental phobia to develop. Similarly, Kleinknecht et al.[22] identified personal experience associated with painful procedures as a main source of adverse reactions to dentistry.

Bernstein et al.[18] found negative remarks about early dental experiences to be significantly more frequent among high fear respondents (70%) than among low fear respondents (45%). The picture of high fear antecedents that emerged from this study was one of painful early dental experiences from unpleasant and professionally threatening dentists. Among the high fear respondents, 42% mentioned pain during early appointments as a factor in their present negative reaction to dentistry, and 50% negatively evaluated the dentist's professional behavior and personal characteristics.

An association between dental anxiety and unpleasant childhood dental experiences was found by Cohen et al.[23] American students with high anxiety scores were much more likely to remember their childhood dental experiences as being negative. Personal past experience was quoted as a major factor governing dental anxiety among English dental patients.[25]

In a study conducted on 160 anxious dental patients in Sweden, dental fear usually commenced during childhood (85%), with the dominating causative factor being a previous traumatic dental experience. For fear of early origin, the dentist's professional behavior was most important, whereas for fear acquired in adult years, pain was important.[30] A similar correlation between the development of dental anxiety and a former painful experience was reported by Davey.[38]

Although there is some evidence that anxious patients tend to increase their report of pain experienced during dental treatment as time elapses after the actual encounter,[33] it seems that direct experience in the dental chair is a major factor in the development of dental anxiety.

B. EFFECT OF VICARIOUS LEARNING

Fear and anxiety can be acquired, not only by direct learning, but also by vicarious learning from role models (family, peers, and society). The learning process can be a result of observation, identification with, or indirect suggestions by the role models.

In some studies, subjects were nonresponsive on the matter of perceived dental anxiety in members of their immediate family.[17] However, many of the studies which quoted direct, aversive experience with a dentist as the main reason for developing dental fear, also pointed out the importance of indirect modeling.[22,36,39] For example, Kleinknecht et al.[22] showed that negative attitudes learned from others were often given by individuals as an explanation for their own negative attitudes about dentistry.

Several studies reported a positive correlation (among other factors) between dental anxiety and "frequency of mother's visit to dentists,"[23] and between dental anxiety scores and vicarious anxiety scores (scores of patient's perceptions of dental anxiety experienced by significant others, e.g., parents, siblings, and peers).[19]

Another method used to assess the effect of role models on dental anxiety was to check for a relationship between parental anxiety and the behavior of children in the dental operatory. Such a correlation was shown among children undergoing dental treatment[40] and in prediction of behavior management problems in children.[41] Parental dental anxiety was also found to be positively associated with the caries status of their children.[42]

Dental anxiety and avoidance behavior can be acquired as a result of social learning. Among irregularly attending patients who reached the stage of full mouth extractions, widespread dental anxiety was reported, but no correlation was made between its level and the number of negative experiences.[35] This group reported a higher average age for the first dental visit (19 years) and a higher percentage of full denture wearers in their social environment (75%). It was suggested that, in this group, anxiety was largely a result of social learning, transmitted because of negative experiences of parents, friends, and peers.

C. CORRELATION BETWEEN DENTAL FEAR/ANXIETY/PHOBIA AND PERSONALITY TRAITS (PSYCHODYNAMIC ASPECTS)

Dental anxiety is a response to a specific situation (confronting dental treatment) and, as such, comprises parameters of both state and trait anxiety. It is, therefore, useful to attempt to outline specific personality traits which, when present, increase the patient's proneness for apprehension in the dental setting.

One such study was conducted among English dental patients attending two different dental practices: a regular clinic using local anesthesia, and a "dental phobic" clinic using sedation anesthesia.[43] In the study, measures of dental fear and anxiety were highly correlated with neuroticism as measured by the Eysenck Personality Questionnaire, a finding which basically agrees with Lautch[37] and Klepac et al.[26]

Higher neuroticism among anxious dental patients was also reported by Schuurs et al.[44] Anxious patients were found to be rigid, less decisive, and less stable (i.e., more neurotic); they had lower self-esteem, felt loss of control in many situations, and were less inclined to act. An additional study[45] showed that a positive correlation existed between the external part of the Health Locus of Control and scores of dental anxiety.

Factors such as general anxiety, neuroticism, and a high tendency toward phobic reactions have also been identified as a cause of dental fear.[30] About 50% of patients referred for treatment due to extreme dental anxiety and avoidance received psychiatric treatment, 31% received psychopharmacological medication, and 64% reported various psychosomatic conditions such as tension, headache, and stomachache.

A positive correlation was found between dental anxiety and changes in the Mood Adjective Check List (reflecting various moods such as pleasantness and relaxation).[21,31] Positive correlations were also found between dental anxiety and other fears, such as fear of pain, mutilation (e.g., injury, blood, disfigurement),[46] flying, enclosures, illness, etc.[47]

V. COMPONENTS OF DENTAL FEAR/ ANXIETY/PHOBIA

What are the major factors quoted as anxiety provoking by anxious and by nonanxious dental patients? The initial study in this area was published by Gale in 1972.[48] A total of 130 dental patients (with high and low dental fear) were asked to rate the amount of fear associated with 25 dental situations. The results were similar for both groups. Although there was a significant difference between the groups as to the overall fear ratings, both ranked the same six situations as being the most fearful:

- dentist is pulling your tooth
- dentist is drilling your tooth
- dentist tells you that you have bad teeth
- dentist holds the syringe and needle in front of you
- dentist is giving you a shot
- dentist places a probe in a cavity

Most of the situations have a direct association with an immediate physical threat (extraction, drilling, injection, etc.). Others are related to future, anticipated harm (bad teeth, watching the needle). The next ranked item reported ("dentist laughs as he looks in your mouth") is associated with a threat to self-esteem and was ranked differently by the two groups (rank order of 7 in the low fear group and 10 in the high fear group).

Berggren and Meynert[30] reported similar findings among patients in a specialized dental fear clinic. The most feared situations were slow and high speed drilling, preparation of anesthetic, extraction of tooth, receiving anesthetic, and waiting in the dental chair, all associated with anticipation and direct physical threat.

In another study conducted by Bernstein et al.,[18] the most highly ranked negative aspects of dentistry were pain during appointment, dentist's personal and professional behaviors and characteristics, and injection. While two of these aspects relate directly to physical threat (pain, injection), the third (dentist) bears clear relevance to an interpersonal relationship in the dental office, which by itself can be a significant factor in initiating or reducing dental anxiety. This is in agreement with the findings of Berggren and Meynert[30] in which phobic patients claimed the "worst dentist" to be critical of the patient, distant, and inconsiderate.

The assumption that dental fear contains a component of physical threat as well as a component of threat to one's self-esteem was also raised by Stouthard and Hoogstraten.[49] The categories ranked highest in the hierarchy of fear arousal were those of "comments by the dentist on oral state" and of "actual dental treatment."

VI. ASSESSMENT OF DENTAL FEAR

The response complex of fear and anxiety consists of three major components,[50] all of which are expressed (in different degrees) by the anxious dental patient:

1. Verbal report of the experience (telling the dentist of being afraid of treatment)
2. Physiological experience (sweating, trembling, muscle tension, acceleration of heart rate)
3. Behavioral effects, such as avoidance and performance inefficiency

The measures which attempt to assess dental fear and anxiety are based on these components. The most frequently used means are based on self-report questionnaires in which the patient is asked directly about the fear ("how do you feel when…?")[51] or the feelings of the patient are indirectly assessed from other parameters (number of appointments cancelled or missed due to fear;[20,24] regular or irregular attendance to dental treatment[28,34]).

Other measures include an assessment of the patient's behavior by an outside observer,[41,52-59] and the use of physiological measures such as heart rate or galvanic skin response.[60-64]

A. SELF-REPORT QUESTIONNAIRES

A common questionnaire used to assess anxiety in different settings is the State-Trait Anxiety Inventory (STAI) developed by Sielberger et al.[65] In the questionnaire, a distinction is made between state and trait anxiety by designing 20 statements to measure trait anxiety, and another 20 statements to measure state anxiety ("how you feel right now"). The STAI has occasionally been used to assess anxiety in the dental setting.[24,66]

Several questionnaires have been developed specifically for use in dentistry. One of the major and most widely used self-report questionnaires of dental anxiety is the Dental Anxiety Scale (DAS) developed by Corah.[51] This measure of trait anxiety is simple, short, and easy to administer. It consists of four items in which the patient is asked to rate on a five-point scale the following variables (reprinted with permission):

1. If you had to go to the dentist tomorrow how would you feel about it?
   a. I would look forward to it as a reasonably enjoyable experience.
   b. I wouldn't care one way or the other.
   c. I would be a little uneasy about it.
   d. I would be afraid that it would be unpleasant and painful.
   e. I would be very frightened of what the dentist might do.
2. When you are waiting in the dentist's office for your turn in the chair, how do you feel?
   a. Relaxed.
   b. A little uneasy.
   c. Tense.
   d. Anxious.
   e. So anxious that I sometimes break out in a sweat or almost feel physically sick.
3. When you are in the dentist's chair waiting while he gets his drill ready to begin working on your teeth, how do you feel? (Same alternatives as number 2.)
4. You are in the dental chair to have your teeth cleaned. While you are waiting and the dentist is getting out the instruments which he will use to scrape your teeth around the gums, how do you feel? (Same alternatives as number 2.)

The DAS provides a range of scores from a minimum of 4 to a maximum of 20 and has shown a high predictive validity rate.[67] Generally the highly fearful or phobic patient scores 13 or higher on the scale.[68] Since its development, the DAS has been uscd extensively in many research projects performed on anxious patients.[14,19,21,23,28,30,31,43-45,60-62,69-75]

Various studies have shown general agreement in mean scores on DAS between Swedish and American populations[21,30,73] and between DAS scores and regular or irregular attendance for treatment.[28] The questionnaire has recently been modified to also assess anxiety in edentulous individuals.[76]

Several other questionnaires have successfully measured dental anxiety. The Geer Fear Scale (GFS)[21,77] was found to be a good predictor of treatment outcome in fearful patients. It correlates significantly with DAS with regard to fearful dental patients following treatment for dental fear. No such correlation was found in a group of extremely fearful patients before treatment.[73]

The Dental Fear Survey (DFS) developed by Kleinknecht et al.[22] is also widely used to assess dental anxiety. The DFS uses a representative five-point scale (1 — no reaction of fear; 5 — great fear or reaction) to assess dental avoidance, somato–visceral arousal during dental treatment, and naturalistic and clinical behaviors involved in receiving dental care. The following parameters are included (reprinted with permission):

Avoidance of dentistry:

1. Have avoided calling for appointment
2. Have cancelled or not appeared

Felt physiological responses:

3. Muscle becomes tense
4. Breathing increases
5. Perspiration increases
6. Nausea
7. Heart rate increases
8. Mouth salivates

Fearfulness of stimuli:

9. Making an appointment
10. Approaching office
11. Waiting room
12. Dental chair
13. Smell of office
14. Seeing dentist
15. Seeing needle
16. Feeling needle
17. Seeing drill
18. Hearing drill
19. Feeling drill
20. Feeling as if you are going to gag
21. Having teeth cleaned
22. Feeling pain even after anesthetic injection
23. Generally how fearful you are of dentistry

How fearful are your:

24. Mother
25. Father
26. Brothers and sisters
27. Childhood friends

Three other open-ended items are included for the respondents to describe past painful and fearful dental experiences and their own interpretation of the ways in which they acquired their present reaction to dentistry.

The DFS has been shown to have predictive validity and be an efficient tool for assessing dental fear.[20,78-80] It has been used in a number of studies concerning dental fear throughout the world.[15,18,22,24]

B. BEHAVIORAL MEASURES

Stress, fear, and anxiety can be indirectly assessed by drawing conclusions from behavior in particular situations. Several behavior measures have been used to assess dental anxiety, especially among children, whose ability (and/or cooperation) in filling out questionnaires is limited.

To assess the effect of maternal anxiety on the behavior of young children in the dental office, Johnson and Baldwin[52] used a behavioral rating scale in which the child's behavior was observed by two independent observers and scored at four rating categories:

1. Definitely negative (refusal of treatment, overt resistance and hostility, extreme fear, forceful crying, massive withdrawal, isolation, or both)
2. Slightly negative (minor negativism or resistance, minimal to moderate reserve, fear, nervousness, or crying)
3. Slightly positive (cautious acceptance of treatment but with some reluctance, questions or delaying tactics, moderate willingness to comply with the dentist, etc.)
4. Definitely positive (good rapport with operator, no sign of fear, interest in procedures and appropriate verbal contact)

Other studies on the behavior of young children in the dental operatory used videotapes of the sessions as a means of measurement.[53-55] Videotapes were then analyzed to create a code scheme of behaviors for the child and for the dentist. The coding scheme for the children included:

1. Movement and physical positioning (ranging from appropriate positioning with child-initiated appropriate movement: reopening mouth without cue, to child-initiated minor movement with positioning no longer appropriate)
2. Verbal behavior (ranging from silence to screaming)
3. Comfort (ranging from pleasantness to discomfort and tension)

Other behavior rating tools include the behavior scale described by Rud and Kissling,[58] and the Behavior Profile Rating Scale developed by Melamed et al.[56,57] Melamed et al.[56] weighed the child's behavior, not only by its absolute meaning (crying, choking, verbal complaints, etc.), but also by its relative duration. The scale includes recording the frequency of behaviors that led to disruption of the treatment procedures on the basis of 3-min intervals (i.e.,

41. **Holst, A., Schröder, U., Ek, L., Hallonsten, A.-L., and Crossner, C.-G.,** Prediction of behavior management problems in children, *Scand. J. Dent. Res.*, 96, 457, 1988.
42. **Lahti, S., Tuutti, H., and Honkala, E.,** The relationship of parental dental anxiety and child's caries status, *J. Dent. Child.*, 56, 191, 1989.
43. **Frazer, M. and Hampson, S.,** Some personality factors related to dental anxiety and fear of pain, *Br. Dent. J.*, 165, 436, 1988.
44. **Schuurs, A. H. B., Duivenvoorden, H. J, Makkes, P. C., Thoden van Velzen, S. K., and Verhage, F.,** Personality traits of patients suffering extreme dental anxiety, *Community Dent. Oral Epidemiol.*, 16, 38, 1988.
45. **Neverlien, P. O.,** Dental fear and locus of control: a pilot study, *Community Dent. Oral Epidemiol.*, 16, 127, 1988.
46. **McNeil, D. W. and Berryman, M. L.,** Components of dental fear in adults?, *Behav. Res. Ther.*, 27, 233, 1989.
47. **Fiset, L., Milgrom, P., and Melnick, S.,** dentification of the relationship between dental and non-dental fears, utilization of the dentist, *J. Dent. Res.*, 67, 169, Abstr. No. 453, 1988.
48. **Gale, E. N.,** Fears of the dental situation, *J. Dent. Res.*, 51, 964, 1972.
49. **Stouthard, M. E. A. and Hoogstraten, J.,** Ratings of fears associated with twelve dental situations, *J. Dent. Res.*, 66, 1175, 1987.
50. **Beech, H. R., Burns, L. E., and Sheffield, B. F.,** *A Behavioural Approach to the Management of Stress*, John Wiley & Sons, Chichester, 1984.
51. **Corah, N. L.,** Development of a dental anxiety scale, *J. Dent. Res.*, 48, 596, 1969.
52. **Johnson, R. and Baldwin, D. C.,** Relationship of maternal anxiety to the behavior of young children undergoing dental extraction, *J. Dent. Res.*, 47, 801, 1968.
53. **Weinstein, P., Getz, T., Ratener, P., and Domoto, P.,** The effect of dentists' behaviors on fear-related behaviors in children, *J. Am. Dent. Assoc.*, 104, 32, 1982.
54. **Weinstein, P., Getz, T., Ratener, P., and Domoto, P.,** Dentists' responses to fear- and nonfear-related behaviors in children, *J. Am. Dent. Assoc.*, 104, 38, 1982.
55. **Weinstein, P., Getz, T., and Domoto, P.,** Temporal patterns of the behavior of young children in the dental chair, *J. Pedodontics*, 9, 188, 1985.
56. **Melamed, B. G., Weinstein, D., Hawes, R., and Borland, M.,** Reduction of fear-related dental management problems with use of filmed modeling, *J. Am. Dent. Assoc.*, 90, 822, 1975.
57. **Melamed, B. G., Bennett, C. G., errell, G., Ross, S. L., Bush, J. P., Hill, C., Courts, F., and Ronk, S.,** Dentists' behavior management as it affects compliance and fear in pediatric patients, *J. Am. Dent. Assoc.*, 106, 324, 1983.
58. **Rud, B. B. and Kisling, E.,** The influence of mental development on children's acceptance of dental treatment, *Scand. J. Dent. Res.*, 81, 343, 1973.
59. **Holst, A. and Crossner, C.-G.,** Direct ratings of acceptance of dental treatment in Swedish children, *Community Dent. Oral Epidemiol.*, 15, 258, 1987.
60. **Corah, N. L., Gale, E. N., and llig, S. J.,** The use of relaxation and distraction to reduce psychological stress during dental procedure, *J. Am. Dent. Assoc.*, 98, 390, 1979.
61. **Corah, N. L., Gale, E. N., and Illig, S. J.,** Psychological stress reduction during dental procedures, *J. Dent. Res.*, 58, 1347, 1979.
62. **Carlsson, S. G., Linde, A., Berggren, U., and Harrison, J. A.,** Reduction of dental fear: psychophysiological correlates, *Community Dent. Oral Epidemiol.*, 14, 253, 1986.
63. **Simpson, W. J., Ruzicka, R. L., and Thomas, N. R.,** Physiologic responses of children to initial dental experience, *J. Dent. Child.*, 41, 465, 1974.

Meldman, M. J, The dental phobia test, *Psychosomatics*, 13, 371, 1972.

Spielberger, C. D., Gorsuch, R., and Lushene, R., *The State Trait Anxiety Inventory (STAI)*, Consulting Psychologists Press, Riverside, CA, 1970.

Wardle, J., Fear of dentistry, *Br. J. Med. Psychol.*, 55, 119, 1982.

Corah, N. L., Gale, E. N., and Illig, S. J., Assessment of a dental anxiety scale, *J. Am. Dent. Assoc.*, 97, 816, 1978.

recording the child's behavior every 3 min). Thus a child who cried only once, for less than 3 min at the beginning of the session, would be rated lower than a child who repeated this behavior several times.

Behavioral measures are occasionally used for the anxious adult patient. In several studies the dentist was asked to rate the cooperation and treatability of anxious adult patients compared to average patients.[74] This was done on a six-point scale, where a rating of 1 indicated "much better," a rating of 3 indicated "equal to," and a rating of 5 indicated "much worse" than average patients. A rating of 6 stood for "impossible to treat." Similar ratings were also used in adult dental phobic patients.[73]

C. PHYSIOLOGICAL MEASURES

Physiological changes are perhaps more subjective, but also less readily available measures of dental stress and anxiety. Commonly used measures include parameters such as electromyograms, heart rate, galvanic skin response, and palmar sweat index.[20,60-64,81] These are relatively easy to apply, noninvasive, physiological measures of stress. An EMG-feedback device to measure and display muscle tension may also be used.[70]

These methods provide a relatively objective measure of the physiological changes that occur during stress. However, they can occasionally act as stress-inflicting factors themselves. The use of additional measuring devices may increase threat appraisal of patients who are already under stress. The attempt to use electrodes connected to unknown, potentially "threatening" instruments may serve as an additional stress-inflicting stimulus.

Several other physiological changes can potentially serve as noninvasive parameters of stress in the dental situation. A good example is the effect of stress on salivary flow and composition[82-89] (see also Chapter 9.I). Saliva is body fluid which is easy to obtain and which is intuitively connected with the oral cavity and oral treatment. As such, it may be a less threatening physiological measure, effective for the evaluation of stress in the dental situation.

VII. TREATMENT

Patients suffering from dental fear/anxiety/phobia pose a special challenge to the dental practitioner. Treatment modalities include measures from all relevant fields: behavior modification, hypnosis, and the use of various relevant pharmaceutical agents. A detailed presentation of the treatment modes is presented in Section 3, Chapters 10 to 13.

VIII. SUMMARY

Fear and anxiety are the most common behavioral dysfunctions related to dental care, with prevalence generally estimated as high as 20%. Patients postpone dental care or avoid it altogether, thereby causing severe deterioration of their oral health.

The antecedents of dental fear are many: early aversive encounters in the dental office, vicarious learning through models, and individual personality traits are the most common factors which predispose dental anxiety. Its major components include a direct association with and an anticipation of immediate physical threat, as well as threat to one's self-esteem.

Proper identification and assessment of dental fear include the use of self-report questionnaires, and behavioral and physiological measures.

REFERENCES

1. **May, R.,** Anxiety and stress, in *Selye's Guide to Stress Research*, Vol. 2, Selye, H., Ed., Scientific and Academic Editions, New York, 1983.
2. **Hinsie, L. E. and Campbell, R. J.,** *Psychiatric Dictionary*, 5th ed., Oxford University Press, New York, 1981.
3. The American Psychiatric Association, *The Diagnostic and Statistical Manual*, III, 1980, 225.
4. **Spielberger, C. D.,** Current trends in theory on research on anxiety, in *Anxiety — Current Trends in Theory and Research*, Vol. 1, Spielberger, C. D., Ed., Academic Press, New York, 1972, 3.
5. **Friedson, E. and Feldman, J. J.,** The public looks at dental care, *J. Am. Dent. Assoc.*, 57, 325, 1958.
6. **Crockett, B.,** Dental survey: Southeastern State College, *J. Okla. Dent. Assoc.*, 51, 25, 1963.
7. Svenska Institutet för Opinionsundersökningar (SIFO): Tandlökarbesök, Intervjuundersökning för Tandvörnet, Stockholm, 1962.
8. **Seeman, K. and Molin, C.,** Psychopathology, feelings of confinement and helplessness in the dental chair, and relationship to the dentist in patients with disproportionate dental anxiety (DDA), *Acta Psychiatr. Scand.*, 54, 81, 1976.
9. **Lindsay, S. J. E., Humphris, G., and Barnby, G. J.,** Expectations and preferences for routine dentistry in anxious adult patients, *Br. Dent. J.*, 163, 120, 1987.
10. **Ayer, W. A. and Corah, N. L.,** Behavioural factors influencing dental treatment, in *Social Sciences and Dentistry: A Critical Bibliography*, Vol. 2, Cohen, L. K. and Bryant, P. S., Eds., Quintessence Publishing Co. for Federation Dentaire Internationale, Kingston-upon-Thames, England, 1984, 267.
11. **Milgrom, P., Weinstein, P., Kleinknecht, R., and Getz, T.,** *Treating Fearful Dental Patients*, Reston Publishing Co., Reston, Va, 1985.
12. **Gatchel, R. J, Ingersoll, B. D., Bowman, L., Robertson, M. C., and Walker, C.,** The prevalence of dental fear and avoidance: a recent survey study, *J. Am. Dent. Assoc.*, 107, 609, 1983.
13. **Milgrom, P., Fiset, L., Melnick, S., and Weinstein, P.,** The prevalence and practice management consequences of dental fear in a major US city, *J. Am. Dent. Assoc.*, 116, 641, 1988.
14. **Locker, D. and Liddell, A. M.,** Correlates of dental anxiety among older adults, *J. Dent. Res.*, 70, 198, 1991.
15. **Domoto, P. K., Weinstein, P., Melnick, S., Ohmura, M., Uchida, H., Ohmachi, K., Hori, M., Okazaki, Y., Shimamoto, T., Matsumura, S., and Shimono, T.,** Results of a dental fear survey in Japan: implications for dental public health in Asia, *Community Dent. Oral Epidemiol.*, 16, 199, 1988.

16. **Chellappah, N. K., Vignehsa, H., Milgrom, P., and Lo, G. L.,** Prevalence of dental anxiety and fear in children in Singapore, *Community Dent. Oral Epidemiol.*, 18, 269, 1990.
17. **Liddell, A. and May, B.,** Some charcteristics of regular and irregular attenders for dental check-ups, *Br. J. Clin. Psychol.*, 23, 19, 1984.
18. **Bernstein, D. A., Kleinknecht, R. A., and Alexander, L. D.,** Antecedents of dental fear, *J. Public Health Dent.*, 39, 113, 1979.
19. **Rankin, J. A. and Harris, M. B.,** Dental anxiety: the patient's point of view, *J. Am. Dent. Assoc.*, 109, 43, 1984.
20. **Kleinknecht, R. A. and Bernstein, D. A.,** The assessment of dental fear, *Behav. Ther.*, 9, 626, 1978.
21. **Berggren, U. and Carlsson, S. G.,** Psychometric measures of dental fear, *Community Dent. Oral Epidemiol.*, 12, 319, 1984.
22. **Kleinknecht, R. A., Klepac, R. K., and Alexander, L. D.,** Origins and characteristics of fear of dentistry, *J. Am. Dent. Assoc.*, 86, 842, 1973.
23. **Cohen, L. A., Snyder, T. L., and LaBelle, A. D.,** Correlates of dental anxiety in a university population, *J. Public Health Dent.*, 42, 228, 1982.
24. **Bernstein, D. A. and Kleinknecht, R. A.,** Multiple approaches to the reduction of dental fear, *J. Behav. Ther. Exp. Psychiatry*, 13, 287, 1982.
25. **Green, R. M. and Green, A.,** Adult attitudes to dentistry among dental attenders in South Wales, *Br. Dent. J.*, 159, 157, 1985.
26. **Klepac, R. K., Dowling, J., and Hauge, G.,** Characteristics of clients seeking therapy for the reduction of dental avoidance: reactions to pain, *J. Behav. Ther. Exp. Psychiatry*, 13, 293, 1982.
27. **Eli, I. and Kleinhauz, M.,** Oro-related behavioral dysfunctions: a disabling factor in dental care, (in press).
28. **Duivenvoorden H. J., Schuurs, A. H. B., Thoden van Velzen, S. K., Verhage, F Makkes, P. C., and Eijkman, M. A. J.,** Influence of repression upon the measuremen dental anxiety, *Community Dent. Oral Epidemiol.*, 13, 315, 1985.
29. **Kent, G.,** Self-efficacious control over reported physiological, cognitive and behav symptoms of dental anxiety, *Behav. Res. Ther.*, 25, 341, 1987.
30. **Berggren, U. and Meynert, G.,** Dental fear and avoidance: causes, sympto consequences, *J. Am. Dent. Assoc.*, 109, 247, 1984.
31. **Harrison, J. A., Carlsson, S. G., and Berggren, U.,** Research in clinical p outcome methodology: psychophysiology, systematic desensitization and de *Behav. Ther. Exp. Psychiatry*, 16, 201, 1985.
32. **Tullman, G. M., Tullman, M. J., and Rogers, B. J.,** Anxiety in dental p of three phases of State anxiety in three treatment groups, *Psychol. Rep.*
33. **Kent, G.,** Memory of dental pain, *Pain*, 21, 187, 1985.
34. **Schuurs, A. H. B., Duivenvoorden, H. J., Thoden van Velzen, S. K.,** Three factors predicting irregular versus regular dental attendance: empirical data, *Community Dent. Oral Epidemiol.*, 8, 413, 1980.
35. **Bouma, J., Uitenbroek, D. G., Westert, G. P., Schaub, R. M. H** C. M., Pathways to full mouth extraction, *Community Dent. Or* 1987.
36. **Forgione, A. G. and Clark, R. E.,** Comments on an empirical st fear, *J. Dent. Res.*, 53, 496, 1974.
37. **Lautch, H.,** Dental phobia, *Br. J. Psychiatry*, 119, 151, 197
38. **Davey, G. C. L.,** Dental phobias and anxieties: Evidence fo acquisition and modulation of a learned fear, *Behav. Res.*
39. **Shoben, E. J., Jr. and Borland, L.,** An empirical study *Clin. Psych.*, 10, 171, 1954.
40. **Johnson, R.,** Maternal influence on child behavior in 2, 221, 1971.

68. **Corah, N. L.,** Dental anxiety: assessment, reduction and increasing patient satisfaction, *Dent. Clin. North Am.*, 32, 779, 1988.
69. **Scott, D. S. and Hirschman, R.,** Psychological aspects of dental anxiety in adults, *J. Am. Dent. Assoc.*, 104, 27, 1982.
70. **Berggren, U. and Carlsson, S. G.,** A psychophysiological therapy for dental fear, *Behav. Res. Ther.*, 22, 487, 1984.
71. **Berggren, U. and Carlsson, S. G.,** Qualitative and quantitative effects of treatment for dental fear and avoidance, *Anesth. Prog.*, 33, 9, 1986.
72. **Berggren, U.,** Long-term effects of two different treatments for dental fear and avoidance, *J. Dent. Res.*, 65, 874, 1986.
73. **Berggren U. and Carlsson, S. G.,** Usefulness of two psychometric scales in Swedish patients with severe dental fear, *Community Dent. Oral Epidemiol.*, 13, 70, 1985.
74. **Berggren, U. and Linde, A.,** Dental fear and avoidance: a comparison of two modes of treatment, *J. Dent. Res.*, 63, 1223, 1984.
75. **Kunzelmann, K.-H. and Dünninger, P.,** Dental fear and pain: effect on patient's perception of the dentist, *Community Dent. Oral Epidemiol.*, 18, 264, 1990.
76. **Vervoorn, J. M., Duinkerke, A. S. H., Luteijn, F., van de Poel, A. C. M.,** Assessment of dental anxiety in edentulous subjects, *Community Dent. Oral Epidemiol.*, 17, 177, 1989.
77. **Geer, J. H.,** The development of a scale to measure fear, *Behav. Res. Ther.*, 3, 45, 1965.
78. **Kleinknecht, R. A., Thorndike, R. M., McGlynn, F. D., and Harkavy, J.,** Factor analysis of the Dental Fear Survey with cross-validation, *J. Am. Dent. Assoc.*, 108, 59, 1984.
79. **McGlynn, F. D., McNeil, D. W., Gallagher, S. L., and Vrana, S.,** Factor structure, stability, and internal consistency of the Dental Fear Survey, *Behav. Assessment*, 9, 57, 1987.
80. **McGlynn, F. D.,** Dental Fear Survey, in *Dictionary of Behavioral Assessment Techniques*, Hersen, M. and Bellack, A. S., Eds., Pergamon Press, New York, 1988.
81. **Wong, M. and Kaloupek, D. G.,** Coping with dental treatment: the potential impact of situational demands, *J. Behav. Med.*, 9, 579, 1986.
82. **Bates, J. F. and Adams, D.,** The influence of mental stress on the flow of saliva in man, *Arch. Oral Biol.*, 13, 593, 1968.
83. **Silverstein, L. and Iverson, M. A.,** Human salivary response to interpersonal bargaining situations: a psycho-physiological investigation, *Psychol. Rep.*, 37, 771, 1975.
84. **Bassett, J. R., Marshall, P. M., and Spillane, R.,** The physiological measurement of acute stress (public speaking) in bank employees, *Int. J. Psychophysiol.*, 5, 265, 1987.
85. **Kakimoto, Y., Nakamura, A., Tarui, H., Nagasawa, Y., and Yagura, S.,** Crew workload in ASDF C-1 transport flights. I. Change in heart rate and salivary cortisol, *Aviat. Space Environ. Med.*, 59, 511, 1988.
86. **Tarui, H. and Nakamura, A.,** Saliva cortisol: a good indicator for acceleration stress, *Aviat. Space Environ. Med.*, 58, 573, 1987.
87. **Rahe, R. H., Karson, S., Howard, N. S., Jr., Rubin, R. T., and Poland, R. E.,** Psychological and physiological assessment on American hostages freed from captivity in Iran, *Psychosom. Med.*, 52, 1, 1990.
88. **Jemmott, J. B., III and Magloire, K.,** Academic stress, social support, and secretory immunoglobulin A, *J. Pers. Soc. Psychol.*, 55, 803, 1988.
89. **Graham, N. M. H., Bartholomeusz, R. C. A., Taboonpong, N., and La Brooy, J. T.,** Does anxiety reduce the secretion rate of secretory IgA in saliva, *Med. J. Aust.*, 148, 131, 1988.

Chapter 5

THE EXCESSIVE GAGGING REFLEX

A normal, physiological gagging reflex has immediate importance in dental treatment because of the constant chance of swallowing foreign material. The gagging reflex protects the gastrointestinal tract from the possible danger of obstruction and acts as an initial warning sign to the dentist that undesired material is caught in the pharynx area and has to be removed.

In some patients, however, the gagging reflex appears in an exaggerated manner even following minor stimulation. These patients pose a special problem to the dentist. The inability to apply instruments into the patient's mouth makes dental treatment almost impossible.

I. DEFINITIONS

Gagging is usually associated with nausea and vomiting. It is often presented in the dental literature under terms such as gagging reflex, pharyngeal reflex, or retching.

The gagging reflex is defined as "the closing of the glottis and cessation of respiration evoked by stimulation of the sensory nerves of the pharynx or larynx either by the introduction of a solid or liquid or by the inspiration of irritating vapor." The pharyngeal reflex is defined as "the contraction of the pharyngeal muscles associated with gagging," and retching as "a straining, ineffective effort to vomit."[1]

Apparently, while gagging is a relatively brief, passing phenomenon associated with an immediate stimulus (it is impossible to cease respiration for a long period), retching is a more continuous act, associated with longer-lasting stimuli. Gagging, if prolonged, is usually followed by vomiting, whereas retching is usually "less productive" in this respect.

Gagging and retching are often used to describe the same phenomenon. However, while gagging seems a more suitable term to describe a reflex evoked during an actual attempt at treatment, retching seems more applicable to the behavior of certain patients who are unable to tolerate dental appliances.

II. PHYSIOLOGY OF SWALLOWING, GAGGING, AND VOMITING

The gag reflex is normally activated when there is a drastic, immediate need to protect the airway and to remove noxious stimuli from the gastrointestinal tract. It is usually triggered by a stimulus in the posterior oral cavity or pharynx, in order to eructate or eliminate the stimuli.[2] Gagging is associated with other reflexes of the oropharynx (i.e., swallowing and vomiting), all part of the reflexes integrated in the medulla oblongata.

Swallowing is triggered by afferent impulses in the trigeminal, glossopharyngeal, and vagus nerves. The efferent fibers pass to the pharyngeal musculature and the tongue via the trigeminal, facial, and hypoglossal nerves. It is initiated by the voluntary act of propelling the oral contents toward the back of the pharynx. This starts a wave of involuntary contractions in the pharyngeal muscles that pushes the material into the esophagus. Inhibition of respiration and glottic closure are part of the swallowing reflex response.[3]

The neuromuscular response that characterizes the gag reflex involves the sudden and strong contraction of pharyngeal walls, soft palate, and larynx to squeeze or eliminate the stimulus that elicited the gag from the pharynx and to push it back into the mouth.[2] It consists of elevating the palate and retracting the tongue with the contraction of the pharyngeal muscles. The afferent loop of the reflex runs in the glossopharyngeal nerve, while the efferent loop runs in the vagus nerve.[4]

The gag reflex is part of the vomiting complex. Repeated stimulation of the glossopharyngeal wall may produce vomiting in susceptible individuals. Under these circumstances, the afferent impulses pass through the glossopharyngeal nerve to the medulla oblongata, to the nucleus solitarius. From here, there is a secondary relay to the "vomiting center". This center may be excited by impulses both from the glossopharyngeal nerve and from the cortical centers (e.g., emotion). It is also affected by vestibular impulses (motion sickness), through the vagus nerve (inflammatory conditions of the viscera and intestinal tract), and from the spinothalamic tract due to painful somatic conditions.[4]

The gagging reflex is not a protection for the swallowing reflex; it does not protect the airway during swallowing or bringing up the aspirated material. This is accomplished by the coughing reflex. The two reflexes (swallowing and gagging) are quite different, sensorily, with regard to the inflicting stimulus. Normally, gagging is not triggered by food, but by material refluxed from the esophagus or during vomiting.[2]

III. COGNITIVE ASPECTS OF GAGGING

When gagging occurs, the applied stimulus must be recognized as noxious, threatening, or unpleasant. During swallowing, the bolus of food is pushed by the tongue to the oropharynx. Food is not normally considered or recognized as a foreign stimulus,[2] unless there is an emotional response to the food, such as a strong aversion to it. An unpleasant smell, look, and/or memory of a particular food can elicit nausea even without direct stimulation of the oral cavity. Many patients who claim to be unable to put any foreign appliance into their mouth due to excessive gagging reflex (or even to perform routine procedures, such as tooth brushing) find no difficulty in managing solid foods (e.g., bones covered with meat).

As in most other life experiences, thoughts, expectations, and beliefs influence cognition with regard to a specific situation. If a person believes that to breathe efficiently the mouth should remain unblocked, the application of dental instruments and materials may be perceived as threatening, resulting in gagging. One who has gagged in the past, because of situational factors, may believe that he/she is prone to gagging. Clinicians who label this patient as a chronic "gagger" further contribute to this belief.[5]

IV. GAG (RETCH) PATIENTS WITH DENTURES

Most cases of extreme gagging described in the literature refer to patients with full or partial dentures.[5-25] The cases relate to patients who are unable to accept the dental appliance and react with retching at any attempt to insert it into the mouth. Among this population, a large proportion of "gaggers" (43%) claim that their problem started when they received their dentures, while about 26% indicated that they "always" had the problem.[19]

Many cases of chronic retching with dentures relate to a full maxillary denture[11,14,21,22,25] or both full dentures.[10,24] The complaints are usually non-specific and relate to the inability to tolerate the dentures in place.[10,21,22,24] Some report specific stimuli, such as the procedure of impression taking,[14,21,25] a "too long" palatal seal of the denture,[11] or external stimuli (e.g., toothbrushing, tea leaves, a thermometer, etc.)[14,19] as partial explanations to the situation. Among children, wearing of orthodontic appliances and taking impressions have been described as a cause for vomiting during dental treatment.[23]

Although the cause for gagging in patients with removable dental appliances may be mechanical (direct stimulation of the soft palate during impression taking, poor retention, insufficient palatal seal of the dental appliance, etc.), many patients continue to complain of retching and are unable to tolerate dentures despite good construction and adaptation. The sight of a patient with several pairs of dentures, none of which are satisfactorily used, is evidence that other (not necessarily mechanical) aspects may be involved in the process.

A. ANATOMIC FEATURES

Among the explanations suggested as a reason for excessive gagging, a possible existence of abnormal anatomic features, such as a long soft palate or hypersensitivity of the soft palate and tongue, was suggested.[26-29] This was examined by Wright[16-19] in several systematic studies with regard to the factors associated with retching in patients who wear dentures.

According to Wright, no specific anatomic abnormalities could be demonstrated in retching patients with regard to the form of the mouth and pharynx — they did not have longer, laxer palates, larger tongues, or potentially reduced airways compared with their matched controls, nor did they show any abnormally marked or heightened reaction to dentures with regard to posture of the tongue, hyoid bone, or soft palate.[16,18]

Retching patients did not differ from nonretching patients with regard to their ability to identify shapes with their oral cavity or to manipulate test pieces with their mouth, indicating that they possess no greater oral awareness than nonretching patients.[16]

B. PERSONALITY FACTORS

The Eysenck Personality Inventory was used to examine personality variables of gagging patients in several studies. Although initial differences were found in psychoticism scores for men retchers,[16] extraversion scores for women retchers,[17] or neuroticism scores for all the examined gagging population,[14] when calculated according to their equivalent values typical to each age, these findings were not significant. Overall, retching patients were not found to be more neurotic or extraversive than nonretching patients.[14,16,17]

C. FEAR/ANXIETY OF DENTAL TREATMENT

Although no reports concerning patients who retch with dentures directly referred to the issue of dental fear and anxiety, some indirect evidence exists whereby retching may be associated, in some patients, with anxiety regarding treatment.

In the survey by Murphy,[14] only one patient stated that anxiety caused the reflex to commence; however, about 30% of the gagging patients discontinued treatment in the middle. This may be due to a variety of factors, but the high percentage of dropouts may suggest the presence of unadmitted anxiety provoked by the attempt of actual treatment.

In other reports, the patient's poor oral condition points to long-term avoidance of dental treatment which eventually led to the need of dentures. Stoffelmayr[10] described a 30-year-old woman who was in need of dentures, Clarke and Persichetti[22] presented a 51-year-old woman who needed a full maxillary denture, and Fleece et al.[24] described a man whose teeth had been extracted due to periodontal disease at the age of 52.

The notion that an excessive gagging reflex may be a symptom of different psychopathological processes, such as specific fear, repugnance-fear-based disturbances, diffused anxiety, goal directed behavior, and depressive states was also raised by Schroeder et al.[30]

V. GAG PATIENTS WITHOUT DENTURES

Relatively few case reports deal with patients whose gagging during treatment prevents routine dental care while still having their natural dentition.[5,20,31,32] Typically, these patients are unable to tolerate the instruments placed into their oral cavity during attempted treatment and react with gagging at even the most superficial examination. In some patients, the gagging reflex is restricted only to the dental situation,[5] in others it may be elicited even by inserting one's own recording the child's behavior every 3 min). Thus a child who cried only once, for less than 3 min at the beginning of the session, would be rated lower than a child who repeated this behavior several times.

Behavioral measures are occasionally used for the anxious adult patient. In several studies the dentist was asked to rate the cooperation and treatability of anxious adult patients compared to average patients.[74] This was done on a six-point scale, where a rating of 1 indicated "much better," a rating of 3 indicated "equal to," and a rating of 5 indicated "much worse" than average patients. A rating of 6 stood for "impossible to treat." Similar ratings were also used in adult dental phobic patients.[73]

C. PHYSIOLOGICAL MEASURES

Physiological changes are perhaps more subjective, but also less readily available measures of dental stress and anxiety. Commonly used measures include parameters such as electromyograms, heart rate, galvanic skin response, and palmar sweat index.[20,60-64,81] These are relatively easy to apply, noninvasive, physiological measures of stress. An EMG-feedback device to measure and display muscle tension may also be used.[70]

These methods provide a relatively objective measure of the physiological changes that occur during stress. However, they can occasionally act as stress-inflicting factors themselves. The use of additional measuring devices may increase threat appraisal of patients who are already under stress. The attempt to use electrodes connected to unknown, potentially "threatening" instruments may serve as an additional stress-inflicting stimulus.

Several other physiological changes can potentially serve as noninvasive parameters of stress in the dental situation. A good example is the effect of stress on salivary flow and composition[82-89] (see also Chapter 9.I). Saliva is body fluid which is easy to obtain and which is intuitively connected with the oral cavity and oral treatment. As such, it may be a less threatening physiological measure, effective for the evaluation of stress in the dental situation.

VII. TREATMENT

Patients suffering from dental fear/anxiety/phobia pose a special challenge to the dental practitioner. Treatment modalities include measures from all relevant fields: behavior modification, hypnosis, and the use of various relevant pharmaceutical agents. A detailed presentation of the treatment modes is presented in Section 3, Chapters 10 to 13.

VIII. SUMMARY

Fear and anxiety are the most common behavioral dysfunctions related to dental care, with prevalence generally estimated as high as 20%. Patients postpone dental care or avoid it altogether, thereby causing severe deterioration of their oral health.

The antecedents of dental fear are many: early aversive encounters in the dental office, vicarious learning through models, and individual personality traits are the most common factors which predispose dental anxiety. Its major components include a direct association with and an anticipation of immediate physical threat, as well as threat to one's self-esteem.

Proper identification and assessment of dental fear include the use of self-report questionnaires, and behavioral and physiological measures.

REFERENCES

1. **May, R.,** Anxiety and stress, in *Selye's Guide to Stress Research*, Vol. 2, Selye, H., Ed., Scientific and Academic Editions, New York, 1983.
2. **Hinsie, L. E. and Campbell, R. J.,** *Psychiatric Dictionary*, 5th ed., Oxford University Press, New York, 1981.
3. The American Psychiatric Association, *The Diagnostic and Statistical Manual*, III, 1980, 225.
4. **Spielberger, C. D.,** Current trends in theory on research on anxiety, in *Anxiety — Current Trends in Theory and Research*, Vol. 1, Spielberger, C. D., Ed., Academic Press, New York, 1972, 3.
5. **Friedson, E. and Feldman, J. J.,** The public looks at dental care, *J. Am. Dent. Assoc.*, 57, 325, 1958.
6. **Crockett, B.,** Dental survey: Southeastern State College, *J. Okla. Dent. Assoc.*, 51, 25, 1963.
7. Svenska Institutet för Opinionsundersökningar (SIFO): Tandlökarbesök, Intervjuundersökning för Tandvörnet, Stockholm, 1962.
8. **Seeman, K. and Molin, C.,** Psychopathology, feelings of confinement and helplessness in the dental chair, and relationship to the dentist in patients with disproportionate dental anxiety (DDA), *Acta Psychiatr. Scand.*, 54, 81, 1976.
9. **Lindsay, S. J. E., Humphris, G., and Barnby, G. J.,** Expectations and preferences for routine dentistry in anxious adult patients, *Br. Dent. J.*, 163, 120, 1987.
10. **Ayer, W. A. and Corah, N. L.,** Behavioural factors influencing dental treatment, in *Social Sciences and Dentistry: A Critical Bibliography*, Vol. 2, Cohen, L. K. and Bryant, P. S., Eds., Quintessence Publishing Co. for Federation Dentaire Internationale, Kingston-upon-Thames, England, 1984, 267.
11. **Milgrom, P., Weinstein, P., Kleinknecht, R., and Getz, T.,** *Treating Fearful Dental Patients*, Reston Publishing Co., Reston, Va, 1985.
12. **Gatchel, R. J, Ingersoll, B. D., Bowman, L., Robertson, M. C., and Walker, C.,** The prevalence of dental fear and avoidance: a recent survey study, *J. Am. Dent. Assoc.*, 107, 609, 1983.
13. **Milgrom, P., Fiset, L., Melnick, S., and Weinstein, P.,** The prevalence and practice management consequences of dental fear in a major US city, *J. Am. Dent. Assoc.*, 116, 641, 1988.
14. **Locker, D. and Liddell, A. M.,** Correlates of dental anxiety among older adults, *J. Dent. Res.*, 70, 198, 1991.
15. **Domoto, P. K., Weinstein, P., Melnick, S., Ohmura, M., Uchida, H., Ohmachi, K., Hori, M., Okazaki, Y., Shimamoto, T., Matsumura, S., and Shimono, T.,** Results of a dental fear survey in Japan: implications for dental public health in Asia, *Community Dent. Oral Epidemiol.*, 16, 199, 1988.

16. **Chellappah, N. K., Vignehsa, H., Milgrom, P., and Lo, G. L.,** Prevalence of dental anxiety and fear in children in Singapore, *Community Dent. Oral Epidemiol.*, 18, 269, 1990.
17. **Liddell, A. and May, B.,** Some charcteristics of regular and irregular attenders for dental check-ups, *Br. J. Clin. Psychol.*, 23, 19, 1984.
18. **Bernstein, D. A., Kleinknecht, R. A., and Alexander, L. D.,** Antecedents of dental fear, *J. Public Health Dent.*, 39, 113, 1979.
19. **Rankin, J. A. and Harris, M. B.,** Dental anxiety: the patient's point of view, *J. Am. Dent. Assoc.*, 109, 43, 1984.
20. **Kleinknecht, R. A. and Bernstein, D. A.,** The assessment of dental fear, *Behav. Ther.*, 9, 626, 1978.
21. **Berggren, U. and Carlsson, S. G.,** Psychometric measures of dental fear, *Community Dent. Oral Epidemiol.*, 12, 319, 1984.
22. **Kleinknecht, R. A., Klepac, R. K., and Alexander, L. D.,** Origins and characteristics of fear of dentistry, *J. Am. Dent. Assoc.*, 86, 842, 1973.
23. **Cohen, L. A., Snyder, T. L., and LaBelle, A. D.,** Correlates of dental anxiety in a university population, *J. Public Health Dent.*, 42, 228, 1982.
24. **Bernstein, D. A. and Kleinknecht, R. A.,** Multiple approaches to the reduction of dental fear, *J. Behav. Ther. Exp. Psychiatry*, 13, 287, 1982.
25. **Green, R. M. and Green, A.,** Adult attitudes to dentistry among dental attenders in South Wales, *Br. Dent. J.*, 159, 157, 1985.
26. **Klepac, R. K., Dowling, J., and Hauge, G.,** Characteristics of clients seeking therapy for the reduction of dental avoidance: reactions to pain, *J. Behav. Ther. Exp. Psychiatry*, 13, 293, 1982.
27. **Eli, I. and Kleinhauz, M.,** Oro-related behavioral dysfunctions: a disabling factor in dental care, (in press).
28. **Duivenvoorden H. J., Schuurs, A. H. B., Thoden van Velzen, S. K., Verhage, F., Makkes, P. C., and Eijkman, M. A. J.,** Influence of repression upon the measurement of dental anxiety, *Community Dent. Oral Epidemiol.*, 13, 315, 1985.
29. **Kent, G.,** Self-efficacious control over reported physiological, cognitive and behavioural symptoms of dental anxiety, *Behav. Res. Ther.*, 25, 341, 1987.
30. **Berggren, U. and Meynert, G.,** Dental fear and avoidance: causes, symptoms, and consequences, *J. Am. Dent. Assoc.*, 109, 247, 1984.
31. **Harrison, J. A., Carlsson, S. G., and Berggren, U.,** Research in clinical process and outcome methodology: psychophysiology, systematic desensitization and dental fear, *J. Behav. Ther. Exp. Psychiatry*, 16, 201, 1985.
32. **Tullman, G. M., Tullman, M. J., and Rogers, B. J.,** Anxiety in dental patients: a study of three phases of State anxiety in three treatment groups, *Psychol. Rep.*, 45, 497, 1979.
33. **Kent, G.,** Memory of dental pain, *Pain*, 21, 187, 1985.
34. **Schuurs, A. H. B., Duivenvoorden, H. J., Thoden van Velzen, S. K., and Verhage, F.,** Three factors predicting irregular versus regular dental attendance: a model fitting to empirical data, *Community Dent. Oral Epidemiol.*, 8, 413, 1980.
35. **Bouma, J., Uitenbroek, D. G., Westert, G. P., Schaub, R. M. H, and van de Poel, A. C. M.,** Pathways to full mouth extraction, *Community Dent. Oral Epidemiol.*, 15, 301, 1987.
36. **Forgione, A. G. and Clark, R. E.,** Comments on an empirical study of the causes of dental fear, *J. Dent. Res.*, 53, 496, 1974.
37. **Lautch, H.,** Dental phobia, *Br. J. Psychiatry*, 119, 151, 1971.
38. **Davey, G. C. L.,** Dental phobias and anxieties: Evidence for conditioning processes in the acquisition and modulation of a learned fear, *Behav. Res. Ther.*, 27, 51, 1989.
39. **Shoben, E. J., Jr. and Borland, L.,** An empirical study of the etiology of dental fear, *J. Clin. Psych.*, 10, 171, 1954.
40. **Johnson, R.,** Maternal influence on child behavior in the dental setting, *Psychiatry Med.*, 2, 221, 1971.

41. **Holst, A., Schröder, U., Ek, L., Hallonsten, A.-L., and Crossner, C.-G.,** Prediction of behavior management problems in children, *Scand. J. Dent. Res.*, 96, 457, 1988.
42. **Lahti, S., Tuutti, H., and Honkala, E.,** The relationship of parental dental anxiety and child's caries status, *J. Dent. Child.*, 56, 191, 1989.
43. **Frazer, M. and Hampson, S.,** Some personality factors related to dental anxiety and fear of pain, *Br. Dent. J.*, 165, 436, 1988.
44. **Schuurs, A. H. B., Duivenvoorden, H. J, Makkes, P. C., Thoden van Velzen, S. K., and Verhage, F.,** Personality traits of patients suffering extreme dental anxiety, *Community Dent. Oral Epidemiol.*, 16, 38, 1988.
45. **Neverlien, P. O.,** Dental fear and locus of control: a pilot study, *Community Dent. Oral Epidemiol.*, 16, 127, 1988.
46. **McNeil, D. W. and Berryman, M. L.,** Components of dental fear in adults?, *Behav. Res. Ther.*, 27, 233, 1989.
47. **Fiset, L., Milgrom, P., and Melnick, S.,** dentification of the relationship between dental and non-dental fears, utilization of the dentist, *J. Dent. Res.*, 67, 169, Abstr. No. 453, 1988.
48. **Gale, E. N.,** Fears of the dental situation, *J. Dent. Res.*, 51, 964, 1972.
49. **Stouthard, M. E. A. and Hoogstraten, J.,** Ratings of fears associated with twelve dental situations, *J. Dent. Res.*, 66, 1175, 1987.
50. **Beech, H. R., Burns, L. E., and Sheffield, B. F.,** *A Behavioural Approach to the Management of Stress*, John Wiley & Sons, Chichester, 1984.
51. **Corah, N. L.,** Development of a dental anxiety scale, *J. Dent. Res.*, 48, 596, 1969.
52. **Johnson, R. and Baldwin, D. C.,** Relationship of maternal anxiety to the behavior of young children undergoing dental extraction, *J. Dent. Res.*, 47, 801, 1968.
53. **Weinstein, P., Getz, T., Ratener, P., and Domoto, P.,** The effect of dentists' behaviors on fear-related behaviors in children, *J. Am. Dent. Assoc.*, 104, 32, 1982.
54. **Weinstein, P., Getz, T., Ratener, P., and Domoto, P.,** Dentists' responses to fear- and nonfear-related behaviors in children, *J. Am. Dent. Assoc.*, 104, 38, 1982.
55. **Weinstein, P., Getz, T., and Domoto, P.,** Temporal patterns of the behavior of young children in the dental chair, *J. Pedodontics*, 9, 188, 1985.
56. **Melamed, B. G., Weinstein, D., Hawes, R., and Borland, M.,** Reduction of fear-related dental management problems with use of filmed modeling, *J. Am. Dent. Assoc.*, 90, 822, 1975.
57. **Melamed, B. G., Bennett, C. G., errell, G., Ross, S. L., Bush, J. P., Hill, C., Courts, F., and Ronk, S.,** Dentists' behavior management as it affects compliance and fear in pediatric patients, *J. Am. Dent. Assoc.*, 106, 324, 1983.
58. **Rud, B. B. and Kisling, E.,** The influence of mental development on children's acceptance of dental treatment, *Scand. J. Dent. Res.*, 81, 343, 1973.
59. **Holst, A. and Crossner, C.-G.,** Direct ratings of acceptance of dental treatment in Swedish children, *Community Dent. Oral Epidemiol.*, 15, 258, 1987.
60. **Corah, N. L., Gale, E. N., and Ilig, S. J.,** The use of relaxation and distraction to reduce psychological stress during dental procedure, *J. Am. Dent. Assoc.*, 98, 390, 1979.
61. **Corah, N. L., Gale, E. N., and Illig, S. J.,** Psychological stress reduction during dental procedures, *J. Dent. Res.*, 58, 1347, 1979.
62. **Carlsson, S. G., Linde, A., Berggren, U., and Harrison, J. A.,** Reduction of dental fear: psychophysiological correlates, *Community Dent. Oral Epidemiol.*, 14, 253, 1986.
63. **Simpson, W. J., Ruzicka, R. L., and Thomas, N. R.,** Physiologic responses of children to initial dental experience, *J. Dent. Child.*, 41, 465, 1974.
64. **Meldman, M. J,** The dental phobia test, *Psychosomatics*, 13, 371, 1972.
65. **Spielberger, C. D., Gorsuch, R., and Lushene, R.,** *The State Trait Anxiety Inventory (STAI)*, Consulting Psychologists Press, Riverside, CA, 1970.
66. **Wardle, J.,** Fear of dentistry, *Br. J. Med. Psychol.*, 55, 119, 1982.
67. **Corah, N. L., Gale, E. N., and Illig, S. J.,** Assessment of a dental anxiety scale, *J. Am. Dent. Assoc.*, 97, 816, 1978.

68. **Corah, N. L.,** Dental anxiety: assessment, reduction and increasing patient satisfaction, *Dent. Clin. North Am.*, 32, 779, 1988.
69. **Scott, D. S. and Hirschman, R.,** Psychological aspects of dental anxiety in adults, *J. Am. Dent. Assoc.*, 104, 27, 1982.
70. **Berggren, U. and Carlsson, S. G.,** A psychophysiological therapy for dental fear, *Behav. Res. Ther.*, 22, 487, 1984.
71. **Berggren, U. and Carlsson, S. G.,** Qualitative and quantitative effects of treatment for dental fear and avoidance, *Anesth. Prog.*, 33, 9, 1986.
72. **Berggren, U.,** Long-term effects of two different treatments for dental fear and avoidance, *J. Dent. Res.*, 65, 874, 1986.
73. **Berggren U. and Carlsson, S. G.,** Usefulness of two psychometric scales in Swedish patients with severe dental fear, *Community Dent. Oral Epidemiol.*, 13, 70, 1985.
74. **Berggren, U. and Linde, A.,** Dental fear and avoidance: a comparison of two modes of treatment, *J. Dent. Res.*, 63, 1223, 1984.
75. **Kunzelmann, K.-H. and Dünninger, P.,** Dental fear and pain: effect on patient's perception of the dentist, *Community Dent. Oral Epidemiol.*, 18, 264, 1990.
76. **Vervoorn, J. M., Duinkerke, A. S. H., Luteijn, F., van de Poel, A. C. M.,** Assessment of dental anxiety in edentulous subjects, *Community Dent. Oral Epidemiol.*, 17, 177, 1989.
77. **Geer, J. H.,** The development of a scale to measure fear, *Behav. Res. Ther.*, 3, 45, 1965.
78. **Kleinknecht, R. A., Thorndike, R. M., McGlynn, F. D., and Harkavy, J.,** Factor analysis of the Dental Fear Survey with cross-validation, *J. Am. Dent. Assoc.*, 108, 59, 1984.
79. **McGlynn, F. D., McNeil, D. W., Gallagher, S. L., and Vrana, S.,** Factor structure, stability, and internal consistency of the Dental Fear Survey, *Behav. Assessment*, 9, 57, 1987.
80. **McGlynn, F. D.,** Dental Fear Survey, in *Dictionary of Behavioral Assessment Techniques*, Hersen, M. and Bellack, A. S., Eds., Pergamon Press, New York, 1988.
81. **Wong, M. and Kaloupek, D. G.,** Coping with dental treatment: the potential impact of situational demands, *J. Behav. Med.*, 9, 579, 1986.
82. **Bates, J. F. and Adams, D.,** The influence of mental stress on the flow of saliva in man, *Arch. Oral Biol.*, 13, 593, 1968.
83. **Silverstein, L. and Iverson, M. A.,** Human salivary response to interpersonal bargaining situations: a psycho-physiological investigation, *Psychol. Rep.*, 37, 771, 1975.
84. **Bassett, J. R., Marshall, P. M., and Spillane, R.,** The physiological measurement of acute stress (public speaking) in bank employees, *Int. J. Psychophysiol.*, 5, 265, 1987.
85. **Kakimoto, Y., Nakamura, A., Tarui, H., Nagasawa, Y., and Yagura, S.,** Crew workload in ASDF C-1 transport flights. I. Change in heart rate and salivary cortisol, *Aviat. Space Environ. Med.*, 59, 511, 1988.
86. **Tarui, H. and Nakamura, A.,** Saliva cortisol: a good indicator for acceleration stress, *Aviat. Space Environ. Med.*, 58, 573, 1987.
87. **Rahe, R. H., Karson, S., Howard, N. S., Jr., Rubin, R. T., and Poland, R. E.,** Psychological and physiological assessment on American hostages freed from captivity in Iran, *Psychosom. Med.*, 52, 1, 1990.
88. **Jemmott, J. B., III and Magloire, K.,** Academic stress, social support, and secretory immunoglobulin A, *J. Pers. Soc. Psychol.*, 55, 803, 1988.
89. **Graham, N. M. H., Bartholomeusz, R. C. A., Taboonpong, N., and La Brooy, J. T.,** Does anxiety reduce the secretion rate of secretory IgA in saliva, *Med. J. Aust.*, 148, 131, 1988.

Chapter 5

THE EXCESSIVE GAGGING REFLEX

A normal, physiological gagging reflex has immediate importance in dental treatment because of the constant chance of swallowing foreign material. The gagging reflex protects the gastrointestinal tract from the possible danger of obstruction and acts as an initial warning sign to the dentist that undesired material is caught in the pharynx area and has to be removed.

In some patients, however, the gagging reflex appears in an exaggerated manner even following minor stimulation. These patients pose a special problem to the dentist. The inability to apply instruments into the patient's mouth makes dental treatment almost impossible.

I. DEFINITIONS

Gagging is usually associated with nausea and vomiting. It is often presented in the dental literature under terms such as gagging reflex, pharyngeal reflex, or retching.

The gagging reflex is defined as "the closing of the glottis and cessation of respiration evoked by stimulation of the sensory nerves of the pharynx or larynx either by the introduction of a solid or liquid or by the inspiration of irritating vapor." The pharyngeal reflex is defined as "the contraction of the pharyngeal muscles associated with gagging," and retching as "a straining, ineffective effort to vomit."[1]

Apparently, while gagging is a relatively brief, passing phenomenon associated with an immediate stimulus (it is impossible to cease respiration for a long period), retching is a more continuous act, associated with longer-lasting stimuli. Gagging, if prolonged, is usually followed by vomiting, whereas retching is usually "less productive" in this respect.

Gagging and retching are often used to describe the same phenomenon. However, while gagging seems a more suitable term to describe a reflex evoked during an actual attempt at treatment, retching seems more applicable to the behavior of certain patients who are unable to tolerate dental appliances.

II. PHYSIOLOGY OF SWALLOWING, GAGGING, AND VOMITING

The gag reflex is normally activated when there is a drastic, immediate need to protect the airway and to remove noxious stimuli from the gastrointestinal tract. It is usually triggered by a stimulus in the posterior oral cavity or pharynx, in order to eructate or eliminate the stimuli.[2] Gagging is associated with other reflexes of the oropharynx (i.e., swallowing and vomiting), all part of the reflexes integrated in the medulla oblongata.

Swallowing is triggered by afferent impulses in the trigeminal, glossopharyngeal, and vagus nerves. The efferent fibers pass to the pharyngeal musculature and the tongue via the trigeminal, facial, and hypoglossal nerves. It is initiated by the voluntary act of propelling the oral contents toward the back of the pharynx. This starts a wave of involuntary contractions in the pharyngeal muscles that pushes the material into the esophagus. Inhibition of respiration and glottic closure are part of the swallowing reflex response.[3]

The neuromuscular response that characterizes the gag reflex involves the sudden and strong contraction of pharyngeal walls, soft palate, and larynx to squeeze or eliminate the stimulus that elicited the gag from the pharynx and to push it back into the mouth.[2] It consists of elevating the palate and retracting the tongue with the contraction of the pharyngeal muscles. The afferent loop of the reflex runs in the glossopharyngeal nerve, while the efferent loop runs in the vagus nerve.[4]

The gag reflex is part of the vomiting complex. Repeated stimulation of the glossopharyngeal wall may produce vomiting in susceptible individuals. Under these circumstances, the afferent impulses pass through the glossopharyngeal nerve to the medulla oblongata, to the nucleus solitarius. From here, there is a secondary relay to the "vomiting center". This center may be excited by impulses both from the glossopharyngeal nerve and from the cortical centers (e.g., emotion). It is also affected by vestibular impulses (motion sickness), through the vagus nerve (inflammatory conditions of the viscera and intestinal tract), and from the spinothalamic tract due to painful somatic conditions.[4]

The gagging reflex is not a protection for the swallowing reflex; it does not protect the airway during swallowing or bringing up the aspirated material. This is accomplished by the coughing reflex. The two reflexes (swallowing and gagging) are quite different, sensorily, with regard to the inflicting stimulus. Normally, gagging is not triggered by food, but by material refluxed from the esophagus or during vomiting.[2]

III. COGNITIVE ASPECTS OF GAGGING

When gagging occurs, the applied stimulus must be recognized as noxious, threatening, or unpleasant. During swallowing, the bolus of food is pushed by the tongue to the oropharynx. Food is not normally considered or recognized as a foreign stimulus,[2] unless there is an emotional response to the food, such as a strong aversion to it. An unpleasant smell, look, and/or memory of a particular food can elicit nausea even without direct stimulation of the oral cavity. Many patients who claim to be unable to put any foreign appliance into their mouth due to excessive gagging reflex (or even to perform routine procedures, such as tooth brushing) find no difficulty in managing solid foods (e.g., bones covered with meat).

As in most other life experiences, thoughts, expectations, and beliefs influence cognition with regard to a specific situation. If a person believes that to breathe efficiently the mouth should remain unblocked, the application of dental instruments and materials may be perceived as threatening, resulting in gagging. One who has gagged in the past, because of situational factors, may believe that he/she is prone to gagging. Clinicians who label this patient as a chronic "gagger" further contribute to this belief.[5]

IV. GAG (RETCH) PATIENTS WITH DENTURES

Most cases of extreme gagging described in the literature refer to patients with full or partial dentures.[5-25] The cases relate to patients who are unable to accept the dental appliance and react with retching at any attempt to insert it into the mouth. Among this population, a large proportion of "gaggers" (43%) claim that their problem started when they received their dentures, while about 26% indicated that they "always" had the problem.[19]

Many cases of chronic retching with dentures relate to a full maxillary denture[11,14,21,22,25] or both full dentures.[10,24] The complaints are usually non-specific and relate to the inability to tolerate the dentures in place.[10,21,22,24] Some report specific stimuli, such as the procedure of impression taking,[14,21,25] a "too long" palatal seal of the denture,[11] or external stimuli (e.g., toothbrushing, tea leaves, a thermometer, etc.)[14,19] as partial explanations to the situation. Among children, wearing of orthodontic appliances and taking impressions have been described as a cause for vomiting during dental treatment.[23]

Although the cause for gagging in patients with removable dental appliances may be mechanical (direct stimulation of the soft palate during impression taking, poor retention, insufficient palatal seal of the dental appliance, etc.), many patients continue to complain of retching and are unable to tolerate dentures despite good construction and adaptation. The sight of a patient with several pairs of dentures, none of which are satisfactorily used, is evidence that other (not necessarily mechanical) aspects may be involved in the process.

A. ANATOMIC FEATURES

Among the explanations suggested as a reason for excessive gagging, a possible existence of abnormal anatomic features, such as a long soft palate or hypersensitivity of the soft palate and tongue, was suggested.[26-29] This was examined by Wright[16-19] in several systematic studies with regard to the factors associated with retching in patients who wear dentures.

According to Wright, no specific anatomic abnormalities could be demonstrated in retching patients with regard to the form of the mouth and pharynx — they did not have longer, laxer palates, larger tongues, or potentially reduced airways compared with their matched controls, nor did they show any abnormally marked or heightened reaction to dentures with regard to posture of the tongue, hyoid bone, or soft palate.[16,18]

Retching patients did not differ from nonretching patients with regard to their ability to identify shapes with their oral cavity or to manipulate test pieces with their mouth, indicating that they possess no greater oral awareness than nonretching patients.[16]

B. PERSONALITY FACTORS

The Eysenck Personality Inventory was used to examine personality variables of gagging patients in several studies. Although initial differences were found in psychoticism scores for men retchers,[16] extraversion scores for women retchers,[17] or neuroticism scores for all the examined gagging population,[14] when calculated according to their equivalent values typical to each age, these findings were not significant. Overall, retching patients were not found to be more neurotic or extraversive than nonretching patients.[14,16,17]

C. FEAR/ANXIETY OF DENTAL TREATMENT

Although no reports concerning patients who retch with dentures directly referred to the issue of dental fear and anxiety, some indirect evidence exists whereby retching may be associated, in some patients, with anxiety regarding treatment.

In the survey by Murphy,[14] only one patient stated that anxiety caused the reflex to commence; however, about 30% of the gagging patients discontinued treatment in the middle. This may be due to a variety of factors, but the high percentage of dropouts may suggest the presence of unadmitted anxiety provoked by the attempt of actual treatment.

In other reports, the patient's poor oral condition points to long-term avoidance of dental treatment which eventually led to the need of dentures. Stoffelmayr[10] described a 30-year-old woman who was in need of dentures, Clarke and Persichetti[22] presented a 51-year-old woman who needed a full maxillary denture, and Fleece et al.[24] described a man whose teeth had been extracted due to periodontal disease at the age of 52.

The notion that an excessive gagging reflex may be a symptom of different psychopathological processes, such as specific fear, repugnance-fear-based disturbances, diffused anxiety, goal directed behavior, and depressive states was also raised by Schroeder et al.[30]

V. GAG PATIENTS WITHOUT DENTURES

Relatively few case reports deal with patients whose gagging during treatment prevents routine dental care while still having their natural dentition.[5,20,31,32] Typically, these patients are unable to tolerate the instruments placed into their oral cavity during attempted treatment and react with gagging at even the most superficial examination. In some patients, the gagging reflex is restricted only to the dental situation,[5] in others it may be elicited even by inserting one's own finger into the mouth,[31] or by toothbrushing, wearing a collar, specific smells, etc.[20]

In all cases, the reflex poses a severe obstacle to dental care up to significant deterioration of oral health. The main reasons suggested as causing extreme gagging during dental treatment include those based on learning.

A. DIRECT AND INDIRECT LEARNING

Gagging is a reflex, affected both by physical stimulation and by cognitive and behavioral responses. Direct learning by a past experience (e.g., choking on food) may increase the sensitivity involved with similar situations (e.g., dental treatment) which are then seen as a direct existential threat.

Several reports present gagging patients who had former aversive experiences associated with dentistry. Ramsey et al.[5] described patients whose gagging condition originated, in part, from learning experiences (e.g., a patient whose gagging was attributed to a bad experience with an impatient dentist; another anxious patient who would panic if presented with dental stimuli, etc.). Muir and Calvert[23] described two young boys whose inability to undergo dental impressions was associated with considerable anxiety-related difficulties. Wilks and Marks[20] presented (among others) a woman whose nausea was initially provoked at the age of 5 by the sight of her grandfather's dirty dentures. Eli and Kleinhauz[31] described (among others) a man who recalled a traumatic dental experience; during the procedure he was forcibly held by four persons, and the experience threatened his sense of self-control.

Indirect learning through the experience of others (by watching, hearing, etc.) may also influence personal judgment of the situation as threatening. In a case reported by Wilks and Marks,[20] the patient recalled feeling nauseated when she saw her mother without dentures. Muir and Calvert[23] described a boy who was unable to undergo dental impressions; his father was reported to have similar problems.

In some cases, symptomatic gagging can be viewed as a learned avoidance reaction, where gagging is associated with a former traumatic dental experience.[32] These patients may use the gagging response as a way to avoid treatment without admitting fear and anxiety even to themselves. Typically, this group is highly motivated, but their gagging reflects the nonverbal message that although they "want" treatment they are too anxious to receive it.[31] The gagging reflex may be a socially acceptable reason for not receiving dental care. The patients view the gagging problem as a physiological feature and use it as a tool which allows them to avoid admitting the less socially desirable problem of anxiety.[5]

It is, therefore, not surprising that most studies dealing with gag patients report a significantly higher number of male patients.[11,17,19-21,23,24,33] Unlike dental anxiety which is reported to be a more prevalent phenomenon in females,[34-42] gagging appears to be rather a male problem.

In the dental setting men generally tend to claim more control than women, probably due to being less willing to admit their loss of control.[43] Although such socialization pressures may confer some advantages to men when it comes to the ability to control behavioral symptoms of anxiety, they may lead to other, less direct ways of expressing the apprehension, such as developing an excessive gagging reflex.

VI. PATIENT MANAGEMENT WITH EXCESSIVE GAGGING REFLEX

Several treatment approaches have been suggested to manage the patient with an excessive gagging reflex:[44]

1. Attempt to change the mechanical aspect of impression trays and/or dentures[11,25]
2. Pharmacological premedication[45-48]
3. Local analgesia of the soft palate and/or the dorsum of the tongue[11,24]
4. Use of nitrous oxide[49]
5. Desensitize the patient to various aspects of tactile stimuli in the oral cavity[5,13,14,20,21,24,31,32,50]
6. Distraction[5,6,10,11]
7. Relinquish control to the patient[5,20,31]
8. Positive suggestions and reinforcement[11,14,23,31]
9. Relaxation and hypnosis[5,12,15,21-23,31,32,50]

Most authors describe a combination of several approaches, individually tailored for each patient (desensitization with relaxation, distraction with local analgesia, etc.). Generally, it seems that behavioral approaches (desensitization, distraction, positive reinforcement, relaxation) have been fairly efficient in the management of extreme gagging in the dental office. (For more detailed discussions of possible treatment modalities see Section 3, Chapters 10 to 13).

VII. SUMMARY

An excessesive gagging reflex poses a significant obstacle to routine dental health. Although the reflex is generally elicited by an immediate noxious stimulus applied to the oropharynx, its associated cognitive aspects may cause apparently "neutral" stimuli to be recognized as noxious, threatening, or unpleasant by the patient, and evoke the associated response.

The largest group of dental patients described as suffering from an excessive gagging reflex are those who gag (retch) with dentures and are therefore unable to use the appliances. These patients were not found to possess specific anatomic features which could explain their reaction, nor were they more neurotic than other patients.

One possible explanation of the development of an excessive gagging reflex in dental patients might be the presence of dental anxiety in those with a specific personality set-up, which prevents the patient from admitting it even to him/herself. In such cases, gagging serves as an efficient way to avoid treatment. The concomitant deterioration in dental health brings many of these patients to require prosthodontic appliances, causing further adaptation problems.

REFERENCES

1. **Critchley, M., Ed.,** *Butterworths Medical Dictionary*, 2nd ed., Butterworths, London, 1978.
2. **Logemann, J. A.,** Swallowing physiology and pathophysiology, *Otolaryngol. Clin. North Am.*, 21, 613, 1988.
3. **Ganong, W. F., Ed.,** *Review of Medical Physiology*, Lange, Los Altos, CA, 1985.
4. **Gilroy, J. and Meyer, J. S.,** *Medical Neurology*, 3rd ed., McMillan, New York, 1979, 40.
5. **Ramsay, D. S., Weinstein, P., Milgrom, P., and Getz, T.,** Problematic gagging: principles of treatment, *J. Am. Dent. Assoc.*, 114, 178, 1987.
6. **Krol, A. J.,** A new approach to the gagging problem, *J. Prosthet. Dent.*, 13, 611, 1963.
7. **Chastain, F. R.,** A case of excessive gagging, *Am. J. Clin. Hypn.*, 7, 257, 1965.
8. **Faigenblum, M. J.,** Retching, its causes and management in prosthetic practice, *Br. Dent. J.*, 125, 485, 1968.
9. **Savage, R. D. and MacGregor, A. R.,** Behavior therapy in prosthodontics, *J. Prosthet. Dent.*, 24, 126, 1970.
10. **Stoffelmayr, B. E.,** The treatment of a retching response to dentures by counteractive reading aloud, *J. Behav. Ther. Exp. Psychiatry*, 1, 163, 1970.
11. **Kovats, J. J.,** Clinical evaluation of the gagging denture patient, *J. Prosthet. Dent.*, 25, 613, 1971.
12. **Weyandt, T. A.,** Three case reports in dental hypnotherapy, *Am. J. Clin. Hypn.*, 15, 49, 1972.
13. **Singer, I. L.,** The marble technique: a method for treating the "hopeless gagger" for complete dentures, *Quintessence Int.*, 6(2), 31, 1975.
14. **Murphy, W. M.,** A clinical survey of gagging patients, *J. Prosthet. Dent.*, 42, 145, 1979.
15. **Rootenberg, A.,** Hypnosis as a means of treating a very difficult gagger, *J. Dent. Assoc. S. Afr.*, 529, 1979.
16. **Wright, S. M.,** An examination of factors associated with retching in dental patients, *J. Dent.*, 7, 194, 1979.
17. **Wright, S. M.,** An examination of the personality of dental patients who complain of retching with dentures, *Br. Dent. J.*, 148, 211, 1980.
18. **Wright, S. M.,** The radiologic anatomy of patients who gag with dentures, *J. Prosthet. Dent.*, 45, 127, 1981.
19. **Wright, S. M.,** Medical history, social habits, and individual experiences of patients who gag with dentures, *J. Prosthet. Dent.*, 45, 474, 1981.
20. **Wilks, C. G. W. and Marks, I. M.,** Reducing hypersensitive gagging, *Br. Dent. J.*, 155, 263, 1983.

21. **Morse, D. R., Hancock, R. R., and Cohen, B. B.,** In vivo desensitization using meditation-hypnosis in the treatment of tactile-induced gagging in a dental patient, *Int. J. Psychosom.*, 31, 20, 1984.
22. **Clarke, J. H. and Persichetti, S. J.,** Hypnosis and concurrent denture construction for a patient with a hypersensitive gag reflex, *Am. J. Clin. Hypn.*, 30, 285, 1988.
23. **Muir, J. D. and Calvert, E. J.,** Vomiting during the taking of dental impressions. Two case reports of the use of psychological techniques, *Br. Dent. J.*, 165, 139, 1988.
24. **Fleece, L., Linton, P., and Dudley, B.,** Rapid elimination of a hyperactive gag reflex, *J. Prosthet. Dent.*, 60, 415, 1988.
25. **Callison, G. M.,** A modified edentulous maxillary custom tray to help prevent gagging, *J. Prosthet. Dent.*, 62, 48, 1989.
26. **Pastorello, J. R.,** Chronic gagging in the new denture wearer, *J. Am. Dent. Assoc.*, 59, 748, 1959.
27. **Leslie, S. W.,** A new operation to overcome gagging as an aid to denture construction, *J. Can. Dent. Assoc.*, 6, 291, 1940.
28. **Ament, P.,** Removal of gagging: a response to variable behavior patterns, *Int. J. Clin. Exp. Hypn.*, 19, 1, 1971.
29. **Mack, A. O.,** Complete dentures. II. The type of mouth, *Br. Dent. J.*, 116, 426, 1964.
30. **Schroeder, H. E., Schroeder, U., and Santibanez H. G.,** Dentist phobia, *Pavlovian J. Biol. Sci.*, 21, 16, 1986.
31. **Eli, I. and Kleinhauz, M.,** Hypnosis: a tool for an integrative approach in the treatment of the gagging reflex, *Int. J. Clin. Exp. Hypn.*, 33, 99, 1985.
32. **Klepac, R. K., Hauge, G., and Dowling, J.,** Treatment of an overactive gag reflex: Two cases, *J. Behav. Ther. Exp. Psychiatry*, 13, 141, 1982.
33. **Eli, I. and Kleinhauz, M.,** Oro-related behavioral dysfunctions — a disabling factor in dental care, (in press).
34. **Kleinknecht, R. A., Klepac, R. K., and Alexander, L. D.,** Origins and characteristics of fear of dentistry, *J. Am. Dent. Assoc.*, 86, 842, 1973.
35. **Gatchel, R. J., Ingersoll, B. D., Bowman, L., Robertson, M. C., and Walker, C.,** The prevalence of dental fear and avoidance: A recent survey study, *J. Am. Dent. Assoc.*, 107, 609, 1983.
36. **Milgrom, P., Fiset, L., Melnick, S., and Weinstein, P.,** The prevalence and practice management consequences of dental fear in a major US city, *J. Am. Dent. Assoc.*, 116, 641, 1988.
37. **Domoto, P. K., Weinstein, P., Melnick, S., Ohmura, M., Uchida, H., Ohmachi, K., Hori, M., Okazaki, Y., Shimamoto, T., Matsumura, S., and Shimono, T.,** Results of a dental fear survey in Japan: implications for dental public health in Asia, *Community Dent. Oral Epidemiol.*, 16, 199, 1988.
38. **Cohen, L. A., Snyder, T. L., and LaBelle, A. D.,** Correlates of dental anxiety in a university population, *J. Public Health Dent.*, 42, 228, 1982.
39. **Milgrom, P., Weinstein, P., Kleinknecht, R., and Getz, T.,** *Treating Fearful Dental Patients*, Reston, Reston, VA, 1985.
40. **Bernstein, D. A. and Kleinknecht, R. A.,** Multiple approaches to the reduction of dental fear, *J. Behav. Ther. Exp. Psychiatry*, 13, 287, 1982.
41. **Green, R. M. and Green, A.,** Adult attitudes to dentistry among dental attenders in South Wales, *Br. Dent. J.*, 159, 157, 1985.
42. **Klepac, R. K., Dowling, J., and Hauge, G.,** Characteristics of clients seeking therapy for the reduction of dental avoidance: reactions to pain, *J. Behav. Ther. Exp. Psychiatry*, 13, 293, 1982.
43. **Kent, G.,** Self-efficacious control over reported physiological, cognitive and behavioural symptoms of dental anxiety, *Behav. Res. Ther.*, 25, 341, 1987.
44. **Conny, D. J. and Tedesco, L. A.,** The gagging problem in prosthodontic treatment. Part II. Patient management, *J. Prosthet. Dent.*, 49, 757, 1983.
45. **Jaffre, A. P.,** Controlling gagging, *Dent. Surv.*, 40, 47, 1964.

46. **Kramer, R. B. and Braham, R. L.,** The management of the chronic or hysterical gagger, *J. Dent. Child.*, 44, 111, 1977.
47. **Rothschild, N.,** Practical gag reflex control, *Dent. Surv.*, 35, 1354, 1959.
48. **Schole, M. L.,** Management of the gagging patient, *J. Prosthet. Dent.*, 9, 578, 1959.
49. **Kaufman, E., Weinstein, P., Sommers, E. E., and Soltero, D. J.,** An experimental study of the control of the gag reflex with nitrous oxide, *Anesth. Prog.*, 35, 155, 1988.
50. **Eli, I., Kleinhauz, M., and Bar-Gil, B.,** Extreme gag reflex: methods of treatment and control, *Isr. J. Dent. Sci.*, 1, 105, 1984.

Chapter 6

PSYCHOGENIC FACTORS IN BENIGN CHRONIC OROFACIAL PAIN

Pain, chronic or acute, is a complex sensory, emotional, and cognitive experience which has an enormous impact on human behavior. The orofacial region harbors various conditions of prolonged, benign, chronic pain that may originate from pathophysiological mechanisms or may have a more vague, psychogenic etiology. In either case, pain has a reciprocal effect on the emotional and cognitive patterns of the patient with potential behavioral consequences.

I. CLASSIFICATION

Several classification methods have been suggested for chronic pain in the orofacial region. For example, Bell[1] outlined three basic categories of pain syndromes about the mouth and face: somatic pain, which results from noxious stimulation of normal neural structures that innervate body tissues; neurogenous pain, which generates within the nervous system itself; and psychogenic pain, which results from psychic causes. The classification gives utmost attention to the first two parts with only little impact on so-called psychogenic pain, including syndromes defined as chronic facial pain and psychoneurotic pain.

The Classification of Chronic Pain prepared by the International Association for the Study of Pain (IASP)[2] and the Diagnostic and Statistical Manual of Mental Disorders of the American Psychiatric Association (DSM-III-R)[3] are more psychologically oriented classifications of chronic pain conditions.

The DSM-III-R suggests the use of the term "somatoform pain disorder" defined as "preoccupation with pain in the absence of adequate physical findings to account for the pain or its intensity." The pain symptom is defined as being inconsistent with the anatomic distribution of the nervous system, or being inadequately accounted for by organic pathology or pathophysiological mechanisms. The diagnostic criteria include preoccupation with pain for at least 6 months without organic pathology or pathophysiological mechanisms, or resulting social or occupational impairment which is grossly in excess of what would be expected from the physical findings.

The IASP divides psychological pain into muscle tension pain ("virtually continuous pain in any part of the body due to sustained muscle contraction and provoked by emotional causes or by persistent overuse of particular muscles"); delusional or hallucinatory pain ("pain of psychological origin and attributed by the patient to a specific delusional cause"); and hysterical or hypochondrical pain ("pain specifically attributable to the thought process, emotional state or personality of the patient in the absence of an organic or delusional cause or tension mechanism").

The IASP rejects the popular term of "atypical facial pain" as it does not describe a definite syndrome but is used to cover a variety of conditions. Terms such as temporomandibular pain and dysfunction syndrome, atypical odontalgia, and odontalgia not associated with lesions are suggested instead. It is this terminology that will be used in the present chapter.

These two concepts acknowledge that the exact relationship between psychological and physical aspects of a painful experience is not yet fully understood. However, different pain conditions are usually classified as either originating in the mind or in the body.[4] Of course, this is not always necessarily true. Today, it is generally accepted that the reciprocal relationship of mind and body prevents a clear-cut distinction between the two. A person suffering from chronic muscle pain due to hyperactive muscle activity is also affected by stress, anxiety, and depression which concomitantly affect the physiopathological activity of the muscles. On the other hand, an individual suffering from a continuous depressive state may react with muscle tension which initiates the chronic pain cycle. A more useful alternative to the single axis system for classifying pain as having either a physical or a psychological origin, might be to allow both a psychological and a physical diagnosis to be made simultaneously for each patient.[4,5]

Although much information exists about the various conditions causing chronic pain in the orofacial region, little relates to the specific features of pain in particular loci. The locus of chronic pain of psychological origin can have profound implications on the total subjective experience of pain. We may even speculate that the body part in which the pain is located has some psychodynamic significance.[6]

A detailed discussion of the various conditions of chronic orofacial pain is beyond the scope of this chapter. Instead, the chapter deals with some of the most common conditions of chronic benign orofacial pain of psychogenic origin and with the emotional and behavioral aspects of several pain states with a known pathophysiological mechanism. To do this, the classification strategy of Dworkin and Burgess[4] is used.

II. PAIN WITH KNOWN PATHOPHYSIOLOGICAL MECHANISMS

In the orofacial region, the main pathophysiological mechanism of chronic pain lies in the musculoskeletal system and results from hyperactive muscle activity. This type of pain includes the temporomandibular pain and dysfunction syndrome (TMPDS, also known as myofacial pain dysfunction), and muscle tension or contraction headache.

A. TEMPOROMANDIBULAR PAIN AND DYSFUNCTION SYNDROME (TMPDS)

TMPDS is defined as aching in the muscles of mastication and, in some cases, an occasional brief severe pain on chewing, possibly leading to restricted jaw movement.[2] Aside from the known pathophysiological mechanism, stress, anxiety, depression, and somatization are strongly suspected as being related to the syndrome.[4]

TMPDS is rather common in western populations.[7-9] In recent epidemiological studies, up to 39% of American students surveyed[10] and 49% of adults surveyed in Toronto[11] reported symptoms. Such high percentage of those suffering should involve an effort to provide advanced training programs to develop proper treatment frameworks.[7,12]

In spite of its relatively high prevalence, many clinical signs important in the differential diagnosis of TMPDS are not measured with accurate reliability. Clinical signs change spontaneously, making it difficult to find the same sign on successive examination attempts.[13] Successful diagnosis may be further complicated by psychological factors that frequently play a major role in both diagnosis and treatment of TMPDS.

Fricton[14] and Fricton and Chang Chung,[15] summarized the factors contributing to chronic pain of TMPDS origin as

1. Behavioral factors, including regular behaviors or actions that contribute to pain (mainly oral parafunctional habits, such as bruxism, clenching, biting objects, biting tongue or cheek, tongue thrust, etc.)
2. Social factors, including antecedent or consequential events in the social environment, that affect perceptions and learned responses to pain (e.g., social support, social modeling, secondary gain, recent stressful events, prolonged stressful events)
3. Emotional factors, including prolonged negative emotions that complicate management or indirectly perpetuate other contributing factors (e.g., depression, low self-esteem, anxiety)
4. Cognitive factors, including thoughts, attitudes, or mental processes that are counterproductive to successful management (e.g., poor problem-solving skills, lack of proper understanding, senility, unrealistic expectations)
5. Biological factors, including any factors related to individual mechanical biological constitution that predispose the individual to developing an illness (e.g., genetic predisposition, skeletal discrepancies, hormonal changes)
6. Environmental factors, including those stimuli in the physical environment that are not under direct control (e.g., allergens, weather, pollutants)

The authors present a medical model and conceptual framework integrating the physical, behavioral, and psychosocial aspects of the illness, in which the multiple levels of problems recursively affect each other. As an example, they describe a patient who suffered from chronic muscular pain, anxiety, and depression. The patient's chronic pain involved concomitant cognitive (e.g., perception of pain, concern), emotional (e.g., anxiety), and behavioral (e.g.,

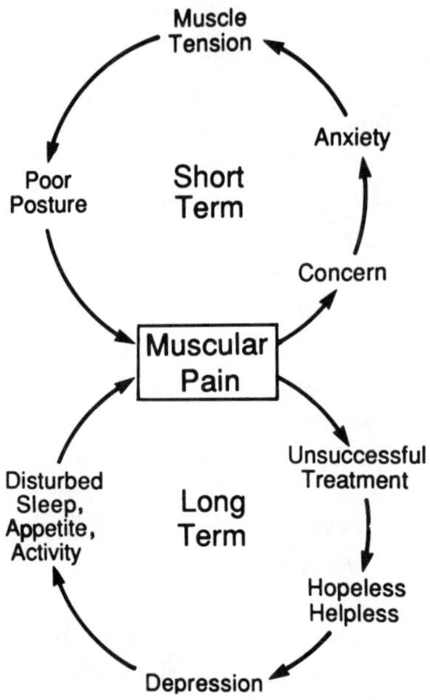

FIGURE 5. Cybernetics and the cyclical manner of factors contributing to chronic muscular pain. The syndrome is considered to have multiple levels of problems that recursively affect each other and the syndrome itself. An aggrevation in one factor (e.g., inadequate sleep) affects a disturbance in another (less daytime energy) and generates positive feedback in other factors that may perpetuate the illness (more pain, depression). Likewise, improving one factor (e.g., self-control of muscle tension) may generate negative feedback in other factors and help to alleviate the illness (relieve pain, improve sleep, reduce depression). (From, Fricton, J. R., Kroening, R. J., and Hathaway, K. M., *TMJ and Craniofacial Pain: Diagnosis and Management*, 1988, 22.)

increased muscle tension, poor posture) factors. The depression involved concomitant cognitive (e.g., feelings of helplessness) and behavioral (e.g., poor sleep) factors. Aggravation of one factor, such as inadequate sleep, leads to less daytime energy, more muscular pain, and further depression. Improving a factor, such as self-control of muscle tension, relieves the pain, improves sleep, and reduces depression (Figure 5).

In several reviews, Rugh[16] and Rugh and Solberg,[17] summarized the influence of psychological factors in the etiology of TMPDS. The relevant points include personality and emotional factors and psychological stress.

1. Personality and Emotional Factors

Although TMPDS patients do not represent a homogenous group with regard to personality characteristics, for many the probability of having a difficult time managing or coping with life situations is increased. Generally, these patients are more anxious and their oral symptoms may be only one aspect of the somatic manifestation of the emotional condition.[16]

Recent studies indicate that TMPDS patients do not differ from control groups on measures such as (1) illness behavior;[18] (2) social dysfunction and depression;[19] (3) Levenson locus of control, mastery, denial, sensation-seeking, need of approval, and acquiescence;[20] and (4) neuroticism, parental bonding attitudes, and emotional disturbance.[19] Psychosocial factors, such as health locus of control and denial, were found to be only slightly correlated to the "core" physical symptoms of TMPDS in nonpatients who report TMPDS symptoms.[21]

Butterworth and Deardoff[22] presented three distinct homogeneous profile subgroups of TMPDS patients: a "no-distress" group (24%) who showed no elevations on the clinical scales of SCL-90R profiles; a moderate distress group (36%) who showed elevations on somatization, depression, and anxiety; and a severe distress group (40%) who demonstrated significant elevations on somatization, obsessive-compulsive behavior, interpersonal sensitivity, depression, anxiety, hostility, phobia, and psychoticism. The authors concluded that there is no specific pain-patient personality or uniform symptom constellation.

2. Effect of Psychological Stress

Many studies have pointed to the effect of psychological stress on TMPDS patients. Stress has been shown to affect muscle activity, leading to increased muscle tension and concomitant pain. TMPDS patients seem to respond to stress with increased masticatory muscle tension which has the potential to cause symptoms of pain and dysfunction. The studies reviewed by Rugh[16] and Rugh and Solberg[17] indicate that TMPDS patients have psychological characteristics which make them more likely to experience emotional difficulties in dealing with life events.

Generally, these patients are more anxious and respond to stress and emotional situations with intense and prolonged masticatory muscle contractions. Emotional factors (anxiety, fear, frustration, anger) elicite the muscular tension and the oral habits which are associated with the etiology of TMPDS. Furthermore, these patients do not show the usual habituation to stressful conditions found in control groups, and they continue to react with increased muscular tension.[16,17] Electromyographic activity was found to be significantly greater in TMPDS patients compared to control subjects during baseline and stress conditions.[23]

In a conceptual stress model, Harber et al.[24] demonstrated the effect of stress on all craniomandibular disorders (Figure 6). According to the model, stress results in muscle hyperactivity, expressed in various forms of parafunctional activities (clenching, grinding, etc.), which can lead to any one of the cardinal symptoms of TMPDS (trismus, TMJ sounds, and/or pain in TMJ and muscles). The symptoms, in turn, affect perception and cognition such that the patient notices the symptom(s) and seeks professional help. Pain symptoms also become stronger with positive or negative reinforcement. When present, nega-

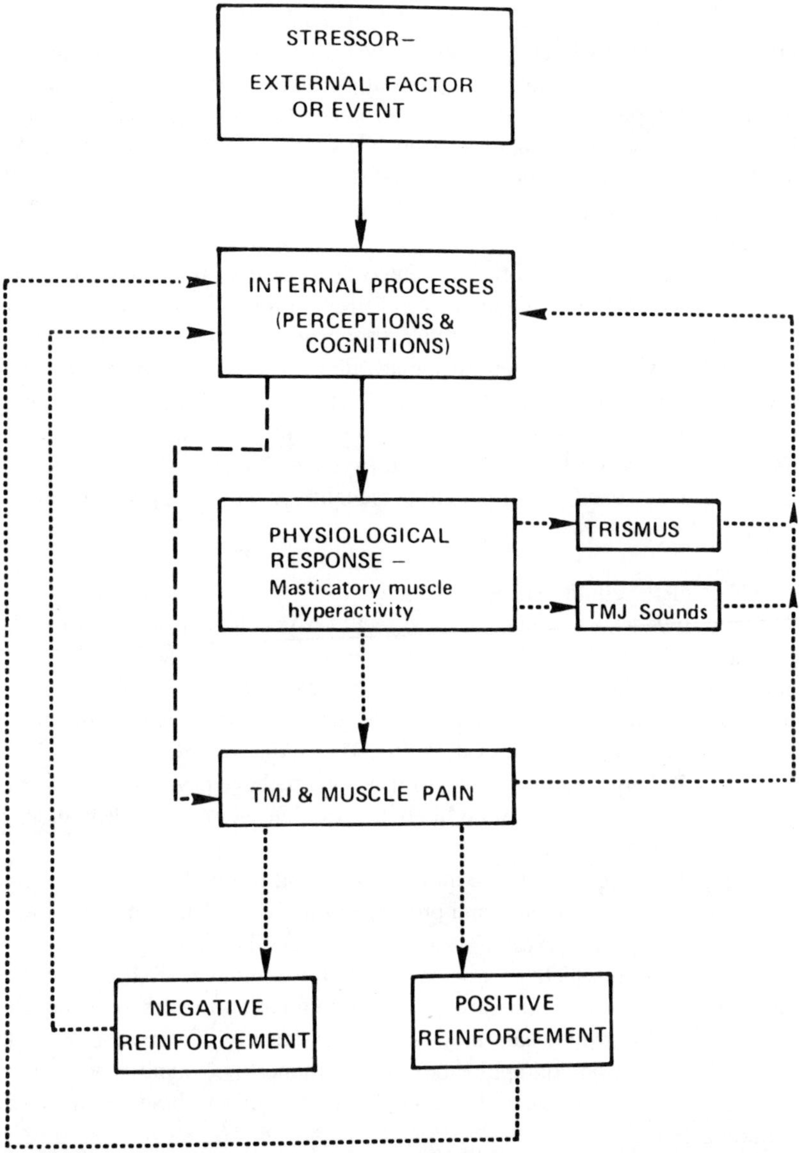

FIGURE 6. Conceptual model of the effect of psychological stress on craniomandibular disorders. (From *J. Oral Rehabil.*, 10, 191, 1983.)

tive reinforcement affects the internal processes of perceptions and cognitions and eventually the physiological responses (more muscle hyperactivity, more pain, more reinforcement, etc.). Finally, it is possible for pain to occur as a direct result of perceptions and cognitions in the absence of abnormal physiological activity or pathological conditions. This situation most often refers to conversion reactions and occurs in association with a high frequency of negative reinforcement. In such cases, the reinforcement of pain behavior maintains the pain patterns even though the abnormal physiological problem no longer exists.

Recently, an association between pain, depression, and impairment of activity in TMPDS patients suffering from muscle pain (but not in patients suffering from joint or combined muscle-joint pain) was reported.[25,26] Marbach et al.[20] reported more past pain-related illness, more life-threatening physical problems, and more recent events involving injury and nonpain-related physical illness in TMPDS patients when compared to controls. Feinman and Harris[27] showed that 78% of patients suffering from TMPDS (facial arthromyalgia) had suffered an adverse life event, such as family health problems, bereavement, change of location, or marital difficulty prior to the onset of the pain. In addition, 80% of the patients also complained of other symptoms (headaches and/or migraines, aches in neck and back, dermatitis or pruritis, spastic colon, and dysfunctional uterine bleeding). The role of recent stressful life events in the onset of TMJ pain in TMPDS patients has also been confirmed by Speculand et al.[28]

In spite of the apparent importance of psychological factors in the etiology of TMPDS, there is evidence that general practitioners have low sensitivity to the psychological conditions of these patients.[29] Although some studies suggested that dentists were able to assess the presence of underlying psychiatric pathology in a large proportion of patients suffering from atypical odontalgia, the high rate of such disorders indicates the need for a regular liaison between dentists working in pain clinics and the psychiatric services.[30]

Clinical awareness, as well as the development of simple, popular psychological screening methods for TMPDS patients, should contribute to the efficiency of treatment in such cases. Standard, simple ways to measure pain and psychological morbidity in dental practice include the use of questionnaires, such as The McGill Pain Questionnaire and the Hospital Anxiety and Depression Scale (HAD).[31] Another simple psychological questionnaire has recently been suggested by Gale and Dixon.[32]

B. TENSION HEADACHE

Although headaches are not directly associated with the oral cavity, continuous, recurrent headaches may have a significant effect on the orofacial region.

A tension headache is a continuous head pain, usually symmetrical, associated with muscle tension, anxiety, and "depression". It usually responds to treatment of anxiety and depression, including antidepressant medication. The system is apparently musculoskeletal. Exacerbating factors include emotional stress, anxiety, depression, physical exercise, and alcohol.[2] De Benedittis et al.[33] reported a relationship between stressful life events and the onset of chronic primary headache. A sudden increase in the frequency and magnitude of stressful life events, associated with a cognitive-emotional appraisal of their negative impact on life patterns, brings about the onset of symptoms.

The underlying pathophysiological mechanism is presumed to be similar to that in TMPDS — prolonged muscle contraction, muscle hyperactivity, or muscle spasm.[4]

III. PAIN WITH NO PATHOPHYSIOLOGICAL MECHANISMS (NONDELUSIONAL AND NONHALLUCINATORY)

Pain of psychological origin includes conditions generally referred to as atypical facial pain, atypical odontalgia, glossodynia, oral dysesthesia, etc. Different terms are used to describe a variety of conditions.[2] In many cases, the various pain conditions are interrelated and difficult to separate (pain in the face is often reported together with pain inside the oral cavity, pain in the tongue is often reported together with burning sensation in the oral tissues, etc.).

The following subsections address two main groups of chronic pain conditions, atypical odontalgia (used here to cover various conditions of benign chronic pain of psychological origin not originating in musculoskeletal pathophysiology, often referred to in the literature as atypical facial pain) and glossodynia (used to cover more specific conditions of benign chronic pain inside the oral cavity, including burning sensation in the tongue and mucosa).

A. ATYPICAL ODONTALGIA

The IASP defines atypical odontalgia (AO) as severe throbbing in the tooth without major pathology, generally sited in the teeth and gingivae, widespread or well localized. Associated symptoms include emotional problems, complaints of temporomandibular pain and dysfunction syndrome, oral dysesthesia, and often excessive concern with oral hygiene.[2]

In the present chapter, the term will also be used to cover other conditions of pain in the face with no known pathophysiological mechanisms. Such conditions are often referred to in the literature as "atypical facial pain" or "psychogenic facial pain".

1. Prevalence and Social Impact

Conditions of chronic pain in the orofacial region are widespread in western societies and have a significant social impact. Although some authors claim that the impact of oral health problems on a person's life is minimal,[34,35] it is difficult to overlook the high prevalence of orofacial pain.

Locker and Grushka[36] reported that about 40% of the population in Toronto experienced some dental pain in a 4-week period prior to their survey. Although most of the respondents indicated that the pain originated in the dentin (pain in the teeth due to hot or cold fluids), a relatively high percentage indicated other sources of oral pain (pain in the jaws, face, etc.). The social and psychological implications of such conditions are complex. While less than 10% reported severe behavioral impacts, such as work disability, bed rest, and reduced social contacts, up to 70% of the subjects who reported pain stated that they were also worried and concerned about their oral or dental health.

Similar results have also been reported regarding an industrial Eastern population. Nearly one half of the surveyed workers in Kuala Lumpur reported having orofacial pain 1 month prior to the survey. Here too, the most common type of pain originated in the dentin, with approximately 1% of the respondents being absent from work because of the pain.[37]

In an epidemiological study conducted in Seattle, the prevalence of facial pain in the 6 months prior to the survey was 12%. About 9% of the respondents who reported facial pain also reported limitation in one or more of their usual activities (work, school, or housework).[38] In the Swedish city of Umea, about 24% of the general population reported symptoms of facial pain and headache at some time.[39]

A high prevalence of AO has also been reported among patients suffering from various chronic pain conditions. In a general pain clinic in Australia, 10% of the patients suffered from pain in the head and neck, about 1% had symptoms of intraoral pain.[40]

2. Demographic Characteristics

Most studies describing patients with symptoms of AO report a higher percentage of women than men.[27,30,40-46] Average age is between 40 and 55.[40-44,46,47] In Mock et al.,[45] 76% of AO patients were women, with two peaks in age range: 30 to 40 and 50 to 60 years old.

The high prevalence of AO among women may be due to the high response rate of middle-aged women in general epidemiological surveys concerning pain complaints as compared to men.[36,38] However, the overwhelmingly higher percentage of women seeking treatment for AO suggests that other, supposed psychodynamic causes may be responsible for the phenomenon.

3. Personality Traits, Emotional Factors and Possible Psychopathology

In the past, facial pain of psychogenic origin has been associated with traits of hysteria, obsession, anxiety, and depression.[48,49] Lascelles[44] found that the majority of AO patients had a background of depressive illness. This "illness" was atypical in that classical features of depressive states (melancholia, retardation, weight loss, and self-reproach) were replaced by intense fatigue, agitation, and sleep disorders.

More recent studies also reported a high percentage of psychiatric illness in AO patients.[27,30,40,42,47,50,51] Remick et al.[42] found that 69% of surveyed patients suffered from psychiatric illness, as defined by the DSM-III-R criteria. In a continuing report, the same group of researchers[47] found 76% of their patients to suffer from or have a suspected psychiatric disorder. The most common psychiatric disorders were affective disorders (18%) and somatoform disorders (about 12%), followed by psychosis (about 8%), adjustment disorders (about 7%), and personality disorders (about 5%).

The high probability of a psychiatric finding in AO patients has also been reported by Goss et al.[40] The authors found that 4 of 15 patients suffering from intraoral pain had histories of major psychiatric problems (paranoid schizophrenia, paranoia with dementia, obsessive hypochondria, and long-standing depressive illness). The most common disorder among the remaining group was an obsessional personality.

Among 34 AO patients reviewed by Hampf et al.,[50] only 2 were found to be mentally healthy, 12 were psychotic (e.g., schizophrenia, major depression, paranoia, atypical psychosis), 16 had pathologic personality disorders, and 4 suffered from a mild psychiatric disorder (the classification was performed according to the DMS-III criteria).

In a Psychiatric Pain Clinic in Glasgow, 41% of the referred dental patients with chronic pain were diagnosed as having affective disorders (e.g., depressive and dysthymic disorders), 30% had somatoform disorders (e.g., psychogenic pain disorder, polysymptomatic hysteria, psychological factors affecting physical condition), and 7% had nonaffective psychosis (e.g., schizophrenia).[30]

In a study by Feinmann and Harris[27] on AO patients, 42% suffered from depressive neurosis and 21% from nondepressive neurosis. Similarly to TMPDS patients, a high percentage of patients with symptoms of AO suffered from stressful life events prior to the pain development.

Using the General Health Questionnaire (GHQ-28), Merskey et al.[52] found that 30% of the patients from an oral medicine facial pain clinic had probable psychiatric illnesses. The authors pointed out that this rate is relatively low when compared to other chronic pain populations,[19,52] suggesting that dentists are prone to referring patients with facial pain for another opinion if the situation appears to have nothing to do with teeth and is not amenable to surgical intervention. While this statement may be partly true (dentists usually have little training in psychology and often feel helpless in treating patients with so-called "behavioral dysfunctions"), utmost attention must be used to avoid misdiagnosis and/or mistreatment by inefficient (and often damaging) surgical interventions.

4. Misdiagnosis and Mistreatment

Many studies indicate the danger of misdiagnosis and mistreatment of patients with AO.[40,42,44-46,53-56]

In one of the first extensive studies on patients with AO, Lascelles[44] pointed out that many patients undergo a significant amount of dental treatment in their quest for relief from pain. In a group of 53 patients suffering from AO, 31 had had some kind of dental surgery, 3 had had all of their teeth extracted, 3 had undergone surgical attempts to interrupt the pain pathways, 9 patients had undergone operations in their nose and paranasal sinuses, and 3 had had their tonsils and adenoids removed in an effort to alleviate the pain. The high number of operative treatments seems amazing in view of the fact that the majority of these patients revealed a background of depressive illness which might have had a significant effect on their condition.

More recent data show the high percentage of surgical treatment (including tooth extractions) performed on these patients, often with no relief from their pain.[42,45,46,55] Remick et al.[42] reported that of 58 AO patients, 21 (36%) accounted for 65 different dental and surgical treatments, with only 1 patient showing less pain as a result. Discomfort was worse in 3 patients after treatment, and in the vast majority (80%) it was unchanged. The ineffective dental and surgical treatments performed included 11 treatments involving tooth extraction (up to 4 extractions in 1 patient); 10 cases of endodontic therapy; 3 of surgical exploration; 2 of apicoectomy; 2 of occlusal adjustment; and some cases of Caldwell-Luc (n = 2), TMJ athroplasty (n = 1), and laryngeal biopsy (n = 1). Of the 21 patients, 17 underwent two or more procedures. It is interesting to note that 69% of the patients in this group suffered from some specific psychiatric illness.

Mock et al.[45] reported that 73% of the AO patients they attended had had some form of treatment to alleviate their symptoms. More than 50% had had endodontic treatment or extractions. In all cases, symptoms either persisted or became more severe after treatment.

Describing several groups of patients suffering from orofacial dysesthesia (atypical facial pain, glossodynia, and geographic tongue), Hampf[55] found that 56% of the patients had had one or more extractions because of their symptoms, 36% had received endodontic treatment, and 55% went through other irreversible invasive surgical treatments.

Goss et al.[40] reported on the large number of dental and medical practitioners who had been consulted by the AO patients before referral to a general pain clinic. On the average, each patient had seen four specialists. These multiple consultations resulted in a considerable amount of treatment: 1 patient was completely edentulous, 5 were edentulous in up to two quadrants, and 10 of 15 patients had had various surgical procedures including exploration of the edentulous alveolus in the painful region. In this group, a high proportion of common personality disorders (obsessional personality) was found.

The amount of misdiagnosis and ineffective surgical treatment in AO patients contradicts the view raised by Merskey et al.[52] regarding the relatively high tendency of dentists to refer patients with AO for another opinion. Apparently, some dentists fail to diagnose the possible psychogenic etiology of the phenomenon and attempt to treat the pain with more familiar, operative procedures. The high rate of treatable psychiatric disorders associated with AO indicates the need for regular and close liaison between dentists working in pain clinics and professionals in the psychiatric field.[30] Dentists must be able to screen psychiatric disorders in order to identify the patients who are in need of more professional help and to encourage more care in the administation of surgical procedures.

B. GLOSSODYNIA

Most of the studies dealing with glossodynia refer to a more general syndrome defined as stomatodynia, or the burning mouth syndrome. The situation is associated with an unexplained, prolonged sensation of pain and/or burning inside the oral cavity, often accompanied by other phenomena, such as dryness, parasthesia, and changes in the sensations of taste and smell. As most patients indicate the tongue as the main locus of symptoms, the term glossodynia, which has been accepted by the IASP taxonomy committee, is used here.

IASP defines glossodynia as burning pain in the tongue, which most often involves the tip and lateral borders of glossal mucosa, palate, lips, and sometimes other buccal mucosa, and is often associated with odd taste, dry mouth, uncomfortable bite, or denture intolerance.[2]

Some refer to glossodynia as a variant of the condition generally known as atypical facial pain,[57] while others see it as a distinct clinical entity.[58-64] Although similarities between the two conditions are apparent, significant differences can be observed.

1. Prevalence

The prevalence of glossodynia in the general population has not been thoroughly investigated. Most of the data deal with populations of patients suffering from glossodynia who have been under treatment in specialized clinics.

In a relatively rare survey of glossodynia in dental patients from a general practitioner, Basker et al.[65] reported that a prolonged burning sensation had been experienced at some time by 5.1% of those surveyed. Only 2.6% reported the sensation present at the time of the survey. The complaint was reported by 4.2% of women and only 0.8% of men. The authors suggested that the problem may affect up to 2.6% of the general population at any time.

2. Demographic Characteristics

Glossodynia is sometimes considered as a variant of atypical facial pain (referred to here as atypical odontalgia) because of the resemblance between the demographic characteristics of patients suffering from the two syndromes.

Similar to AO, the typical glossodynia patient is a middle-aged woman. Nearly all authors report a strikingly higher percentage of women suffering from glossodynia,[57,58,60-62,64-70] ranging as high as 90%[57,67,69] with a mean age between 55 and 60 years.[57-62,64,66,68-70]

3. Site and Duration of Symptoms

Symptoms usually occur in more than one site in the mouth.[65,67,68] The most common site of sensation is the tongue.[57,62,65,67,68] Other areas include lips, palate,[57,62,67] buccal mucosa, upper and lower denture-bearing tissues, throat, and pharyngeal cavity.[62,65,68]

According to Main and Baskar,[68] the tongue and upper denture-bearing tissues are affected in up to 68% of cases, lips in up to 35%, lower denture-bearing tissues in up to 25%, buccal mucosa in up to 20%, oropharynx in up to 8%, and floor of the mouth in 4%.

According to Grushka,[70] the prevalence of oral sites at which burning sensation was reported (among 102 subjects complaining of glossodynia) is as follows: tip of tongue (78%), anterior two thirds of tongue (58%), ventral side of tongue (17%), posterior third of tongue (11%), floor of mouth (13%), anterior third of hard palate (49%), posterior two thirds of hard palate (26%), soft palate (6%), oropharynx (13%), mucosal portion of lower lip (49%), cutaneous portion of lower lip (24%), mucosal portion of upper lip (39%), cutaneous portion of upper lip (18%), lower alveolar ridges (25%), upper alveolar ridges (24%), and buccal mucosa (14%).

Some authors report that without exception, all patients describe the burning sensation as occurring bilaterally.[62,67] Most of the patients suffer from the syndrome for a relatively long time, ranging from months up to 18 years.[57,65,67,70] The onset was reported to be gradual for 63% of the subjects and sudden for the others.[70]

4. Physiological Aspects

Although many patients (33%) relate the onset of symptoms to previous dental procedures (e.g., extractions) or a previous illness (10%), up to 57% cannot relate it to any prior event.[70] Several causes have been proposed as possible etiologic factors for glossodynia. These include:

1. Local irritation by environmental factors, such as denture base[65,68,71]
2. Oral parafunction[62,72]
3. Deficiency states (especially vitamin deficiency)[65,68,69]
4. Hormonal changes occurring in menopause[65,68]
5. Change in salivary composition[73]
6. Candidiasis[74]
7. Diabetes[65,75]

More than one possible causative factor for the syndrome has been suggested.[62,74] In a prospective study of etiological factors in 150 glossodynia patients, Lamey and Lamb[62] found that one tenth of the patients had features of climacterium and more than three fourths were postmenopausal. Problems with dentures, parafunctional habits, and allergies were found to be important in the syndrome. Vitamin deficiencies (especially vitamin B) as well as several cases of impaired glucose tolerance and undiagnosed diabetes mellitus were also found. Some patients suffered from salivary gland dysfunction, and in one third, species of Candida were isolated.

In several studies, Grushka et al.[58-60.70] compared patients suffering from glossodynia with age- and sex-matched control subjects. Little support was provided for some of the earlier proposed etiological factors, such as dentures, oral habits, candidiasis, and nutritional deficiency.[70] Furthermore, different sensory modalities (tests of touch, two-point discrimination, warmth scaling, and oral stereognostic ability) showed no significant differences between the two groups. One significant difference, however, was a decreased pain tolerance among the glossodynia patients at the tongue tip, a site of clinical pain in a majority of subjects tested. The authors suggested that some specific changes occur in the peripheral or central sensory functions.[59]

Additionally, glossodynia patients displayed significant alterations in sensory dysfunction, at the taste threshold for sweet as well as at the suprathreshold levels for sweet and sour.[60] As taste and saliva mutually influence each other,[76] the changes in the patients' sense of taste may suggest salivary changes which concomitantly cause the reported symptoms.

Furthermore, statistically significant differences in tongue temperature were observed between glossodynia patients and age- and sex-matched controls. The lowest temperatures were measured in the apex lingual area and were significantly lower in the study group. Thermoesthesiometry tests were suggested as possible diagnosis for glossodynia.[77]

5. Emotional Factors, Personality Traits, and Psychosocial Aspects

A psychogenic etiology for glossodynia has been suggested in the past.[62,74,78-86] Several recent investigations also suggest the presence of a strong psychological component in the symptoms of these patients. Van der Ploeg et al.[67] reported glossodynia patients as scoring clearly higher than the normal population on state and trait anxiety, depression, somatic reactions to stress, neuroticism, and neurosomaic lability. Browning et al.[61] found psychiatric disorders in 44% of glossodynia patients compared to only 16% in a control group. Hampf et al.[50] reported that 7 of 10 glossodynia patients suffered from a pathologic personality disorder and 3 from a mild psychiatric disorder (according to DMS-III criteria). Lamey and Lamb[64] indicated that 39% of their study population had clinically significant anxiety and 13% had depression.

The definite cause effect of glossodynia has not yet been determined. It is not fully understood whether the emotional status of glossodynia patients is causative in their pathology, or whether it is the result of the chronic pain they experience.

Grushka et al.[58] compared the pain experience and the personality profiles of glossodynia patients and their age- and sex-matched controls. The results indicated that the magnitude of the pain was similar to a toothache, that self-reports seemed to be valid, and that patients showed elevations in some personality characteristics, changes which tended to increase with pain. These patients differed from the control group in that they were more concerned with bodily function, more depressed, more emotionally repressed, more angry, more distrustful, more anxious, and more socially isolated. The MMPI profiles of these subjects were consistent with those found in subjects with chronic pain. The authors claimed that the personality disturbances associated with glossodynia occur as a result of the chronic pain and are not its cause.

A similar notion was suggested by Zilli et al.[57] In their study, 75% of the patients were depressed, 41% were anxious, and 16% were inwardly irritable.

However, the GHQ scores of the patients (a questionnaire used to assess the respondent's inability to carry out normal healthy functions and the presence of current new distressing symptoms) showed little difference from scores obtained in other pain clinics.

The idea that, at least in some patients, the psychological findings may be the consequence of the chronic pain condition rather than its cause, can also be indirectly supported by the fact that a significant percentage of glossodynia patients showed no psychiatric morbidity[61] or depression.[64]

6. Possible Etiology

Apparently, in spite of the generally uniform demographic and clinical features of glossodynia patients, the etiology is not homogeneous. Physical as well as psychological factors play a significant role in the syndrome and determine both the patient's emotional status and the possible outcome of treatment.

Some recent studies suggest that the population of glossodynia patients can be divided into those responsive to treatment and those who resist it. When the psychological profiles of cured vs. noncured glossodynia patients were compared, the latter were found to be more unstable, more intelligent, more apprehensive, and more tense.[63] Among 16 glossodynia patients who resisted any form of oral treatment (out of 100 treated patients), all reported symptoms in other organs. Only one patient was judged as purely somatic (formalin allergy), while the others were classified as a combination of somatic and psychological causes (8 patients) or purely psychological causes (6 patients).[66]

Many of the studies describing glossodynia (and/or AO) patients refer to selected populations treated in specialized clinics. These are not necessarily representative of the general population and their deductions may be misleading. In their review of neglected factors in chronic pain treatment outcome studies, Turk and Rudy[87] questioned the methodological adequacy of such publications. The authors point out that many of the studies lacked proper control groups, described only brief-duration follow-up periods, and presented vague criteria for establishing the success of the therapeutic interventions.

The critique raised by Turk and Rudy is relevant to many of the publications dealing with glossodynia and AO, a fact which impairs our ability to deduct exact conclusions as to the etiology of the syndromes. Apparently, glossodynia has a multifactorial etiology. Physical changes, combined with specific personality type, lead to the initiation of symptoms. Individual response to the pain determines whether cure is possible (by either pharmacological, physical, or psychological means) or the condition will turn into a chronic, persistent pathology.

The presence (or absence) of depression in chronic pain patients has been shown to affect the patient's treatment response.[88] Therefore, early identification of any possible psychological factors may significantly contribute to the understanding and treatment of these patients.

C. ORAL "GALVANISM"

Recently, an increased interest emerged from patients as well as from dentists, in a so-called syndrome of "oral galvanism."[72,89-93] The syndrome is supposed to describe a situation of chronic pain or atypical taste sensations inside the oral cavity due to metal taste and galvanic currents caused by metal restorations (mainly amalgam and nonprecious alloys).

Oral galvanism is a term that covers various symptoms and disorders.[72,92,93] In spite of what appears to be a physiological etiology (galvanic currents), the syndrome has characteristics similar to those of AO and can often be considered as a variant.

Although several studies attempted to define intraoral conditions associated with symptoms of galvanism (intraoral galvanic currents, saliva conductivity, salivary buffer capacity, contact allergy to dental materials, etc.),[92,94-96] no definite conclusions can be drawn from the presented data. Patients with symptoms defined as oral galvanism have significantly fewer teeth with amalgam fillings[94] and have no signs of a possible presence of contact allergy to dental materials.[95] Most patients have a normal salivary secretion rate and pH, and their saliva conductivity values are within a normal reference interval.[94] A large proportion of patients show parafunctions and functional disturbances of the masticatory system.[92,96]

An extensive clinical study[97] found that metallic taste was encountered by 5% of the general dental patients and was associated with bruxism and grinding. It is possible that the phenomenon of metallic taste which occurs normally in some patients and usually passes with time, develops in others to a general syndrome of AO with fixation on the symptom of galvanic currents.

Attempts to treat the condition by removing and replacing the metallic constructions do not usually solve the problem.[89] Although such treatment was initially evaluated to be successful in about 80% of the patients, about half reported recurrences, more often after removal of metallic constructions than after dental treatment. Therefore, a more thorough consideration of the patient is recommended.

IV. PAIN WITH NO KNOWN PATHOPHYSIOLOGICAL MECHANISMS (DELUSIONAL OR HALLUCINATORY)

Delusional or hallucinatory pain is a pain of psychological origin, attributed by the patient to a specific delusional cause. It may occur in any part of the body, including the face and neck. The attribution of the pain to a specific delusional cause (e.g., to worms inside the teeth or gums) is an essential characteristic. It may be exacerbated by psychological stress and relieved by treatment, causing remission of illness. The etiology is basically manic-depressive, schizophrenic, or psychotic. The pain may last for weeks in manic-depressive or schizo-affective psychoses, or even months or years in established schizophrenia.[2]

Fortunately, these patients are rare in general dental practice. In cases where delusional or hallucinatory causes are suspected as being involved in the patient's symptoms, professional consultation is strongly suggested.

V. TREATMENT

A detailed discussion of treatment modalities is presented in Part 3 of this book and refers mainly to dysfunctions having a behavioral or emotional aspect (e.g., anxiety, stress, depression, etc.).

Treatment approaches that have been suggested for patients with benign chronic orofacial pain include behavior modication techniques,[98] biofeedback,[85,99,100,101] relaxation, and hypnosis.[85,99,102]

In the treatment of chronic pain, numerous other techniques have also been described in the literature, such as the use of antidepressant drugs and/or tranquilizers,[41,43,49,99,103-106] vitamin therapy, antimycotic agents or hormone replacement (in glossodynia),[69] removal of local irritants and/or denture replacement, and others. These were considered to be beyond the scope of this book and will not be described.

VI. SUMMARY

Benign, chronic orofacial pain is often a source of massive frustration to the patient and dentist. Although some of its possible etiological factors (oral parafunctions, muscle tension) are more clearly understood than others, the mutual linkage between physiological factors and psychosocial aspects of the pain experience makes their separation impossible.

Syndromes, such as temporomandibular pain and dysfunction syndrome, atypical odontalgia, and glossodynia are relatively widespread in western societies and have significant personal and social impact. They are affected by various behavioral, social, emotional, cognitive, biological, and environmental factors. If not properly related to, the syndromes can occasionally be misdiagnosed and/or mistreated.

REFERENCES

1. **Bell, W. E.,** *Orofacial Pains: Classification, Diagnosis, Management*, Yearbook Medical Publishers, Chicago, 1989.
2. **Merskey, H., Ed.,** Classification of chronic pain: descriptions of chronic pain syndromes and definitions of pain terms, *Pain* (Suppl.) 3, 1, 1986.
3. American Psychiatric Association, Diagnostic and Statistical Manual of Mental Disorders, 3rd ed. Rev. (DSM-III-R), Washington, D. C., 1987.
4. **Dworkin, S. F. and Burgess, J. A.,** Orofacial pain of psychogenic origin: current concepts and classification, *J. Am. Dent. Assoc.*, 115, 565, 1987.

5. **Dworkin, S. F.,** Integrating behavioral and pharmacological therapeutic modalities, *Anesth. Prog.*, 33, 29, 1986.
6. **Lipsitt, D. R.,** Pain in the neck, face, and head. Role of the consultation liaison psychiatrist, *Psychiatric Clin. North Am.*, 10, 69, 1987.
7. **Rugh, J. D. and Solberg, W. K.,** Oral health status in the United States: Temporomandibular disorders, *J. Dent. Educ.*, 49, 398, 1985.
8. **Greene, C. S. and Marbach, J.,** Epidemiological studies of mandibular dysfunction: a critical review, *J. Prosthet. Dent.*, 48, 184, 1982.
9. **Carlsson, G. E., Kopp, S., and Wedel, A.,** Analysis of background variables in 350 patients with TMJ disorders as reported in self-administered questionnaire, *Community Dent. Oral Epidemiol.*, 10, 47, 1982.
10. **Pullinger, A. G., Seligman, D. A., and Solberg, W. K.,** Temporo-mandibular disorders. Part I. Functional status, dentomorphologic features, and sex differences in a nonpatient population, *J. Prosthet. Dent.*, 59, 228, 1988.
11. **Locker, D. and Slade, G.,** Prevalence of symptoms associated with temporomandibular disorders in a Canadian population, *Community Dent. Oral Epidemiol.*, 16, 310, 1988.
12. **Marbach, J. J. and Lipton, J. A.,** Biopsychosocial factors of the temporomandibular pain dysfunction syndrome: relevance to restorative dentistry, *Dent. Clin. North Am.*, 31, 473, 1987.
13. **Dworkin, S. F., LeResche, L., DeRouen, T., and Von Korff, M.,** Assessing clinical signs of temporomandibular disorders: reliability of clinical examiners, *J. Prosthet. Dent.*, 63, 574, 1990.
14. **Fricton, J. R.,** Establishing the problem list: An inclusive conceptual model for chronic illness, in *TMJ and Craniofacial Pain: Diagnosis and Management,* Fricton, J. R., Kroening, R. J., and Hathaway, K. M., Eds., Ishiyaku EuroAmerica, St. Louis, 1988, 21.
15. **Fricton, J. R. and Chang Chung S.,** Contributing factors: a key to chronic pain, in *TMJ and Craniofacial Pain: Diagnosis and Management,* Fricton, J. R., Kroening, R. J., and Hathaway, K. M., Eds., Ishiyaku EuroAmerica, St. Louis, 1988, 27.
16. **Rugh, J. D.,** Psychological factors in the etiology of masticatory pain and dysfunction, in *The President's Conference on the Examination, Diagnosis and Management of Temporomandibular Disorders*, Laskin, D., Greenfield, W., Gale, E., Rugh, J., Neff, P., Alling, C., and Ayer, W., Eds., American Dental Association, Chicago, 1983, 85.
17. **Rugh, J. D. and Solberg, W. K.,** Psychological implications in temporomandibular pain and dysfunction, *Oral Sci. Rev.*, 7, 3, 1976.
18. **Speculand, B., Goss, A. N., Hughes, A., Spence, N. D., and Pilowsky, I.,** Temporomandibular joint dysfunction: pain and illness behaviour, *Pain*, 17, 139, 1983.
19. **Salter, M., Brooke, R., Merskey, H., Fichter, G. F., and Kapusianyk, D. H.,** Is the temporo-mandibular pain and dysfunction syndrome a disorder of the mind?, *Pain*, 17, 151, 1983.
20. **Marbach, J. J., Lennon, M. C., and Dohrenwend, B. P.,** Candidate risk factors for temporomandibular pain and dysfunction syndrome: psychosocial, health behavior, physical illness and injury, *Pain*, 34, 139, 1988.
21. **Kleinknecht, R. A., Mahoney, E. R., and Alexander, L. D.,** Psychosocial and demographic correlates of temporomandibular disorders and related symptoms: an assessment of community and clinical findings, *Pain*, 29, 313, 1987.
22. **Butterworth, J. C. and Deardorff, W. W.,** Psychometric profiles of craniomandibular pain patients: identifying specific subgroups, *J. Craniomandibular Pract.*, 5, 225, 1987.
23. **Dahlström, L., Carlsson, S. G., Gale, E. N., and Jansson, T. G.,** Stress-induced muscular activity in mandibular dysfunction: effects of biofeedback training, *J. Behav. Med.*, 8, 191, 1985.
24. **Haber, J. D., Moss, R. A., Kuczmierczyk, A. R., and Garrett, J. C.,** Assessment and treatment of stress in myofascial pain-dysfunction syndrome: a model for analysis, *J. Oral Rehabil.*, 10, 187, 1983.

25. **Lundeen, T. F., Sturdevant, J. R., and George, J. M.,** Stress as a factor in muscle and temporomandibular joint pain, *J. Oral Rehabil.*, 14, 447, 1987.
26. **Lundeen, T. F., George, J. M., and Sturdevant, J. R.,** Stress in patients with pain in the muscles of mastication and the temporo-mandibular joints, *J. Oral Rehabil.*, 15, 631, 1988.
27. **Feinmann, C. and Harris, M.,** Psychogenic facial pain. Part I. The clinical presentation, *Br. Dent. J.*, 156, 165, 1984.
28. **Speculand, B., Hughes, A. O., and Goss, A. N.,** Role of recent stressful life events experience in the onset of TMJ dysfunction pain, *Community Dent. Oral Epidemiol.*, 12, 197, 1984.
29. **Oakley, M. E., McCreary, C. P., Flack, V. F., Clark, G. T., Solberg, W. K., and Pullinger, A. G.,** Dentists' ability to detect psychological problems in patients with temporo-mandibular disorders and chronic pain, *J. Am. Dent. Assoc.*, 118, 727, 1989.
30. **Hughes, A. M., Hunter, S., Still, D., and Lamey, P.-J.,** Psychiatric disorders in a dental clinic, *Br. Dent. J.*, 166, 16, 1989.
31. **Zakrzewska, J. M. and Feinmann, C.,** A standard way to measure pain and psychological morbidity in dental practice, *Br. Dent. J.*, 24, 337, 1990.
32. **Gale, E. N. and Dixon, D. C.,** A simplified psychologic questionnaire as a treatment planning aid for patients with temporomandibular joint disorders, *J. Prosthet. Dent.*, 61, 235, 1989.
33. **De Benedittis, G., Lorenzetti, A., and Pieri, A.,** The role of stressful life events in the onset of chronic primary headache, *Pain*, 40, 65, 1990.
34. **Davis, P.,** Compliance structures and the delivery of health care: the case of dentistry, *Soc. Sci. Med.*, 10, 329, 1976.
35. **Westert, G. P., Oosterhaven, S. P., and Schaub, R. M. H.,** Spontaneous recall as an indicator of the impact of dental complaints, *Community Dent. Oral Epidemiol.*, 15, 306, 1987.
36. **Locker, D. and Grushka, M.,** The impact of dental and facial pain, *J. Dent. Res.*, 66, 1414, 1987.
37. **Jaafar, N., Razak, I. A., and Zain, R. B.,** The social impact of oral and facial pain in an industrial population, *Ann. Acad. Med. Singapore*, 18, 553, 1989.
38. **Von Korff, M., Dworkin, S. F., LeResche, L., and Kruger, A.,** An epidemiologic comparison of pain complaints, *Pain*, 32, 173, 1988.
39. **Agerberg, G. and Carlsson, G. E.,** Functional disorders of the masticatory system. I. Distribution of symptoms according to age and sex as judged from investigation by questionnaire, *Acta Odontol. Scand.*, 30, 597, 1972.
40. **Goss, A. N., McNamara, J., and Rounsefell, B.,** Dental patients in a general pain clinic, *Oral Surg. Oral Med. Oral Pathol.*, 65, 663, 1988.
41. **Feinmann, C.,** Psychogenic facial pain: presentation and treatment, *J. Psychosom. Res.*, 27, 403, 1983.
42. **Remick, R. A., Blasberg, B., Barton, J. S., Campos, P. E., and Miles, J. E.,** Ineffective dental and surgical treatment associated with atypical facial pain, *Oral Surgery, Oral Medicine, Oral Pathol.*, 55, 355, 1983.
43. **Feinmann, C. and Harris, M.,** Psychogenic facial pain. Part II. Management and prognosis, *Br. Dent. J.*, 156, 205, 1984.
44. **Lascelles, R. G.,** Atypical facial pain and depression, *Br. J. Psychiatry*, 112, 651, 1966.
45. **Mock, D., Frydman, W., and Gordon, A. S.,** Atypical facial pain: a retrospective study, *Oral Surg. Oral Med. Oral Pathol*, 59, 472, 1985.
46. **Moore, D. S. and Nally, F. F.,** Atypical facial pain: an analysis of 100 patients with discussion, *J. Can. Dent. Assoc.*, 7, 396, 1975.
47. **Blasberg, B., Remick, R. A., Conklin, R., and Keller, F. D.,** Atypical facial pain in the elderly, *Gerodontology*, 3, 77, 1984.
48. **Lesse, S.,** Atypical facial pain of psychogenic origin, *J. Nerv. Ment. Disorders*, 124, 347, 1956.

49. **Rees, R. T. and Harris, M.,** Atypical odontalgia, *Br. J. Oral Surg.*, 16, 212, 1978.
50. **Hampf, G., Vikkula, J., Ylipaavalniemi, P., and Aalberg, V.,** Psychiatric disorders in orofacial dysaesthesia, *Int. J. Oral Maxillofacial Surg.*, 16, 402, 1987.
51. **Hampf, G., Ekholm, A., and Salo, T.,** Sensibility threshold, mental health, and endocrine markers in patients with chronic orofacial pain, *Int. J. Psychosom.*, 36, 37, 1989.
52. **Merskey, H., Lau, C. L., Russell, E. S., Brooke, R. I., James, M., Lappano, S., Neilsen, J., and Tilsworth, R. H.,** Screening for psychiatric morbidity. The pattern of psychological illness and premorbid characteristics in four chronic pain populations, *Pain*, 30, 141, 1987.
53. **Mastrocola, R., Gross, A., and Hall, R. E.,** Atypical facial pain of psychogenic origin, *Gen. Dent.*, 35, 207, 1987.
54. **Kreisberg, M. K.,** Atypical odontalgia: differential diagnosis and treatment, *J. Am. Dent. Assoc.*, 104, 852, 1982.
55. **Hampf, G.,** Dilemma in treatment of patients suffering from orofacial dysaesthesia, *International J. Oral Maxillofacial Surg.*, 16, 397, 1987.
56. **Brooke, R. I.,** Atypical odontalgia: a report of twenty-two cases, *Oral Surg. Oral Med. Oral Pathol.*, 49, 196, 1980.
57. **Zilli, C., Brooke, R. I., Lau, C. L., and Merskey, H.,** Screening for psychiatric illness in patients with oral dysesthesia by means of the General Health Questionnaire — twenty-eight item version (GHQ-28) and the Irritability, Depression and Anxiety Scale (IDA), *Oral Surg. Oral Med. Oral Pathol.*, 67, 384, 1989.
58. **Grushka, M., Sessle, B. J., and Miller, R.,** Pain and personality profiles in burning mouth syndrome, *Pain*, 28, 155, 1987.
59. **Grushka, M., Sessle, B. J., and Howley, T. P.,** Psychophysical assessment of tactile, pain and thermal sensory functions in burning mouth syndrome, *Pain*, 28, 169, 1987.
60. **Grushka, M., Sessle, B. J., and Howley, T. P.,** Psychophysical evidence of taste dysfunction in burning mouth syndrome, *Chem. Senses*, 11, 485, 1986.
61. **Browning, S., Hislop, S., Scully, C., and Shirlaw, P.,** The association between burning mouth syndrome and psychosocial disorders, *Oral Surg. Oral Med. Oral Pathol.*, 64, 171, 1987.
62. **Lamey, P.-J. and Lamb, A. B.,** Prospective study of aetiological factors in burning mouth syndrome, *Br. Med. J.*, 296, 1243, 1988.
63. **Lamb, A. B., Lamey, P.-J., and Reeve, P. E.,** Burning mouth syndrome: psychological aspects, *Br. Dent. J.*, 165, 256, 1988.
64. **Lamey, P.-J. and Lamb, A. B.,** The usefulness of the HAD scale in assessing anxiety and depression in patients with burning mouth syndrome, *Oral Surg. Oral Med. Oral Pathol.*, 67, 390, 1989.
65. **Basker, R. M., Sturdee, D. W., and Davenport, J. C.,** Patients with burning mouths: a clinical investigation of causative factors, including the climacteric and diabetes, *Br. Dent. J.*, 145, 9, 1978.
66. **Hammarén, M. and Hugoson, A.,** Clinical psychiatric assessment of patients with burning mouth syndrome resisting oral treatment, *Swed. Dent. J.*, 13, 77, 1989.
67. **van der Ploeg, H. M., van der Wal, N., Eijkman, M. A. J., and van der Waal, I.,** Psychological aspects of patients with burning mouth syndrome, *Oral Surg. Oral Med. Oral Pathol.*, 63, 664, 1987.
68. **Main, D. M. G. and Basker, R. M.,** Patients complaining of a burning mouth: further experience and clinical assessment and management, *Br. Dent. J.*, 154, 206, 1983.
69. **Lamey, P.-J., Hammond, A., Allam, B. F., and McIntosh, W. B.,** Vitamin status of patients with burning mouth syndrome and the response to replacement therapy, *Br. Dent. J.*, 160, 81, 1986.
70. **Grushka, M.,** Clinical features of burning mouth syndrome, *Oral Surg. Oral Med. Oral Pathol.*, 63, 30, 1987.

71. **Kaaber, S., Thulin, H., and Nielsen, E.,** Skin sensitivity to denture base materials in the burning mouth syndrome, *Contact Dermatitis*, 5, 90, 1979.
72. **Jontell, M., Haraldson, T., Persson, L.-O., and Ohman, S.-C.,** An oral and psychosocial examination of patients with presumed oral galvanism, *Swed. Dent. J.*, 9, 175, 1985.
73. **Glick, D., Ben-Aryeh, H., Gutman, D., and Szargel, R.,** Relation between idiopathic glossodynia and salivary flow rate and content, *Int. J. Oral Surg.*, 5, 161, 1976.
74. **Zegarelli, D. J.,** Burning mouth: an analysis of 57 patients, *Oral Surg. Oral Med. Oral Pathol.*, 58, 34, 1984.
75. **Brody, H. A., Prendergast, J. J., and Silverman, S., Jr.,** The relationship between oral symptoms, insulin release, and glucose intolerance, *Oral Surg. Oral Med. Oral Pathol.*, 31, 777, 1971.
76. **Spielman, A. I.,** Interaction of saliva and taste, *J. Dent. Res.*, 69, 838, 1990.
77. **Cekic-Arambasin, A., Vidas, I., and Stipetic-Mravak, M.,** Clinical oral test for the assessment of oral symptoms of glossodynia and glossopyrosis, *J. Oral Rehabil.*, 17, 495, 1990.
78. **Gilpin, S. F.,** Glossodynia, *J. Am. Med. Assoc.*, 106, 1722, 1936.
79. **Ziskin, D. E. and Moulton, R.,** Glossodynia: a study of idiopathic orolingual pain, *J. Am. Dent. Assoc.*, 33, 1423, 1946.
80. **Kutscher, A. H., Silvers, H. F., Stein, G., Ziskin, D. E., and Karshan, M.,** Therapy of idiopathic orolingual paresthesias, *N. Y. State J. Med.*, 52, 1401, 1952.
81. **Kutscher, A. H., Schoenberg, B., and Carr, A. C.,** Death, grief, and the dental practitioner: thanatology as related to dentistry, *J. Am. Dent. Assoc.*, 81, 1373, 1970.
82. **Schoenberg, B., Carr, A. C., Kutscher, A. H., and Zegarelli, E. V.,** Chronic idiopathic orolingual pain, *N. Y. State J. Med.*, 71, 1832, 1971.
83. **Zucker, A. H.,** A psychiatric appraisal of tongue symptoms, *J. Am. Dent. Assoc.*, 85, 649, 1972.
84. **Harris, M.,** Psychogenic aspects of facial pain, *Br. Dent. J.*, 136, 199, 1974.
85. **Brooke, R. I. and Seganski, D. P.,** Aetiology and investigation of the sore mouth, *J. Can. Dent. Assoc.*, 10, 504, 1977.
86. **Lowenthal, U. and Pisanti, S.,** The syndrome of oral complaints: etiology and therapy, *Oral Surg. Oral Med. Oral Pathol.*, 46, 2, 1978.
87. **Turk, D. C. and Rudy, T. E.,** Neglected factors in chronic pain treatment outcome studies — referral patterns, failure to enter treatment, and attrition, *Pain*, 43, 7, 1990.
88. **Dworkin, R. H., Richlin, D. M., Handlin, D. S., and Brand, L.,** Predicting treatment response in depressed and non-depressed chronic pain patients, *Pain*, 24, 343, 1986.
89. **Yontchev, E., Hedård, B., and Carlsson, G. E.,** Outcome of treatment of patients with orofacial discomfort complaints, *Int. J. Oral Maxillofacial Surg.*, 16, 312, 1987.
90. **Agerberg, G.,** Signs and symptoms of mandibular dysfunction in patients with suspected oral galvanism, *Acta Odontol. Scand.*, 45, 41, 1987.
91. **Hampf, G., Ekholm, A., Salo, T., Ylipaavalniemi, P., Aalberg V., Tuominen, S., and Alfthan, G.,** Pain in oral galvanism, *Pain*, 29, 301, 1987.
92. **Hugoson, A.,** Results obtained from patients referred for the investigation of complaints related to oral galvanism, *Swed. Dent. J.*, 10, 15, 1986.
93. **Haraldson, T.,** Oral galvanism and mandibular dysfunction, *Swed. Dent. J.*, 9, 129, 1985.
94. **Yontchev, E. and Emilson, C.-G.,** Salivary and microbial conditions in patients with orofacial discomfort complaints, *Acta Odontol. Scand.*, 44, 215, 1986.
95. **Yontchev, E., Meding, B., and Hedegård, B.,** Contact allergy to dental materials in patients with orofacial complaints, *J. Oral Rehabil.*, 13, 183, 1986.
96. **Yontchev, E., Carlsson, G. E., and Hedegård, B.,** Clinical findings in patients with orofacial discomfort complaints, *Int. J. Oral Maxillofacial Surg.*, 16, 36, 1987.

97. Participants of CSP Nos. 147/242 and Morris, H. F., Veterans Administration cooperative studies project no. 147: association of metallic taste with metal ceramic alloys, *J. Prosthet. Dent.*, 63, 124, 1990.
98. **Pillemer, F. G., Masek, B. J., and Kaban, L. B.,** Temporo-mandibular joint dysfunction and facial pain in children: an approach to diagnosis and treatment, *Pediatrics*, 80, 565, 1987.
99. **Gessel, A. H.,** Electromyographic biofeedback and tricyclic antidepressants in myofascial pain-dysfunction syndrome: psychological predictors of outcome, *J. Am. Dent. Assoc.*, 91, 1048, 1975.
100. **Dahlström, L. and Carlsson, S. G.,** Treatment of mandibular dysfunction: the clinical usefulness of biofeedback in relation to splint therapy, *J. Oral Rehabil.*, 11, 277, 1984.
101. **Hudzinski, L. G. and Walters, P. J.,** Use of a portable electromyogram integrator and biofeedback unit in the treatment of chronic nocturnal bruxism, *J. Prosthet. Dent.*, 58, 698, 1987.
102. **Grzesiak, R. C.,** Strategies for multidisciplinary pain management, *Compendium of Continuing Education in Dentistry*, 10, 444, 1989.
103. **Stauffer, J. D.,** Antidepressants and chronic pain, *Journal of Family Practice*, 25, 167, 1987.
104. **France, R. D.,** The future for antidepressants: treatment of pain, *Psychopathology*, 20 (Supplement 1), 99, 1987.
105. **Kreisberg, M. K.,** Tricyclic antidepressants: analgesic effect and indications in orofacial pain, *Journal of Cranio-mandibular Disorders*, 2, 171, 1988.
106. **Hersh, E. V.,** Tricyclic antidepressant drugs: pharmacologic implications in the treatment of chronic orofacial pain, *Compendium Continuing Educ. Dent.*, 8, 688, 1987.

Chapter 7

THE ELDERLY DENTAL PATIENT

Increasing interest and effort have been devoted in the last decade to exploring and understanding the unique problems of the elderly dental patient. This growing population poses special challenges to the dental practitioner from technical, physiological, social, and behavioral aspects.

The elderly patient undergoes physiological changes which are part of normal aging. The effect of aging on dental conditions, such as coronal caries, root caries, tooth loss, attrition, abrasion, erosion, periodontal disease, oral mucosa, salivary glands, and oral cancer have been widely reviewed in the literature[1-9] and will not be discussed here.

The present chapter summarizes some of the psychological and social factors which affect the elderly dental patient. For more extensive discussions on this subject, the reader is referred to the comprehensive work by Kiyak and associates.[4,10-18]

I. DEMOGRAPHIC CONSIDERATIONS

Enormous changes, occurring during the last decades in western industrialized communities, have resulted in increased standards of living and increased life expectancy. People live longer, stay active longer, and expect to enjoy life longer. It is not surprising that an increasing number of dentists are concerned with the future dental needs of this population.[19,20]

The increase in life expectancy, together with a decline in birth rates, results in changes in population proportions in favor of the elderly. For example, in 1980, the number of Americans over the age of 60 was found to be higher than the number of children under the age of 10.[21]

It is not only the absolute numbers of older people which are increasing, it is also their relative age. More and more people reach ages over 75. The oldest group, 85 and older, is projected to increase by 110% from 1982 to 2000. Thus, by the year 2000, we may expect to see not only more elderly patients, but proportionally more of the oldest segment of the elderly population.[3]

Today, elderly patients are retaining more and more of their natural dentition. The percentage of edentulism among 65 to 74 year olds decreased from 55.4% to 33.8% between the years 1957 and 1980, and will probably continue to decline despite the aging of the population.[2]

In 1982, Ettinger and Beck[22] attempted to define the social and cultural differences between the "old elderly" (at the time of the study being 75 years and older), and the "new elderly" (then, between 60 and 64 years old). The old elderly grew up during the early part of the century, when dentistry was still perceived as a luxury. The "focal infection" theory, popular at the time, resulted in a high rate of extractions. Local anesthesia was not yet well developed, a fact which often led to unavoided pain and stress. Negative attitudes toward teeth and dentistry were popular and led to avoidance of treatment and early edentulism.

The new elderly had a different dental experience.[22] They benefitted from the technological advancement in dental treatment which came before many of them were rendered edentulous. This group is defined as healthier, better educated, more politically aware, more demanding of social services, having greater economic security and having more natural teeth. Although possible diversity still exists among this population with regard to former dental experiences, values concerning their natural dentition, and treatment expectations, the future elderly dental patient will probably show an increase in the demand for dental care.

II. NEED AND UTILIZATION OF DENTAL SERVICES

There is almost no dispute in the literature that the elderly are in need of significant dental care. Numerous reports relate to the poor oral health of this population.[23-37] The relatively high prevalence of periodontal problems, oral cancer, root caries, and tooth loss as compared to younger populations[1-3,6,8] points to the existence of a real need.

The orofacial area is crucial to survival and to the patient's well-being. It plays a significant role in the acquisition of the important needs of love and belonging, communication, and esteem throughout our life, including old age. Oral impairment can be a symbol of final social exclusion of the elderly and, as such, may carry deep emotional significance.

Therefore, it is striking to find that only low percentages of the elderly receive any professional dental care. Professional evaluations suggest that while about 70% of older adults require dental treatment, only 25 to 40% perceive this need, and only 20 to 35% seek care.[10,14,34,38-40] In spite of the fact that the elderly usually use medical care to a much higher extent than younger populations, they show the lowest utilization rates for dental services (with the possible exception of children under the age of 6).[10,14]

Several reviews[4,10,15,16,18,41,42] address the issue of utilization of dental care by the elderly and raise several points.

A. FINANCIAL COSTS

Dental care involves substantial financial costs which are a burden on many users. This may be a major problem, especially among the elderly, since their financial resources are often significantly lower than the rest of the population. Therefore, financial costs have been mentioned as the main barrier to the use of dental care by the elderly.[43,44] For example, Bomberg and Ernst[45] found that 30% of elderly respondents felt that dental care was too expensive for them.

Kiyak,[4,10,15,16,18] however, reported several studies in which the availability of insurance, allowing free or reduced-cost services, increased utilization only slightly. Although in some studies the presence of insurance did increase utilization, the elderly still had the lowest use rates of any age group.

Tobias and Smith[40] found that while 75% of elderly residents of local authority sheltered housing did show a normal need for treatment, only 1% claimed that dental charges were too high. Similar results were also reported by MacEntee et al.[46]

In spite of these findings, financial costs probably play some role in the use of dental services by the elderly. A study conducted in England[47] suggested that the incidence of patient charges imposes a significant disincentive to use dental care. In the study, elderly attenders who were not exempt from charges were compared to exempt patients. The former were found four times more likely to receive emergency care only, 340 times more likely to receive only an examination, and, when receiving treatment, to receive 40% less treatment than exempt patients.

B. PERCEIVED NEED

The variable of perceived need plays an important role in the use of dental services by the elderly. The elderly respondents often rate oral health among their least important health concerns.[43]

A survey conducted by the American Dental Association in 1978[48] showed that nearly half of the respondents over the age of 60 had not sought dental care in more than 3 years. Only 12% of this group blamed the costs involved as a reason for the situation, while approximately 80% indicated that they felt no need.

The low perceived need of dental care emerges from numerous studies carried out among different communities of elderly. In studies conducted on elderly residents of a sheltered accommodation in West Essex, only 22% perceived a need for dental treatment despite high normative need (78%).[39,40] Among a representative sample of nonedentulous Canadian adults (65 years and over), only 58% perceived the need for dental treatment, although actual need reached 96%. The survey found that the mean delay since the last use of dental services among this population was 10 years. Of those surveyed, 73% had not been to the dentist in the past 5 years and gave "no need" as their main reason. Significant gaps between normative and perceived need of dental care among the elderly have also been shown by others.[33,34,36,46]

In a study by Kiyak,[14] 116 elderly users of low-cost dental services in the Seattle/King County area and 142 nonusers of similar socioeconomic status were interviewed. Among the nonusers, only 13% mentioned concerns with costs, while 71% felt no need for care.

The cost of dental services is not usually cited as a barrier even by respondents in the lowest income groups.[4] Although variables such as education or occupation may differentiate between regular and infrequent users of dental services, these factors do not necessarily imply a greater availability of financial resources but represent a greater awareness of and concern with oral health.

C. PATIENT ATTITUDES

Attitudes toward oral health and dental care are important in the use of dental services of all ages. Most research regarding attitudes of the elderly toward dental care was conducted on the generation defined by Ettinger and Beck[22] as the "old elderly". Among this group, misconceptions about dental care are very common, such as the belief that teeth are lost as a natural consequence of aging and that at advanced age the teeth are no longer worth saving.[49]

Aged respondents generally hold significantly more negative attitudes toward oral health and attribute less importance to dental care than young people.[50] They realize that dental care is needed, but it is not a top priority relative to their other needs. For example, among healthy elderly subjects, oral health was not included in a personal listing of health issues, and dental health was ranked among the least important items within a prepared alphabetized list of oral concerns.[43] In another study concerning the elderly, 14% of the participants felt that oral health was not important.[45]

The elderly tend to view illness and pain as an unavoidable consequence of aging. While this attitude acts, in some cases, as a basis for healthy coping in everyday life, it can also be a barrier to seeking routine medical and dental care.[18] Manne and Mehra[51] provided indirect support for this possibility. Their data showed a negative relation between satisfaction with dentures among geriatric patients and their technical accuracy: dissatisfied respondents had technically superior dentures compared to satisfied respondents. They suggested that dissatisfaction (a possible sign of perceived need of treatment) may benefit the patient's oral health.

At present, the elderly population is gradually transforming to the "new elderly" as described by Ettinger and Beck in 1982.[22] Unlike the former generation of elderly, the new elderly are more likely to disagree with statements, such as "problems with my teeth and gums do not affect my lifestyle," "it does not make sense to visit the dentist for regular examinations since they can fix problems as they occur," or "the money spent on dental care could be better used on other essentials (or on extras)." The new elderly are significantly different in attitude and utilization behavior from the old elderly. Although they still have a less positive attitude toward dentistry than a younger group (ages 18 to 60 at the time of the study), many of their attitudes are similar.[22] Therefore, a gradual change may be expected in the elderly patient's attitudes toward treatment, which will hopefully increase his/her perceived needs and use of dental care.

Indeed, a more recent study[40] showed that in spite of the low perceived need of treatment (28%), a relatively high pecentage of elderly (77%) believed that "appearance of their teeth" was very important to them. The positive attitudes of the elderly to dental health are a good indication of the use of dental services.

D. ATTITUDES OF CARE PROVIDERS

What are the attitudes of care providers toward elderly patients? Are they different than those toward younger patients? Do attitudes affect the dentist's behavior and, as a result, the nature and quality of treatment provided? The treatment of elderly patients embraces many popular myths. One such myth among dentists is that the elderly are too delicate to withstand certain procedures and that they may become exhausted even during routine appointments.[49]

Several studies showed a mixed tendency for neutral or negative attitudes toward the elderly patient among dental students.[52,53] For example, English dental students generally viewed people 65 and over as more ineffective, less autonomous, and less personally acceptable than did U.S. students.[52]

Although dentists usually perceive the elderly patient's behavior as positive, many indicate that the elderly are the least satisfying group to treat[54] and show inaccurate perceptions concerning this population.[13]

When 332 Washington State dentists were surveyed to explore the nature and extent of their contact with elderly patients and their attitudes toward the aged, more than 50% showed inaccurate perceptions.[13] For example, between 65 and 85% of the dentists agreed with incorrect statements, such as "health status shows a sharp decline upon retirement," "people are likely to become lonely and isolated as they grow older," or "most people eventually become a financial burden to their children."

Regardless of these misconceptions, the same group of dentists expressed fairly favorable feelings toward the elderly. Positive scores were generally given for friendliness, generosity, cooperativeness, and pleasantness. The least positive was flexibility.

The most negative stereotypes were quoted by dentists with the greatest and lowest proportion of elderly in their practices. Dentists with 25 to 50% of their practice comprising elderly patients were most favorable toward this group. In addition, dentists whose elderly patients paid for treatments themselves or with private insurance held fewer stereotypes and more favorable views of the elderly.

Kiyak et al.[13] concluded that the tendency to stereotype increases if dentists have had little practice, experience, and/or familiarity with elderly patients on public assistance. Although attitudes are not necessarily predictive of behavior, the patient's ability to pay for treatment may be a better predictor of the behavior of the dentists than the patient's age.[12,15]

The kind of practice also affects dentists' attitudes toward elderly patients.

In England, dentists in large dental practices (three or more) showed fewer misconceptions about the elderly than those in small practices.[55] The larger practices were found to be more accessible to the elderly and disabled. Thus, it is possible that increased contact with the elderly contributed to a more favorable view of this population by the dentist.

Misconceptions about the necessity of dental care for the elderly are also found among other care providers. For example, among directors of private old-age homes in Finland, only one fifth of the respondents considered dental care more necessary than the other facilities (i.e., hairdressing and pedicure) which are usually available in institutions. Five respondents considered dental treatment as less necessary than other facilities.[56]

E. SOCIAL NETWORK

The utilization of dental care by the elderly has been found to be affected by various aspects of the social network. Rickardsson and Hanson[57] developed a model that includes the parameters of social networks, social support, and social influence. According to this model, social networks are defined by three different criteria: social anchorage (to what degree the individual belongs, or feels that he/she belongs, to formal and informal groups in the social network), contact frequency (how often the individual meets with his/her family, neighbors, etc.), and social participation (how actively he/she is involved in activities of formal and informal groups).

Social support is regarded as a function of the individual's interactions with his social networks and is classified under emotional support (reflecting the individual's opportunity for care, encouragement of personal value, and feeling of confidence and trust). Informational support relates to the individual's access to guidance, advice, and information. Material support reflects the individual's access to practical services and material resources. Social influence describes to what extent the individual is able to control and manipulate his environment, using his own resources and the resources to which he/she is given access through his social network and support.

In their research with a representative sample of 68-year-old men (n = 621) in the city of Malmo, Sweden, Rickardsson and Hanson[57] found that well-developed social networks and social support were associated with regular care. Social class, social anchorage, and social participation were independently associated with regular dental care, while inadequate social network and social support were associated with negative health behavior and health problems.

Social anchorage and social participation, together with social support and social influence, are resources that enable a person to cope with stressful situations (major and minor) in daily life. The authors concluded that these resources facilitate preventive health actions, including regular dental services. As such, social networks and social support are important determinants of regular dental care.

III. PSYCHIATRIC FACTORS AFFECTING DENTAL CARE

Getting old also means having to deal with changes occurring in the sensory-perceptual, psychomotor, and cognitive areas. Some changes are due to normal aging, while others are caused by secondary processes (disease, environmental conditions).[17,18] In each instance, the changes affect the patient as well as his/her dentist, who must be aware of the special requirements of this population.

Depression, dementia, paranoia, and anxiety are the main psychiatric problems affecting dental care of the elderly.[50,58,59] Although psychiatric illnesses are not inherent to normal aging, the aging process brings an increased risk of such illnesses. For example, a progressive reduction in cerebrocortical neurons diminishes physiological reserves and enhances vulnerability to insult.[58] Additionally, the elderly use more drugs which are often associated with confusion.[59]

The estimated rate of depression in the general population is between 10 and 15%, dementia — 5%, and schizophrenia-like conditions — 1 to 2%. Rates increase as high as 20% when dementia is assessed among those at age 80, and 10% when schizophrenia is assessed among those over the age of 60 who have been admitted to psychiatric hospitals.[50]

Dementia is a nonspecific clinical syndrome characterized by a global deterioration of intellect, cognition, behavior, and emotions. It can be caused by reversible conditions, such as nutritional deficiencies, tumors, general health decline, depression, and use of drugs and alcohol. It can also be the irreversible outcome of syndromes (e.g., Alzheimer's disease) relatively prevalent among the elderly.[50,59] When present, such conditions significantly affect access to dental treatment. In a study conducted on an institutionalized elderly Finnish population, cardiovascular diseases and neurological and mental disorders were found to reduce dental treatability more than other disorders.[60]

Although some believe that the dentist has no responsibility for the primary psychiatric care of the acutely mentally ill elderly patient,[58] others emphasize the importance in recognizing the most frequent conditions and point out that in many cases the elderly patient with cognitive and affective disorders can and should be treated in the dental office.[59]

IV. ORAL PHYSICAL SENSES

The oral cavity is involved in two major sensory systems: taste and olfaction. As in other senses, the capacity to taste and smell is commonly believed to decline with age. Complaints in this respect are often mentioned by the patient to the dentist. Anecdotal, clinical, and basic research reports suggest that some changes do occur with regard to the sensory ability of the elderly.

Decremental changes in taste sensitivity were found to be significantly associated with aging, although the age-related changes were not uniform for all taste qualities, taste performances, or populations of elderly individuals.[61-63] In one study, for example, changes were observed in threshold sensitivity for salt and quinine.[64] In another study, elderly subjects found the characteristic tastes of caffeine and citric acid less intense than did younger subjects, while no differences were observed with regard to the tastes of sucrose and salt.[65]

Complaints concerning taste weakening can be due to impairment of taste function, but it can also result from changes only casually associated with aging. Distortions in remembered experiences from the past and the use of various medications can influence the subjective experience of taste.[61] Furthermore, the elderly are more likely to use medications with potential effects on taste. For example, changes in the taste system with age may be related to nutrient intake (vitamins A, thiamine, B-6, B-12, folacin, zinc and copper)[66] or to drugs with potential xerostomic effects used by more than 50% of the elderly population.[67]

Also affecting the experience of taste is the gradual olfactory loss with age.[62,63,68] The elderly have higher olfactory thresholds, perceive suprathreshold odors as being weaker, and do not recognize and identify common odors.[69,70] They are also more prone to olfactory adaptation and are slower to recover threshold sensitivity.[71]

As with all physical senses, taste and smell are also affected by the cognitive and emotional context of the applied stimulus. This may possibly explain some of the differences in taste detection threshold between institutionalized and noninstitutionalized elderly.[72] Similarly, noninsitutionalized elderly showed relatively low rates of complaints regarding the pleasures of food and drink when compared to the institutionalized.[70] These changes, however, may originate from the different health status of the two populations.

Another point of consideration is the increasing evidence of an association between several pathologies that cause cognitive impairment (such as schizophrenia, Alzheimer's disease, and Parkinson's disease) and impairment of olfactory.[73-82] As these diseases are more common among the elderly, the increased incidence of cognitive impairment in old age may increase the incidence of olfactory impairment. Some researchers hypothesize that the olfactory tracts might provide a portal of entry to the brain for any putative pathogenic agent(s) that might be responsible for the induction of the cognitive impairment.[73,74,76]

V. PAIN

Misconceptions and myths are very common regarding the experience of pain in the elderly. While the elderly are "known" to be frequent sufferers and complainers of chronic pain, many believe that their sensitivity to acute pain decreases with age. Whether such beliefs are true or not, changes occurring in the sensory, emotional, cognitive, and behavioral systems may influence pain perception and expression in old age.[83]

A. ACUTE PAIN

Many studies have attempted to determine whether the perception of acute pain stimuli changes with age.[83-85]

Chapman[85] found it difficult to draw conclusions from the collected data for several reasons: different methods of stimulation were used, cultural differences exist between the young and old, and responses could be biased due to the exaggerated cautiousness of the elderly during laboratory tasks.

Harkins et al.[84] summarized that pain threshold is probably unaffected by advanced age and that the stereotype that the elderly feel less pain should be discarded. The diversity in results may be due to the different types of painful stimuli used in the different test settings.

With regards to dental pain, LeResche and Dworkin[83] concluded that pain perception is unaffected by age because age-related changes occur in cutaneous peripheral receptors but not in tooth pulp. In spite of the general notion that physiological changes occurring with age in the dentin-pulp complex make the tooth less sensitive to acute pain stimuli, changes in acute dental pain threshold using electrical tooth pulp stimulation were not demonstrated across different age groups.[86-88]

Harkins and Chapman[86,87] showed that age does not influence sensation thresholds for the perception of electrical tooth pulp stimulation either in men or in women. However, significant age differences were observed in the ability of subjects to discriminate among noxious stimuli of two different intensities. The elderly were less accurate than the young subjects in discriminating between two suprathreshold electrical dental shocks, even though equivalent thresholds were obtained between age groups. The authors concluded that the elderly have a central nervous deficit for discrimination between noxious stimuli which is not confounded by age-related, peripheral sensory changes in apparently healthy teeth. They also reported that at lower levels of perceived stimulus intensity, the elderly subjects were less willing to report the sensation as pain. However, at the upper end of the response continuum, they were more willing to report stimuli as painful than the younger subjects. It is possible that changes in pain perception with age are complex and may include interaction between response bias, subjective estimation of intensity, and age.

If the elderly are really less willing to report low intensity stimuli as painful, a possible alternative to convey the feelings of pain to the dentist may be through the nonverbal channel of facial expression. However, physical changes in the face that occur with age (wrinkling of skin, loss of subcutaneous fat, loss of elastic fibers, loss of hair, etc.), as well as psychiatric disorders which are more prevalent in the elderly, can influence the facial expression of pain by the elderly.[89] The failure of the dentist to decode (and relate to) such signs can lead to anxiety and frustration on the part of the patient.

B. CHRONIC PAIN

Chronic pain is often associated with old age. Many elderly patients suffer from degenerative neurological, vascular, and musculoskeletal changes that can produce persisting pain.[85] However, the common preconception that pain is a natural and inevitable part of the aging process may mislead the clinician to underdiagnose disease states that are causing the pain.[83]

Osteoarthritis, temporal arthritis, tic douloureux, back pain, posttherapeutic neuralgia, and certain types of abdominal pain are often encountered in aged patients.[90] Furthermore, many conditions of benign chronic orofacial pain (e.g., atypical odontalgia, glossodynia) are most prevalent among the older age groups (see Chapter 6).

Several factors, especially relevant to the aged, affect the diagnosis and treatment of chronic pain.

1. Depression

Depression is a common problem among the elderly. Economic pressures, hopelessness about the future, loss of loved ones, and poor health can all initiate depression.[83,85] When present, depression influences conditions of chronic pain and vice versa. The high rate of depression among people over the age of 65[50] indicates that it has to be taken into consideration (as a reason and/or outcome) when dealing with chronic pain in the elderly.

2. Cognitive Impairment

More people are prone to suffer from dementia with increasing age.[50] When cognitive impairment occurs, the individual becomes bewildered and confused by the loss of memory, attention span, and mental abilities. If this happens in conjunction with injury or disease, pain complaints may be used to express (or to hide) the increasing psychological disability.[84,85]

3. Personality

Although basic personality patterns continue throughout life, some personality disorders may come with aging. As the older person turns inward and withdraws from outward concerns, there may be a preoccupation with bodily functions. Obsessive-compulsive, dependent, and narcissistic traits are accentuated and influence the presentation of a pain syndrome.[84]

4. Use of Medications

Most of the elderly use prescription drugs. The majority (80 to 90%) use at least one drug regularly, and in many cases, up to five or six.[10] This group of patients is often over-medicated, either because their systems clear drugs more slowly, or because too many drugs have been prescribed.[85] Additional medication for treatment of chronic pain may be ineffective or inadvisable. All medications used by the patient have to be considered.

VI. PREVENTIVE CARE

Concurrently with the presumption that tooth loss and periodontal disease are the natural concomitants of aging, preventive care is often neglected. Today, there is no doubt that older people, whether institutionalized or living independently in the community, can learn techniques which would improve oral hygiene, prevent further disease, and have an impact on their psychological well-being.[4,15,91,92]

Kiyak[4,15] summarized several principles especially relevant in the administration of effective preventive oral care to the elderly:

1. Since learning and recall occur more slowly as one gets older, any information presented must be repeated several times and reinforced both visually and orally.
2. Because of changing learning styles with aging, active learning techniques are particularly suited for the elderly, with special emphasis on a self-monitoring approach. A self-monitoring checklist is kept by the patient to record his/her behavior between sessions and allows the participant to become more involved in the change program.
3. Because of sensory changes with aging, written material must be presented in large-format print with contrasting figure-ground relations.
4. Because fatigue occurs more rapidly, frequent and brief sessions are far superior to a few long sessions.
5. Motivation can be significantly enhanced with regular feedback to participants regarding their success in achieving predetermined oral health goals. Verbal reinforcements were found effective in this respect in a community setting and with depressed elderly in nursing homes.[91,93]

VII. SUMMARY

The proportion of elderly dental patients is constantly increasing among the general population, which calls for devoting more attention to the special needs of this group. In spite of a high objective need of treatment, the use of dental services by the elderly is mainly affected by their low perception of need for dental care and general attitudes toward dental care as "luxurious" and nonessential. Other variables include the tendency for negative attitudes from care providers, as well as financial costs of treatment.

While providing dental care to the elderly, the dentist has to consider the specific psychiatric and physiological problems of these patients. With increasing age, a gradual increase occurs in the prevalence of various disorders, such as dementia, depression, and chronic pain conditions, which may affect the dental care of the aged patients.

REFERENCES

1. **Beck, J. D.,** The epidemiology of dental diseases in the elderly, *Gerodontology*, 3, 5, 1984.
2. **Weintraub, J. A. and Burt, B. A.,** Oral health status in the United States: tooth loss and edentulism, *J. Dent. Educ.*, 49, 368, 1985.
3. **Beck, J. D. and Hunt, R. J.,** Oral health status in the United States: problems of special patients, *J. Dent. Educ.*, 49, 407, 1985.
4. **Kiyak, H. A.,** Management of oral problems in the elderly, *Ann. Rev. Gerontol. Geriatr.*, 4, 106, 1984.
5. **Baum, B. J.,** Research on aging and oral health: an assessment of current status and future needs, *Spec. Care Dent.*, 1, 156, 1981.
6. **Beck, J., Cons, N., Field, H., and Walker, J.,** The Iowa Survey of Oral Health: 1980, University of Iowa College of Dentistry and Iowa Dental Association, Iowa City, 1982.
7. **Page, R. C.,** Periodontal diseases in the elderly: a critical evaluation of current information, *Gerodontology*, 3, 63, 1984.
8. **Banting, D. W.,** Dental caries in the elderly, *Gerodontology*, 3, 55, 1984.
9. **Baum, B. J.,** Salivary gland function during aging, *Gerodontics*, 2, 61, 1986. .
10. **Kiyak, H. A.,** Utilization of dental services by the elderly, *Gerodontology*, 3, 17, 1984.
11. **Kahana, E. F. and Kiyak, H. A.,** Attitudes and behavior of staff in facilities for the aged, *Res. Aging*, 6, 395, 1984.
12. **Kiyak, H. A.,** Impact of patients' and dentists' attitudes on older persons' use of dental services, *Gerodontics*, 4, 331, 1988.
13. **Kiyak, H. A., Milgrom, P., Ratener, P., and Conrad, D.,** Dentists' attitudes toward and knowledge of the elderly, *J. Dent. Educ.*, 46, 266, 1982.
14. **Kiyak, H. A.,** An explanatory model of older persons' use of dental services: implications for health policy, *Med. Care*, 25, 936, 1987.
15. **Kiyak, H. A.,** Recent advances in behavioral research in geriatric dentistry, *Gerodontology*, 7, 27, 1988.
16. **Kiyak, H. A.,** Psychosocial factors in dental needs of the elderly, *Spec. Care Dent.*, 1, 22, 1981.
17. **Kiyak, A. and Bennett, J.,** Special problems of the geriatric patient, in *Behavioral Aspects In Dentistry*, Ingersoll, B., Ed., Appleton-Century Crofts, New York, 1982, 135.
18. **Kiyak, H. A.,** Psychological and social factors in the dental care of the elderly, *Int. Dent. J.*, 33, 281, 1983.
19. **Drummond, J. R., Newton, J. P., and Yemm, R.,** Dentistry for the elderly: a review and an assessment of the future, *J. Dent.*, 16, 47, 1988.
20. **Gordon, S. R.,** Older adults: demographics and need for quality care, *J. Prosthet. Dent.*, 61, 737, 1989.
21. Community Action Stirs Senior Potential, US Department of Health and Human Services, Administration on Aging, *Aging*, 307, 10, 1980.
22. **Ettinger, R. L. and Beck, J. D.,** The new elderly: what can the dental profession expect?, *Spec. Care Dent.*, 2, 62, 1982.
23. **Grabowski, M. and Bertram, U.,** Oral health status and need of dental treatment in the elderly Danish population, *Comm. Dent. Oral Epidemiol.*, 3, 108, 1975.
24. **Smith, J. M. and Sheiham, A.,** How dental conditions handicap the elderly, *Comm. Dent. Oral Epidemiol.*, 7, 305, 1979.
25. **Banting, D. W.,** A study of dental care cost, time and treatment requirements of older persons in the community, *Can. J. Public Health*, 63, 508, 1972.
26. **Manderson, R. D. and Ettinger, R. L.,** Dental status of the institutionalized elderly population of Edinburgh, *Comm. Dent. Oral Epidemiol.*, 3, 100, 1975.
27. **Osborne, J., Maddick, I., Gould, A., and Ward, D.,** Dental demands of old people in Hampshire, *Br. Dent. J.*, 146, 351, 1979.

28. **Rise, J. and Heloe, L. A.,** Oral conditions and need for dental treatment in an elderly population in Northern Norway, *Comm. Dent. Oral Epidemiol.*, 6, 6, 1978.
29. **Ritchie, G. M.,** A report of dental findings in a survey of geriatric patients, *J. Dent.*, 1, 106, 1973.
30. **Ekelund, R.,** Oral mucosal disorders in institutionalized elderly people, *Age Ageing*, 17, 193, 1988.
31. **Stockwell, A. J.,** Survey of the oral health needs of institutionalised elderly patients in Western Australia, *Comm. Dent. Oral Epidemiol.*, 15, 273, 1987.
32. **Ekelund, R.,** Dental state and subjective chewing ability of institutionalized elderly people, *Comm. Dent. Oral Epidemiol.*, 17, 24, 1989.
33. **Schou, L., Wight, C., Clemson, N., Douglas, S., and Clark, C.,** Oral health promotion for institutionalised elderly, *Comm. Dent. Oral Epidemiol.*, 17, 2, 1989.
34. **Hoad-Reddick, G., Grant, A. A., and Griffiths, C. S.,** The dental health of an elderly population in North-west England: results of a survey undertaken in the Halton Health Authority, *J. Dent.*, 15, 139, 1987.
35. **MacEntee, M. I. and Scully, C.,** Oral disorders and treatment implications in people over 75 years, *Comm. Dent. Oral Epidemiol.*, 16, 271, 1988.
36. **Diu, S. and Gelbier, S.,** Oral health screening of elderly people attending a Community Care Centre, *Comm. Dent. Oral Epidemiol.*, 17, 212, 1989.
37. **Vigild, M.,** Dental caries and the need for treatment among institutionalized elderly, *Comm. Dent. Oral Epidemiol.*, 17, 102, 1989.
38. **Branch, L. G., Antczak, A. A., and Stason, W. B.,** Toward understanding the use of dental services by the elderly, *Spec. Care Dent.*, 6, 38, 1986.
39. **Tobias, B.,** Dental aspects of an elderly population, *Age Ageing*, 17, 103, 1988.
40. **Tobias, B. and Smith, J. M.,** Barriers to dental care, and associated oral status and treatment needs, in an elderly population living in sheltered accommodation in West Essex, *Br. Dent. J.*, 163, 293, 1987.
41. **Krout, J. A.,** Knowledge and use of services by the elderly: A critical review of the literature, *Int. J. Aging Hum. Dev.*, 17, 153, 1983.
42. **Gooch, B. F. and Berkey, D. B.,** Subjective factors affecting the utilization of dental services by the elderly, *Gerodontics*, 3, 65, 1987.
43. **Marinelli, R. D., Sreebny, L. M., and Kamen, S.,** Perception of dental needs by the well elderly, *Spec. Care Dent.*, 2, 161, 1982.
44. **Warren, K. L.,** Increasing access to dental care for the older patient: a special challenge, *Spec. Care Dent.*, 2, 248, 1982.
45. **Bomberg, T. J. and Ernst, N. S.,** Improving utilization of dental care services by the elderly, *Gerodontics*, 2, 57, 1986.
46. **MacEntee, M. I., Dowell, T. B., and Scully, C.,** Oral health concerns of an elderly population in England, *Comm. Dent. Oral Epidemiol.*, 16, 72, 1988.
47. **Birch, S.,** Hypothesis: charges to patients impair the quality of dental care for elderly people, *Age Ageing*, 18, 136, 1989.
48. American Dental Association, *Family Dental Survey*, American Dental Association Publications, Chicago, 1978.
49. **Evans, R. W.,** The aging dental patient: myth and reality, *Gerodontology*, 3, 271, 1984.
50. **Kiyak, H. A. and Miller, R. R.,** Age differences in oral health attitudes and dental service utilization, *J. Public Health Dent.*, 42, 29, 1982.
51. **Manne, S. and Mehra, R.,** Accuracy of perceived treatment needs among geriatric denture wearers, *Gerodontology*, 2, 67, 1983.
52. **Sheiham, A., Ettinger, R. L., and Beck, J. D.,** English dental students' attitudes toward the aged, *Gerodontics*, 2, 142, 1986.
53. **Steele, L. P.,** Dental students' attitudes and knowledge about elderly people, *Gerodontics*, 3, 61, 1987.

54. **Strayer, M. S., DiAngelis, A. J., and Loupe, M. J.,** Dentists' knowledge of aging in relation to perceived elderly patient behavior, *Gerodontics*, 2, 223, 1986.
55. **Hamilton, F. A., Sarll, D. W., Grant, A. A., and Worthington, H. V.,** Dental care for elderly people by general dental practitioners, *Br. Dent. J.*, 168, 108, 1990.
56. **Ekelund, R.,** National survey of oral health care in Finnish private old people's homes, *Comm. Dent. Oral Epidemiol.*, 17, 158, 1989.
57. **Rickardsson, B. and Hanson, B. S.,** Social network and regular dental care utilisation in elderly men: results from the population study "Men born in 1914", Malmo, Sweden, *Swed. Dent. J.*, 13, 151, 1989.
58. **Levenson, A. J.,** Psychiatric implications in the treatment of the geriatric dental patient, *Spec. Care Dent.*, 3, 4, 1983.
59. **Kiyak, H. A.,** The dentist's role, *Spec. Care Dent.*, 3, 8, 1983.
60. **Ekelund, R.,** General diseases and dental treatability of the institutionalized elderly Finnish population, *Comm. Dent. Oral Epidemiol.*, 16, 159, 1988.
61. **Weiffenbach, J. M.,** Taste changes with aging, *Int. J. Tech. Aging*, 1, 136, 1988.
62. **Weiffenbach, J. M.,** Taste perception mechanisms, *Front. Oral Physiol.*, 6, 151, 1987.
63. **Weiffenbach, J. M.,** Taste and smell perception in aging, *Gerodontology*, 3, 137, 1984.
64. **Weiffenbach, J. M., Baum, B. J., and Burghauser, R.,** Taste thresholds: quality specific variation with human aging, *J. Gerontol.*, 37, 372, 1982.
65. **Murphy, C. and Gilmore, M. M.,** Quality-specific effects of aging on the human taste system, *Percept. Psychophys.*, 45, 121, 1989.
66. **Chauhan, J., Hawrysh, Z. J., Gee, M., Donald, E. A., and Basu, T. K.,** Age-related olfactory and taste changes and inter-relationships between taste and nutrition, *J. Am. Diet Assoc.*, 87, 1543, 1987.
67. **Levy, S. M., Baker, K. A., Semal, T. P., and Kohout, F. J.,** Use of medications with dental significance by a noninstitutionalized elderly population, *Gerodontics*, 4, 119, 1988.
68. **Tylenda, C. A. and Baum, B. J.,** Oral physiology and the Baltimore longitudinal study of aging, *Gerodontology*, 7, 5, 1988.
69. **Cain, W. S. and Stevens, J. C.,** Uniformity of olfactory loss in aging, *Ann. N. Y. Acad. Sci.*, 561, 29, 1989.
70. **Stevens, J. C.,** Food quality reports from noninstitutionalized aged, *Ann. N. Y. Acad. Sci.*, 561, 87, 1989.
71. **Stevens, J. C., Cain, W. S., Schiet, F. T., and Oatley, M. W.,** Olfactory adaptation and recovery in old age, *Perception*, 18, 265, 1989.
72. **Spitzer, M. E.,** Taste acuity in institutionalized and non-institutionalized elderly men, *J. Gerontol.*, 43, 71, 1988.
73. **Reyes, P. F., Golden, G. T., Fagel, P. L., Fariello, R. G., Katz, L., and Carner, E.,** The prepiriform cortex in dementia of the Alzheimer type, *Arch. Neurol.*, 44, 644, 1987.
74. **Nann, D. M. A., Tucker, C. M., and Yates, P. O.,** Alzheimer's disease: an olfactory connection, *Mech. Ageing Dev.*, 42, 1, 1988.
75. **Quinn, N. P., Rossor, M. N., and Marsden, C. D.,** Olfactory threshold in Parkinson's disease, *J. Neurol. Neurosurg. Psychiatry*, 50, 88, 1987.
76. **Brun, A.,** Structural changes in ageing and dementia of Alzheimer's type with special reference to recent etiologic and therapeutic theories, *Prog. Clin. Biol. Res.*, 317, 285, 1989.
77. **Dunn, T. P. and Weller, M. P.,** Olfaction in schizophrenia, *Percept. Mot. Skills*, 69, 833, 1989.
78. **Doty, R. L.,** Influence of age and age-related diseases on olfactory function, *Ann. N. Y. Acad. Sci.*, 561, 76, 1989.
79. **Doty, R. L., Riklan, M., Deems, D. A., Reynolds, C., and Stellar, S.,** The olfactory and cognitive deficits of Parkinson's disease: evidence for independence, *Ann. Neurol.*, 25, 166, 1989.

80. **Talamo, B. R., Rudel, R., Kosik, K. S., Lee, V. M., Neff, S., Adelman, L., and Kauer, J. S.,** Pathological changes in olfactory neurons in patients with Alzheimer's disease, *Nature (London)*, 337, 736, 1989.
81. **Doty, R. L., Deems, D. A., and Stellar, S.,** Olfactory dysfunction in parkinsonism: a general deficit unrelated to neurologic signs, disease stage, or disease duration, *Neurology*, 38, 1237, 1988.
82. **Doty, R. L., Reyes, P. F., and Gregor, T. P.,** Presence of both odor identification and detection deficits in Alzheimer's disease, *Brain Res. Bull.*, 18, 597, 1987.
83. **LeResche, L. and Dworkin, S. F.,** Evaluating orofacial pain in the elderly, *Gerodontics*, 1, 81, 1985.
84. **Harkins, S. W., Kwentus, J., and Price, D. D.,** Pain and the elderly, in *Advances in Pain Research and Therapy*, Vol. 7, Benedetti, C., Chapman, C. R., and Moricca, G., Eds., Raven Press, New York, 1984, 103.
85. **Chapman, C. R.,** Pain perception in the elderly patient: an overview of issues, *Gerodontology*, 3, 71, 1984.
86. **Harkins, S. W. and Chapman, C. R.,** The perception of induced dental pain in young and elderly women, *J. Gerontol.*, 32, 428, 1977.
87. **Harkins, S. W. and Chapman, C. R.,** Detection and decision factors in pain perception in young and elderly men, *Pain*, 2, 253, 1976.
88. **Mumford, J. M.,** Pain perception threshold and adaptation of normal human teeth, *Arch. Oral Biol.*, 10, 957, 1965.
89. **LeResche, L.,** Facial behaviors related to pain in the elderly, *Gerodontology*, 3, 83, 1984.
90. **Butler, R. N. and Gastel, B.,** Care of the aged: perspectives on pain and discomfort, in *Pain and Discomfort*, Ng, L. K. G. and Bonica, J. J., Eds., Elsevier/North Holland, Amsterdam, 1980, 297.
91. **Price, S. C. and Kiyak, H. A.,** A behavioral approach to improving oral health among the elderly, *Spec. Care Dent.*, 1, 267, 1981.
92. **Fiske, J., Gelbier, S., and Watson, R. M.,** The benefit of dental care to an elderly population assessed using a socio-dental measure of oral handicap, *Br. Dent. J.*, 168, 153, 1990.
93. **Kiyak, H. A. and Mulligan, K.,** Studies of the relationship between oral health and psychological well-being, *Gerodontics*, 3, 109, 1987.

Chapter 8

PSYCHOSOCIAL FACTORS IN ADAPTATION TO DENTURES

In spite of the decline in the rate of edentulism among the elderly,[1] growing old is still associated with tooth loss (partial or full). Therefore, dental treatment for this population includes a relatively high prevalence of removable dentures.

There are many technical problems which can cause dentures to be unsatisfactory (insufficient retention, improper occlusion, incorrect vertical dimension, excessive pressure on the soft tissues, incorrect intermaxillary relations, etc.). However, while the technical aspect can be solved in most cases, some patients find it difficult emotionally to adapt to the new situation and pose a difficult problem for the dentist to handle.

I. THE EDENTULOUS PATIENT

A. THE MEANING OF TOOTH LOSS

Teeth are an integral part of our body and, as such, are not easy to part with. Their immediate function in supplying the individual with basic survival needs (nutrition) is enhanced in western culture by social functions and connotations. Theoretical, psychological, and dental research has shown the effect of the edentulous state on the mental and emotional condition of the elderly.[2-5]

In western societies, teeth symbolize youth, potency, strength, and virility. Aging is associated with tooth loss,[2-5] usually represented by a sunken face, reduced vertical dimension, unsupported lips, clicking of the remaining teeth, and disordered speech. Together with the decline in edentulousness, tooth loss is now often regarded as a pronounced social, psychological, and functional handicap.[6,7] Usually, about 70% of patients express regret over losing their natural dentition and about 60% consider dentures to be a handicap.[6]

D'Augustine et al.[3] referred to the differences between the general aging changes which occur in appearance, and the loss of teeth and insertion of full dentures. Most physical changes occur gradually, and although apparent, one often chooses to ignore them. There is a tendency to rationalize and attribute the changes to environmental rather than personal reasons. If the loss of teeth is gradual, these changes may also be ignored. However, when the edentulous state is reached and a full denture is inserted, the reality of the situation can no longer be disregarded. Because one's attention is now focused on this undeniable symbol of old age, all of the formerly unnoticed or ignored changes suddenly become apparent

It is, therefore, not surprising that tooth loss and denture wearing are relatively important life events which require adjustment. In a study conducted in Sweden,[8] 316 people were asked to rate 48 life events as to the degree of adjustment needed to cope with each one of them. Death of a child or a spouse ranked the highest (rank order 48 and 47, respectively), getting dentures ranked 33, and losing one or more teeth ranked 28 out of 48. The latter two events ranked higher than events such as "change of sexual habits," "addition of new member of household" (e.g., relative), "trouble with colleagues," "change in workplace," "retirement," or "marriage." The results demonstrate that loss of teeth and the provision of dentures are perceived as requiring a relatively high amount of psychosocial readjustment in relation to other life events.

B. BODY IMAGE

The body plays a significant role in self-image. Generally, people are resistant to changes in their appearance and often deny their new condition. If such changes are imposed on them, they are often unwilling to accept devices which will aid rehabilitation.[9]

The effect of body image on the denture selection has been studied by Lefer et al.[10] Patients were asked to select size, color, and set-up of teeth to be constructed for them. Four set-ups were presented to the patients: a conventional, nonindividualistic one, an aggressive-looking one, a "beauty contest girl" one, and a passive-looking one. All patients underwent a psychiatric interview in an attempt to predict the set-up of choice.

Most patients who were given the choice selected the conventional and nonindividualistic set-up. These patients were generally evaluated as being rigid, perfectionists, and fearful of making mistakes. The second most selected set-up was the passive-looking one. Patients who selected this were greatly concerned about the feelings that others had about them, looked at others to make demands upon them, and viewed their spouses as dominating people who criticized freely. The aggressive looking set-up was chosen by individuals with a one-upmanship way of relating to others, who strove, yet feared to compete, and prided themselves upon their independence from others.

The study suggested that the choice of denture appearance reflects self-image. Although the patient's choice did not reflect the dentist's choice (in a control group half of the patients received the passive look and one third the aggressive look), most patients were pleased with the method. It was concluded that when the patient was able to fulfill his/her undefined psychological needs with regard to body image, satisfaction of the restoration increased.

C. EXPECTATIONS

Many prosthodontic failures are the result of mismatches between the patient's expectations for dentures and the dentist's goal for the same treatment.[11] The patient often expects dentures that improve on nature to the point of being artificial in color, size, shape, and symmetry. Often there is little correlation between the physical structure of face and body and the choice of denture esthetics by the patient.[10] It has been suggested that patients who are unhappy with their own teeth may expect dentures to improve on nature. Furthermore, possible negative associations with the aging process, that dentures frequently evoke, may cause the patient to seek a younger image, not simply more attractive teeth.[11]

The patient's expectations of his/her dentures often differ significantly from the dentist's perceptions of what is good for the patient. A significant difference was found regarding the preferred appearance of teeth among dentists, dental students, and patients.[12] Preferences differed for proportions of length and width of the teeth, and with respect to the symmetry of maxillary anterior teeth. While patients found horizontal symmetry pleasing, most dentists and dental students rejected the artificial appearance caused by this look.

Unrealistically high expectations of dentures have also been expressed by long-term denture wearers (average of 22 years).[13] Especially high expectations were expressed by patients with regard to dentures vs. natural teeth ("dentures should be like or better than natural teeth"), stability ("dentures should fit perfectly and not move"), and ability to chew with dentures vs. natural teeth ("I should be able to eat and chew as well with dentures as with natural teeth"). Expectations regarding appearance were more realistic, but most of the patients still expected dentures to have the appearance of natural teeth.

While unrealistically high expectations affect patient satisfaction with new dentures, realistic and positive attitudes contribute to the patient's future adaptation. Patients who are positive about the functional aspects and/or expect no problems before receiving new dentures are more often satisfied after receiving the appliances.[14] Those who think negatively about dentures prior to receiving them are more often dissatisfied.[15]

Hirsch et al.[16] asked patients who were about to receive dentures to rate four different denture set-ups in order of preference. They were then randomly assigned to receive their first, second, third, or last choice. In spite of the differences in fulfilling the patients' preferences, the groups did not differ in adaptation to dentures. There was, however, a significant difference in the pre-post changes in the rating of patients receiving their first, second, third, and fourth choice set-ups. The lower the patient's initial rating of the set-up, the higher his rating of the same set-up after actually receiving the dentures.

The authors explained this reversal in terms of the cognitive dissonance theory, which states that individuals experience cognitive dissonance or discomfort when exposed to inconsistencies about themselves or their environment. Thus, patients who were given dentures which they had not rated as their first esthetic choice would be expected to experience cognitive dissonance, increasing in relation to their pre-rating of the dentures they received. To reduce dissonance, the individual tends to reorganize his cognitive evaluation of the situation by finding "extra attractions" for the dentures received. For example, patients who did not receive their expected dentures simply found new reasons for liking what they did receive.

D. EFFECT OF PERSONALITY ON DENTURE SATISFACTION

Are there special personality traits which make one dissatisfied with his/her dentures? Several authors have attempted to deal with this question, but the answer is still unclear.

Langer et al.[17] and Seifert et al.[18] attempted to define the various factors that determine an individual's satisfaction with complete dentures. No significant correlation was found between the clinical fit of the dentures and patient satisfaction, or between the patient's intelligence and satisfaction with the dentures.

A correlation was found between patient satisfaction and his/her personality.[18] In this study, personality ratings were made by the director and a psychologist of an old-age home. A patient was considered to have a positive personality when he/she showed a positive approach to life, could accept failings of others, and had adjusted well to the environment. A patient was considered to be negative when he/she was hypercritical of the home and its residents and felt that he/she was being exploited. A patient was listed as disturbed when the interviewer believed that he/she was not truthful and had something to hide. According to these definitions, most of the patients who were satisfied with their dentures had a "positive" personality.

In later studies, other, more accurate methods were used to measure personality. The Cornell Medical Index (CMI) is one method to assess patient reaction to dentures. The CMI was originally designed to collect medical data and to increase the accuracy of clinical diagnoses. It was also found to be helpful in detecting emotional disorders. Nairn and Brunello[19] found that patients who complained more about their dentures scored higher as being neurotic according to the CMI. A direct relationship between patient satisfaction with new dentures and a rise above the established critical level of CMI score was also shown by Bolender et al.,[20] who demonstrated a correlation between emotional problems and denture problems in the patients.

The association between CMI score and patient satisfaction with dentures was not confirmed in a study by Guckes et al.[21] No difference was found in this study between patient's denture satisfaction scores and patient groups as determined by CMI scores. The same patients were also evaluated according to the Eysenck Personality Inventory (EPI) which measures the traits of extraversion-introversion and neuroticism-stability. The less satisfied group had a significantly higher EPI neuroticism score. It was concluded that many patients who are difficult to satisfy are somewhat more neurotic than those who are easy to satisfy.

A shortened version of the Minnesota Multiphasic Personality Inventory (MMPI) was used by Smith[22] to measure personality traits that included depression, hysteria, and anxiety in patients about to receive dentures. Although there was a high prevalence of these traits among those investigated, no significant relationship was found between them and the degree of patient satisfaction with dentures, nor was satisfaction affected by denture quality.

Reeve and associates[6,23-25] made use of the Cattell 16 PF Questionnaire to acquire personality profiles for different patients. The vast majority of complete denture patients were referred to the University Clinic after having already completed treatment elsewhere, and appeared to have psychological problems as well as denture difficulties. These patients were found to be difficult to please, fussy, moralistic and proper, and somewhat stubborn. In addition, women showed signs of instability, lack of willpower and self-integration, insecurity, anxiety, and tenseness.

Following new denture construction, 58% of the patients were satisfied. The dissatisfied group differed significantly from the satisfied group in being emotionally less stable, more apprehensive, worried, depressed, and troubled; more casual, careless of protocol, and untidy; and more tense, driven, overwrought, and fretful.

Similar results were shown with regard to satisfied vs. dissatisfied partial denture patients.[24] The personality profile for the dissatisfied group was found to be significantly more unstable, more casual, tough-minded, suspicious, and self-sufficient. This suggests that, as a group, they would not accept advice readily and would lack perseverance.

In more recent studies,[14,15] patient personality was evaluated by Wilde's Neurotic Liability Scale and the Health Locus of Control Scale. The former measures the extent to which an individual reacts neurotically in a stress situation, whereas the latter measures the extent to which an individual believes he/she has personal control over what happens. Neither measure showed a significant relationship with regard to patient satisfaction with new dentures.

Several other theories have been used to explain the so-called "difficult denture patient." Chamberlain and Chamberlain[26] stressed the importance of depression in the treatment of full denture patients. Silverman et al.[27] suggested that a relationship exists in geriatric patients between their self-image and the extent of denture acceptance.

Pitts[28] proposed that the difficult denture patient resembles the syndrome identified in the psychotherapeutic literature as the patient who is a "help-rejecting complainer". These patients systematically reject treatment and all attempts to help from the therapist, even though the help was originally sought by the patient. The author suggested that both the "help-rejecting complainer" and the "difficult denture patient" are working through the same mechanism:

- Both types are driven by a need to seek treatment from someone they will ultimately reject.
- A self-fulfilling prophecy of failure develops into a cycle leading to failure.
- Due to lack of trust and a desire to feel important, the patient creates an atmosphere that leads to discord, hostility, anger, and frustration.
- The discord leads to the establishment of a relationship that demands extra time and energy from the helper.

- The helper is ultimately manipulated into a no-win situation that ends with the helper dismissing the patient, thereby completing the patient's self-fulfilling prophecy.
- Recurrent stress in the patient's life recycles the drive and the need for treatment and attention starts all over again.

It seems difficult to conclude which specific personality traits are correlated with patient satisfaction or dissatisfaction with dentures. The difficult-to-please patient varies in several aspects from the easily adapting patient, but the pattern which makes these two groups different has not, as yet, been clearly defined.

E. SOCIAL ADAPTATION

The wearing of dentures is also a social act. One is expected to function with dentures not only at home but at work and social gatherings. The subjective or objective need for acceptable social behavior is a powerful factor in adapting to dentures. A person who interacts with others in everyday life has a "motive" which drives him/her to make an extra effort to adapt. A person who withdraws from society and spends most of his/her time in isolation often finds it more difficult to adapt.

Some studies examined the possible association between social factors and denture satisfaction. Langer et al.[17] investigated factors which influence satisfaction with complete dentures among geriatric patients living in old-age homes. The social adjustment of subjects was determined by a questionnaire which took into consideration the subject's participation in community life and activities and social adjustment to roommates. The relation between social adjustment of subjects and their satisfaction with dentures was present, although weak.

Carlsson et al.[29] also found a weak association among 182 edentulous patients who received complete dentures in a university clinic in Sweden. Social adaptation of the patient was considered poor if he/she felt unhappy in his present job; did not relate to his fellow workers, neighbors, or family; had been provided care by social workers from the welfare bureau, or was known to have problems with alcohol. The patient was considered socially active if an active member in a club, union, or church, or appointed a representative in political or municipal life. In the study, social adaptation was found to be only weakly associated with patient appreciation of dentures.

The data concerning this issue still seem to be too scarce to draw definite conclusions. Social adaptation probably has an effect on morale, which in turn affects the adaptation process. For example, Silverman et al.[27] showed significantly greater denture acceptance among employed subjects compared to those who were unemployed, and a significant relationship between scores on morale questions and the degree of denture acceptance. Apparently, subjects who are employed and have an active social life retain a high morale and a high self-image and show a greater facility in adjusting to new situations, including dentures.

F. ORAL MOTOR PATTERNS

Oral motor patterns, such as function, parafunction, mucosa displaceability, adaptive responses, and TMJ dysfunction play significant roles in adaptation or rejection of dentures.[30]

As most removable dental appliances are adapted among older patients, the success (or failure) of such restorations may be affected by the changes which occur in patient motor performance. With age, the prevalence of altered motor performance, such as lip posture and masticatory muscle function increases.[31] Such alterations may affect the ability of older people to prepare food for swallowing and function with dentures.

II. THE DENTIST-PATIENT RELATIONSHIP

Construction of good dentures requires continuous cooperation between the patient and dentist. The nature of this interaction is of paramount importance in determining the final result, both technically and psychologically.

Friedman et al.[32] summarized the importance of the dentist's behavior as originating in the patient's dependence on the dentist to make a significant change in the patient's life. To adapt to the new situation, the patient must have an alliance with the dentist. Distrust or resentment towards the dentist can adversely affect one's attitude toward new dentures. A warm trusting relationship can do much to create acceptance of the dentures.

A positive correlation between patient-dentist relationship and patient satisfaction with the dentures has been shown.[17,18] Geriatric patients were asked to comment on their relationship with the dentist. The relationship was rated as positive when the patient expressed complete satisfaction with the dentist, stating that the dentist was good, kind, and helpful, that he/she liked the dentist, and that the dentist did everything possible to make good dentures. The rating was negative when the patient stated that the dentist was nervous, impatient, and not good, that the dentist did not like the patient and vice versa. The relationship was judged to be indifferent when the patient stated that the dentist did his/her job and no definition was made concerning the dentist as being "good" or "bad."

The patient-dentist relationship was more strongly correlated with patient satisfaction than were other factors, such as intelligence or patient personality.[18] The greatest degree of patient satisfaction (in a group of patients treated by dentists in their usual manner) was found in those who were treated by a dentist who considered the patient's feelings as the most important guide in selecting denture esthetics.[10]

Hirsch et al.[16] found that the crucial variable in patient acceptance of dentures was their *involvement* in the process of denture selection and not the esthetic quality of the dentures received. Patient satisfaction with new dentures was also associated with the authoritarian personality characteristics of their treating dental students.[33] The results indicated that patient's treated by low authoritarian students reacted much more favorably to the denture set-ups they received than those treated by high authoritarian students. Although the patients were allowed to choose their own preferred set-up of teeth, the personality characteristics of the students had a significant effect on patient satisfaction with the outcome.

The issue of the dentist's authoritarian approach is even more pronounced in a clinical setting where the dentist often takes total responsibility for the correct selection of denture set-up for the patient. It was shown that discrepancies exist between the patient's preference as to the denture appearance and that of the dentist.[10,12] Ignoring the patient's preferences and dealing with the situation in an authoritative manner increases the danger of maladaptation.

III. HABITUATION

Habituation and learning mechanisms play an important role in the interim between insertion of new dentures and the development of satisfactory function. A criterion of successful denture wearing is that the patient should be able to forget about the dentures most of the time; a common complaint of the difficult denture patient is that such a delegation to automatic control does not occur.[34]

Fortunately, most elderly patients do adapt surprisingly well to dentures and continue to use them even when they are wrong technically. For example, Brill et al.[35] described a 63-year-old woman who continued to successfully wear her complete upper denture for 5 years after it fractured into two separate pieces.

In a survey conducted in Sweden,[36] most patients were satisfied with the fit, the esthetic effect of the denture, and the ability to chew and speak 1 year after acquiring new dentures. Patients who were satisfied with the fit were, as a rule, also satisfied with esthetic effect and with their ability to chew and speak.

In a long-term clinical study of complete denture wearers,[37] a discrepancy was found between patient satisfaction with the dentures and the dentist's assessment of their quality. According to the clinical examination, 63% of the subjects needed new dentures or substantial adjustment; however, more than 70% showed excellent adaptation to denture wearing, and only 6% assessed the total denture function as less than adequate.

Similar results were also presented by Smith.[22] Most patients were "very satisfied" (63%) or "fairly satisfied" (24%) with their dentures. This high rate of satisfaction was not related to the clinical evaluation of the dentures. Among the same patients, 36% of the dentures were clinically evaluated as "poor," 36% as "fair." No relationship was shown between the overall technical quality of the dentures and the patient's general satisfaction with them.

As suggested,[16] the relatively high adaptation of patients to their dentures may be explained by the cognitive dissonance theory by which beliefs, values, or behaviors are changed to reduce an uncomfortable state of dissonance.[11,16] Furthermore, denture wearing is a matter of "skilled performance,"[30] and once acquired, the patient relies much less on physical factors for denture control.

IV. PREDICTION OF PATIENT ADAPTATION

Many dentists feel that an overall "impression" of the patient's personality is enough to evaluate the patient who is about to receive complete or partial dentures. This, of course, is inaccurate and often leads to problems.

Watson and Reeve[6] and Reeve et al.[23,25] have attempted to develop methods to predict satisfaction with the outcome of prosthetic treatment. In their studies, clinicians were asked to predict the level of satisfaction of each patient. Concomitantly, patients were asked to fulfill the Cattell 16 PF Questionnaire. It was found that clinical predictions were less accurate than those of the personality questionnaire. In one study, a clinician correctly predicted only 20% of the cases and another only as much as 33%.[23]

In a second study,[25] the overall predictive accuracy was 71% for the personality questionnaire and 65% for clinical assessment. The clinical assessment was less accurate with regard to patients who were dissatisfied with their complete dentures (48%). Similar results were also obtained with regard to satisfaction of preprosthetic surgery patients.[6]

These results suggest that clinicians have difficulty in recognizing the personality characteristics of their patients. The clinical predictions were, on the whole, no better than chance.[25] Although all clinicians felt that personality and behavior in the clinic were the most influential in predicting the outcome of treatment in complete dentures, no significant differences were found in the personality profiles of the potentially satisfied/dissatisfied clinically predicted group. It was concluded that patients do not reveal noticeably different behaviors during treatment.[25]

Clinical prognoses are probably influenced by personal preference, experience, and previous history of denture wearing. The Cattell questionnaire was slightly more effective in this respect, but prediction was still not absolute. It is advisable to avoid classifying the patient in advance according to a personal "hunch." Although some patients may become a problem in the future, understanding, acceptance, and patience can help most to adapt properly.

V. SUMMARY

Adaptation to full or partial dentures is affected not only by the technical fit of the appliances, but also by multiple psychosocial variables. The individual meaning of tooth loss and its effect on body image play a major role in adjustment.

Patients often have unrealistically high expectations of new dentures which do not match the dentist's perceptions as to what is good for the patient. Although some patients' personality traits have been associated with their satisfaction (or dissatisfaction) with the dentures, it is still impossible to predict most of the future "difficult" denture patients. Environmental factors, such as social adaptation and dentist-patient relationship, are crucial in this issue.

Most patients adapt rather well and use their dentures continuously for many years, even when the fit is technically poor. Only a small proportion of patients, whose psychosocial adaptation to new dentures is long and troublesome, needs extra attention from the dentist.

REFERENCES

1. **Weintraub, J. A. and Burt, B. A.,** Oral health status in the United States: tooth loss and edentulism, *J. Dent. Edu.*, 49, 368, 1985.
2. **Swoope, C. C.,** Identification and management of emotional patients, *J. Prosthet. Dent.*, 27, 434, 1972.
3. **D'Augustine, R., Blitz, A. N., and Wechsler, S. M.,** Psychological problems of the edentulous patient, *Clin. Prev. Dent.*, 2(2), 9, 1980.
4. **Friedman, N., Landesman, H. M., and Wexler, M.,** The influences of fear, anxiety, and depression on the patient's adaptive responses to complete dentures, Part I, *J. Prosthet. Dent.*, 58, 687, 1987.
5. **Friedman, N., Landesman, H. M., and Wexler, M.,** The influences of fear, anxiety, and depression on the patient's adaptive responses to complete dentures, Part II, *J. Prosthet. Dent.*, 59, 45, 1988.
6. **Watson, C. J. and Reeve, P. E.,** The effects of combined psychological and controlled clinical management of preprosthetic surgery patients, *Br. Dent. J.*, 159, 286, 1985.
7. **Blomberg, S. and Lindquist, L. W.,** Psychological reactions to endentulousness and treatment with jawbone-anchored bridges, *Acta Psychiatr. Scand.*, 68, 251, 1983.
8. **Bergendal, B.,** The relative importance of tooth loss and denture wearing in Swedish adults, *Community Dent. Health*, 6, 103, 1989.
9. **Kolb, L.,** Disturbances of body image, in *Handbook of Psychiatry*, Basic Books, New York, 1959, 763.
10. **Lefer, L., Pleasure, M. A., and Rosenthal, L.,** A psychiatric approach to the denture patient, *J. Psychosom. Res.*, 6, 199, 1962.
11. **Albino, J. E., Tedesco, L. A., and Conny, D. J.,** Patient perceptions of dental-facial esthetics: shared concerns in orthodontics and prosthodontics, *J. Prosthet. Dent.*, 52, 9, 1984.
12. **Brisman, A. S.,** Esthetics: a comparison of dentists' and patients' concepts, *J. Am. Dent. Assoc.*, 100, 345, 1980.
13. **Davis, E. L., Albino, J. E., Tedesco, L. A., Portenoy, B. S., and Ortman, L. F.,** Expectations and satisfaction of denture patients in a university clinic, *J. Prosthet. Dent.*, 55, 59, 1986.
14. **van Waas, M. A. J.,** The influence of psychologic factors on patient satisfaction with complete dentures, *J. Prosthet. Dent.*, 63, 545, 1990.
15. **van Waas, M. A. J.,** Determinants of dissatisfaction with dentures: a multiple regression analysis, *J. Prosthet. Dent.*, 64, 569, 1990.
16. **Hirsch, B., Levin, B., and Tiber, N.,** Effects of patient involvement and esthetic preference on denture acceptance, *J. Prosthet. Dent.*, 28, 127, 1972.

17. **Langer, A., Michman, J., and Seifert, I.,** Factors influencing satisfaction with complete dentures in geriatric patients, *J. Prosthet. Dent.*, 11, 1019, 1961.
18. **Seifert, I., Langer, A., and Michman, J.,** Evaluation of psychologic factors in geriatric denture patients, *J. Prosthet. Dent.*, 12, 516, 1962.
19. **Nairn, R. I. and Brunello, D. L.,** The relationship of denture complaints and level of neuroticism, *Dent. Pract.* 21, 156, 1971.
20. **Bolender, C. L., Swoope, C. C., and Smith, D. E.,** The Cornell Medical Index as a prognostic aid for complete denture patients, *J. Prosthet. Dent.*, 22, 20, 1969.
21. **Guckes, A. D., Smith, D. E., and Swoope, C. C.,** Counseling and related factors influencing satisfaction with dentures, *J. Prosthet. Dent.*, 39, 259, 1978.
22. **Smith, M.,** Measurement of personality traits and their relation to patient satisfaction with complete dentures, *J. Prosthet. Dent.*, 35, 492, 1976.
23. **Reeve, P., Stafford, G. D., Watson, C. J., and Hopkins, R.,** The use of Cattell's personality profile in patients who have had preprosthetic surgery, *J. Dent.*, 10, 121, 1982.
24. **Watson, C. J., Reeve, P. E., Barnes, E., Lane, A. E., and Bates, J. F.,** The role of personality in the management of partial dentures, *J. Oral Rehabil.*, 13, 83, 1986.
25. **Reeve, P. E., Watson, C. J., and Stafford, G. D.,** The role of personality in the management of complete denture patients, *Br. Dent. J.*, 156, 356, 1984.
26. **Chamberlain, B. B. and Chamberlain, K. R.,** Depression: a psychologic consideration in complete denture prosthodontics *J. Prosthet. Dent.*, 53, 673, 1985.
27. **Silverman, S., Silverman, S. I., Silverman, B., and Garfinkel, L.,** Self-image and its relation to denture acceptance, *J. Prosthet. Dent.*, 35, 131, 1976.
28. **Pitts, W. C.,** Difficult denture patients: observations and hypothesis, *J. Prosthet. Dent.*, 53, 532, 1985.
29. **Carlsson, G. E., Otterland, A., and Wennstrom, A.,** Patient factors in appreciation of complete dentures, *J. Prosthet. Dent.*, 17, 322, 1967.
30. **Zarb, G. A.,** Oral motor patterns and their relation to oral prostheses, *J. Prosthet. Dent.*, 47, 472, 1982.
31. **Baum, B. J. and Bodner, L.,** Aging and oral motor function: evidence for altered performance among older persons, *J. Dent. Res.*, 62, 2, 1983.
32. **Friedman, N., Landesman, H. M., and Wexler, M.,** The influences of fear, anxiety, and depression on the patient's adaptive responses to complete dentures, Part III, *J. Prosthet. Dent.*, 59, 169, 1988.
33. **Hirsch, B., Levin, B., and Tiber, N.,** Effects of dentist authoritarianism on patient evaluation of dentures, *J. Prosthet. Dent.*, 30, 745, 1973.
34. **Newton, A. V.,** The difficult denture patient: a review of psychological aspects, *Br. Dent. J.*, 138, 93, 1975.
35. **Brill, N., Tryde, G., and Schubeler, S.,** The role of learning in denture retention, *J. Prosthet. Dent.*, 10, 468, 1960.
36. **Bergman, B. and Carlsson, G. E.,** Review of 54 complete denture wearers: patients' opinions 1 year after treatment, *Acta Odontol. Scand.*, 30, 399, 1972.
37. **Bergman, B. and Carlsson, G. E.,** Clinical long-term study of complete denture wearers, *J. Prosthet. Dent.*, 53, 56, 1985.

Chapter 9

EFFECTS OF STRESS ON PHYSIOLOGICAL CONDITIONS IN THE ORAL CAVITY

Like many other parts of our body, the oral cavity is affected by conditions of acute and chronic stress. Acute stress and its response are usually associated with an immediate cause (e.g., fear of dental treatment) and tend to diminish when not in the face of the "stressor." Chronic stress and its response persist beyond the time of the immediate stimulus and have long-term effects (e.g., stressful life events).

Acute stress is characterized by several immediate physiological responses, including increased heart rate, elevated blood pressure, and changed galvanic skin response. In the oral cavity, most of the observed changes involve the effect of the stressful situation on salivary fluid.

Chronic stress affects everyone differently. Some people develop heart disease, others peptic ulcers, or complain of recurrent headaches. Wolff[1] suggested that the particular adaptation pattern for individuals is the result of previous life experiences which condition them to react in a specific way. An individual may have a potential "nose reactor" or "colon reactor" without using this particular protective pattern because it was never needed. With the onset of stress, the given protective pattern may become evident, involving the gut, the heart and vascular systems, the nasorespiratory apparatus, the skin, or general metabolism.

One of the body systems potentially affected by chronic stress is the oral cavity and its related systems. The specific target of the stress response in each individual, be it muscle tension or periodontal disease, is still unclear. Nevertheless, the effect of stress (acute and/or chronic) on psychophysiological changes in the oral cavity has been acknowledged for many years.[2,3]

I. EFFECT OF STRESS ON SALIVA

Saliva is probably one of the most studied oral correlates of stress. Being controlled by both sympathetic and parasympathetic fibers, the salivary glands are affected by various factors. While stimulation of the parasympathetic fibers leads to vasodilation and increased secretion of saliva, sympathetic stimulation produces a complex series of reactions with little or no effect.[3-5]

Salivary fluid is sensitive to various disease states, both in its organic and inorganic components.[6,7] Therefore, its use for diagnostic purposes, such as the estimation of systemic levels of lipid-soluble drugs and hormones, is continuously expanding.[6]

Salivary secretion is affected by physiological and psychological factors. In healthy individuals the saliva flow rate is modulated by aging, circadian rhythm (low in the morning, high in the mid-afternoon), circannual rhythm (reduced in summer months), body position (greater in standing position), light (decreased in light), smoking (decreased in smokers), previous stimulation (increased when preceded by gustatory stimulation), and olfactory stimulation (increased).[8] Psychological variables, such as emotions (e.g., depression), cognitions (e.g., anticipation of food) and conditioning (e.g., specific smells in different cultures) also affect the salivary flow.[4,9-12]

The quantity and quality of the salivary fluid influence the conditions and functions of various oral tissues. Salivary functions include lubrication (through mucins, proline-rich proteins, H_2O), antimicrobial activity (through lactoferrin, lysozyme, lactoperoxidase, immunoglobulins, mucins, histatins, cystatins, and the proline-rich proteins), remineralization of tooth tissues (through ions of Ca, P, Pl, Statherin, and proline-rich proteins), buffering (through HCO_3PO_4), food digestion (through amylase, lipase, proteases, nucleases, mucins, and gustin), and protection of the mucosal integrity (through H_2O, electrolytes, and mucins).[13]

Changes occurring in saliva as a result of stress (acute or chronic) can at the same time initiate other psychophysiological changes in the oral cavity, such as periodontal disease or increased carious activity.

A. STRESS AND SALIVARY FLOW

Salivary flow, being relatively easy to measure, was one of the first studied oral correlates of stress. The clinical observation that stressful situations cause a decrease in salivary flow was used in ancient times to determine the truth; Bedouins made suspected criminals lick a hot iron, the Chinese and the North American Indians used rice, and the English used bread and cheese.[3,14,15] It was believed that those who were lying would have a dry mouth and would, therefore, be burned by the hot iron, expectorate dry rice, or be unable to swallow the bread and cheese.

The effect of stress on salivary flow was studied in the early decades of this century. In 1931, Windsor[16] reported salivary flow to be inhibited by periods of sustained attention accompanying the performance of mental tasks.

Patterns of coping with stress are significantly influenced by personality.[17] Therefore, the impact of stress on saliva is highly dependent on individual factors. In 1961, Bogdonoff et al.[18] examined the flow of parotid saliva as related to acute stress in 24 normal subjects who were assessed prior to the experiment as having either an aggressive or a defensive characteristic pattern of meeting challenges. The stressful situation was caused by the imminence of physical harm (presentation, but not use, of a dental drill). Of the 17 subjects rated as aggressive, all had increased salivary flow as a reaction to the stimulus, while 6 of the defensive subjects showed a decrease in the amount of their parotid saliva. The one subject who showed no change described the dental experience as "relaxing" and nonthreatening, a fact which probably led to the lack of effect.

Hafner,[19] in 1974, attempted to replicate the approach of Bogdonoff et al.[18] with an examination of the relationship between acute stress, salivary flow rate, and composition. All subjects completed the Hostility and Direction of Hostility Questionnaire (HDHQ), measuring personality factors termed extra- and intro-punitiveness, and The Eysenck Personality Inventory (EPI). Stressful situations were devised by exposing the subjects to high tones transmitted through headphones or by asking them to perform mental arithmetic while being distracted by the same tones at a reduced volume.

The results showed a decreased flow rate among subjects who scored low in the intro-punitive range and those classified as extra-punitive. No change in salivary flow was observed in subjects who scored high in this scale. A significant negative correlation was found between the decline in salivary flow and neuroticism score (N) according to EPI.

Hafner's data also showed a significant correlation between the total hostility score (T) according to HDHQ and the neuroticism score (N). The T score measures the amount of hostility which enters consciousness — high scores indicating greater awareness of hostile thoughts and impulses. The N scale mainly measures emotionality or intensity of emotional response. It was hypothesized that high T and N scores both indicate greater than normal awareness of emotional responses, including aggressive ones, and that those subjects who are able to use the aggressive methods to cope with stress would be more likely to experience and express such emotions. These subjects showed a slight increase in salivary flow with stress. Those subjects who were less able to recognize or express aggressive emotions during stress would be more likely to adopt a defensive posture and showed a significant decline in salivary flow.

In a further study conducted on depressed and obsessional subjects, Hafner[20] reported a significantly lower mean salivary flow for the depressed group than in a control group or in the obsessional group, indicating the effect of chronic stress on the amount of saliva. All groups, however, reacted to acute stress with a significant decline in salivary flow.

The effect of personality factors on the amount of stimulated salivary secretion was also studied by Corcoran.[21] In this study, 35 subjects were evaluated on the personality dimension of introversion-extroversion. The hypothesis was that introverts are generally more aroused than extroverts, and as a result salivary gland stimulation should influence them to a greater extent (lemon juice or citric acid was used to stimulate salivary secretion). Differences were found in the amount of saliva secreted after lemon juice stimulation between introverts and extroverts, suggesting the existence of possible differences between patients in their reaction to salivary stimulation. A replication by Eysenck and Eysenck,[22] in 1967, similarly showed that introverted subjects react more strongly with salivation to stimulation of the taste buds with lemon juice, thus confirming Corcoran's findings.

In spite of the individual differences in reaction to salivary stimulation, acute stress usually leads to a decrease in the amount of secreted saliva. In

1968, Bates and Adams[23] attempted to evaluate the influence of a stressful situation (professional examinations) on the salivary secretion of dental students. Whole saliva (resting and stimulated saliva) was collected 30 min before examinations and then 1 week later. Significant differences were noted in the amount of stimulated salivary secretion under stress compared to the control situation (less saliva before examinations).

Silverstein and Iverson[24] referred to the issue of acute, social stress and its effect on salivary flow. The social situation chosen was to pose subjects with risk and threat to their sense of well-being through interpersonal bargaining. In this situation, expectations regarding one's capacity to control outcomes, relative to those of his/her bargaining rival, come into play. Not only can expectations be proven erroneous through an opponent's counterplays, but they are also conditional on the degree to which an opponent will yield or seize on an unequal power advantage. The results provided evidence to reduced salivary flow in individuals engaged in the social interaction as opposed to subsequent individualized activity.

In the early 1970's, it became apparent that the measurement of flow alone was not sufficient to understand the full effect of stress on saliva.[4] Today, more sophisticated measures are used to better understand the psychophysiological effect of stressful conditions on saliva.

B. STRESS AND SALIVARY COMPOSITION

Some of the early studies on the effect of emotional states on salivary composition suggested that the pH of saliva changes under emotional stress.[25] A series of clinical studies by Morse and associates[14,26-33] deal with this issue.

Subjects in two of the studies were dental patients undergoing nonsurgical endodontic therapy.[14,27] The stressor was the patient's fear of the upcoming endodontic therapy. Prior to treatment, each subject completed a dental-anxiety questionnaire and supplied a sample of unstimulated pooled saliva. During treatment, patients were instructed to perform different relaxation procedures (e.g., hypnosis, meditation). Another saliva sample and a second dental anxiety questionnaire were obtained after the session was completed. Positive correlations were found between the questionnaire-assessed evaluation of stress and relaxation and the salivary results. The stress-related salivary changes were increased opacity, increased protein, reduced volume, reduced α amylase, and reduced pH. These results were also found when separate salivary gland secretions were used[28] and when the technique of relaxation was performed by a patient well trained in deep relaxation through meditation.[31]

The effect of relaxation on salivary composition was also examined on dental students practicing relaxation.[26,32,33] Correlations were found between relaxation and stress and the level of salivary proteins (increased under stress, unchanged under relaxation). The authors concluded that the salivary changes which occur during stress act as a possible etiological factor in the development of dental caries.[30]

C. STRESS AND SALIVARY CORTISOL

Saliva is often used to determine steroid levels including cortisol, aldosterone, dehydroepiandrosterone, testosterone, progesterone, etc.[6] Steroid analysis in saliva has been described,[34,35] and the use of salivary cortisol as a noninvasive method to measure acute stress response has been suggested.[36-45]

To assess the effect of acute physical stress on the salivary cortisol level, Tarui and Nakamura[39] exposed adult volunteers to relatively high degrees of $+G_z$ acceleration (through centifugation). The $+G_z$ acceleration caused a significant increase in the salivary cortisol of the subjects, with the peak value attained 20 min after centrifugation (3 times its initial level in saliva after acceleration at $+G_z$, while in serum it increased only 1.5 times).

Salivary cortisol is also affected by psychological stimulation. In a further study, Kakimoto et al.[40] used salivary cortisol and heart rate to assess the physiological responses of pilots and co-pilots. The relative change in both responses showed similar patterns and was found to be significantly influenced by whether the pilots or co-pilots were in control of the aircraft (salivary cortisol level of both groups was higher when controlling the aircraft than when not). Differences in flying experience and responsibility also influenced the salivary cortisol: co-pilots showed a much higher activation and change in their salivary cortisol levels (compared to pilots) between periods of controlling and noncontrolling the aircraft. The authors explained these findings by the increased stress of the less experienced pilots when in control of the aircraft.

The salivary cortisol level is significantly affected by situations which bear aspects of social stress and by individual mood states. When bank employees were asked to prepare and deliver a 15 min public lecture, their salivary cortisol was found to be significantly higher both immediately before and after the lecture.[41] In another study, volunteers watching a suspense film were found to show a significant increase in their saliva cortisol.[42] While there were no significant correlations between saliva cortisol release and the subject's trait anxiety or depression, saliva cortisol secretion significantly correlated with state mood scales of "joyfulness" or anxiety. After the film, subjects with higher ratings of "anxious" and lower ratings of "joyfulness" released more cortisol. Similar results were reported by Kirschbaum and Hellhammer.[43]

A relatively rare study on the effect of chronic stress on saliva was conducted by Rahe et al.,[44] which examined 52 Americans held hostage in Iran for 444 days immediately after their release from captivity. The study focused on the stress management capabilities of the group and included psychological testing (Minnesota Multiphasic Personality Inventory — MMPI) and physiological testing (cortisol levels in plasma, urine, and saliva; urinary catecholamine levels, and salivary testosterone).

For all subjects (civilians and military), salivary cortisol and testosterone were found to be highly elevated. Furthermore, while no significant correlations were seen between plasma and urinary cortisol and psychiatric disturbance scores or psychological test scales, consistent and often significant correlations were found between salivary cortisol and the psychiatric disturbance score.

Although the study was conducted on subjects who had undergone severe chronic stress, release from captivity also carries with it aspects of an immediate acute stress. A senior military officer described his reactions after arriving in Europe as a mixture of distress, anxiety, and elation. His distress was over what his military superior would think of his performance as a hostage and his anxiety included concerns as to how to relate again to family and friends. Thus, although providing some insight on the effect of chronic stress on salivary cortisol, the results also indicated the immediate effect of acute social stress.

As there is little storage of saliva in the body (saliva is produced as required), there is no significant lagtime involved in the appearance of cortisol in the saliva, and its measurements reflect more closely the time-dependent changes in the plasma levels of the hormone than urinary hormone measurements. The more immediate response of salivary cortisol, together with its high availability (noninvasive, easy to collect on demand, and volume and time of previous sample do not need to be measured and recorded), makes it a measurement of choice in evaluating human stress.[41]

D. STRESS AND SALIVARY IgA

An important antimicrobial system in saliva is the secretory IgA (S-IgA) that binds to bacteria and fungi, leads to bacterial aggregation in the fluid phase, and may lead to complement-mediated killing.[13] S-IgA is known to play an important role in the mucosal immune defense of the nasal and oral cavities against infections by respiratory viruses. S-IgA antibodies interfere with bacterial and viral adherence to mucosal surfaces, and consequently limit colonization of these surfaces by pathogens.[46-48]

More and more evidence has been collected showing that under stress the level of S-IgA decreases, thus increasing the probability of oral infection and disease. For example, Jemmott et al.[49] evaluated the S-IgA levels in 64 dental students who were facing examinations. S-IgA secretion during the examination period significantly decreased in comparison to pre- and post-examination levels. In addition, personality characteristics differentiated patterns of S-IgA secretion rates. Students characterized by a desire to establish and maintain warm personal relationships secreted more S-IgA at each point than did other subjects. The more relaxed the subject, the higher S-IgA.[50,51]

In another study, Jemmott and Magliore[52] examined the relationship between academic stress, social support and salivary concentration of S-IgA. Whole, unstimulated saliva samples were collected from 15 students 5 days prior to their final examinations, during the actual examinations, and 14 days after the last examinations. A decrease in S-IgA levels was found during the time of examinations. Furthermore, the study showed the effect of social support on the subjects' responses: students who had greater social support (relative to their needs of social support) had consistently higher S-IgA levels compared with their peers reporting less adequate support.

Although some authors claim that assessing S-IgA to measure students' stress during examination periods may not be as useful as expected,[53] the development and use of more sensitive methods to assess S-IgA quantities can increase the effectiveness of this method.

It has been suggested that S-IgA levels may correlate with general personality traits, such as need for power, trait anxiety, or sense of humor. For example, among 27 male college students, those who were found to have a high need for power, a high rate of inhibition, and a high power stress were also found to have relatively low rates of S-IgA. Furthermore, the lower S-IgA rates were significantly associated with reports of more frequent illness.[51]

Lower S-IgA secretion rates were also associated with the anxiety,[54] and the daily mood of the subjects.[55] S-IgA levels were found to be depressed on days with relatively high-negative mood and elevated on days with relatively high-positive mood.[55]

Furthermore, the concentration of S-IgA in saliva was found to correlate with positive emotional states and sense of humor.[56,57] Subjects showed an increase in the amount of their S-IgA levels after viewing a humorous film but not after viewing a didactic film. The subjects' initial levels of S-IgA were found to positively correlate with their scores on a Coping Humor Scale (a measure of subject's reported tendency to make use of humor to cope with stressors).[56]

Martin and Dobbin[57] used saliva samples to determine S-IgA levels in subjects who were also assessed for their sense of humor (by Situational Humor Response Questionnaire, Coping Humor Scale, and Sense of Humor Questionnaire), and their sensitivity to stress due to minor, irritating, day-to-day events (Daily Hassles Scale). Their hypothesis was that sense of humor moderates the relationship between stressors and mood disturbance and, as such, may also moderate the immunosuppressive effects of stress.

The study revealed a weak, but significant, negative relationship between stressors and S-IgA. A negative correlation between frequency of hassles and S-IgA was also shown, suggesting an immunosuppressive effect of hassles. Furthermore, a significant moderating effect was found on humor measures and the relationship between hassles and S-IgA. Subjects with low scores on the humor scales showed a strong negative relationship between hassles and S-IgA, whereas those with high scores on the humor scales revealed virtually no relationship between these two variables.

Undoubtedly, chronic and acute stress can adversely affect the IgA concentration in saliva and can, as such, increase susceptibility to various infections of the oral cavity and the upper respiratory tract. The effect of stress on an increased susceptibilty of subjects to upper respiratory tract infections has been reported.[58-61]

II. STRESS AND SOFT TISSUES IN THE ORAL CAVITY

Several pathologies of the oral soft tissues have been shown to be associated with stress. These include conditions such as acute necrotizing ulcerative gingivitis (ANUG), recurrent herpes labialis (RHL), recurrent aphthous ulcerations (RAU), and periodontal disease. The effect of psychophysiological responses on diseases of the oral soft tissues was summarized in 1984 by Rugh et al.[3] (for a more extensive literature review, the reader is referred to this source).

A. STRESS AND ANUG

ANUG is one of the oral pathologies most often associated with stress. The possible relationship between stress and ANUG was initially described by numerous clinical case reports.[62-65] In an early study, Grupe et al.[66] reported a relatively high occurrence of ANUG (2.2%) among recent army inductees, which could have originated from mental stress.

Goldhaber and Giddon[67] accepted psychophysiological mechanisms as a possible etiology of ANUG. They reported that three times as many students with ANUG had sought psychiatric help than students without ANUG. Other epidemiological studies conducted on students and soldiers under stress further support this notion.[68,69]

To investigate whether there is a specific ANUG-prone personality, Formicola et al.[70] gave the Edwards Personal Preference Profile to 82 naval aviation students. A significant correlation was found between two personalty traits, dominance and abasement, and ANUG. While the former trait indicates the need to be in constant dominance, the latter suggests a lack of ability to humble oneself. These two traits characterize the type of individual who would find it difficult to adjust to the military environment and react with increased stress, increasing the probability of ANUG.

B. RECURRENT HERPES LABIALIS (RHL) AND RECURRENT APHTOUS ULCERATIONS (RAU)

The association between stress and occurrence of the oral conditions of RHL and RAU has been suggested by both clinical observations and epidemiological research.[71-77] Sircus et al.[76] reported an incidence of approximately 19% of RAU among 1738 patients in Great Britain. The study focused on 120 positive cases of RAU and included parameters of psychiatric assessment of 55 patients, some of whom maintained diaries concerning the incidence of the lesions. Of the patients suffering from RAU, 21% indicated that the appearance of lesions was usually preceded by periods of mental stress associated with domestic problems (including financial or sexual). Of the 55 cases which were psychiatrically evaluated, 33% showed a recognizable mental illness. The diagnoses included chronic anxiety, hysteria, obsession, hypochondria, paranoia, and epilepsy. Severe and emotional stress immediately preceded the onset of ulceration in approximately 60% of these patients.

In several epidemiological studies, Ship et al.[72-75] reported that about half of the population surveyed (student bodies of the Schools of Medicine, Dentistry, Dental Hygiene, Veterinary Medicine, Graduate Nursing, and Hospital Nursing of the University of Pennsylvania) had a history of RAU and about 38% had a history of RHL. A strong relationship between emotional factors and RAU was found. The severity of the disease appeared to be related to emotional factors and showed increased activity during times of increased stress, such as major examination periods. As recorded by monthly diaries by those suffering from RAU, subjects responded to periods of examinations with increased disease activity, while a decrease in the number of lesions was noted during periods of vacation.

Katcher et al.[78] attempted to predict the incidence of RHL from psychological measures, such as the Cornell Medical Index, the Johns Hopkins Symptom Index, the Clyde Mood Scale, and a social assets inventory. The social assets measure both variables related to social class (e.g., occupation, ethnicity, nationality, religion, and parents' education) and aspects of the individual's personal history (e.g., early relationship with parents, success in school, and extracurricular and social activity). The questionnaire was intended to be a measure of perceived personal success in acquiring and achieving desirable social attributes.

In the study, 49 nursing students were asked to keep daily calendars for 6 months on the onset of symptoms. A significant positive correlation was shown between incidence of RHL and the unhappy factor of Clyde Mood Scale and a significant negative correlation with the social assets score. Low social assets scores were found to correlate significantly with increased incidence of RHL. Nursing students who judged themselves as more typically unhappy tended to have more incidences of RHL.

However, the use of the Clyde Mood Scale as a possible predictor of RHL incidence did not yield positive results in follow-up studies of similar populations.[79,80] The most useful predictors of RHL incidence were found to be biological and historical measures of previous or current RHL experiences and the illness experience of the subjects as measured by the frequency of upper respiratory infections.[80]

C. STRESS AND PERIODONTAL DISEASE

Rugh et al.[3] summarized numerous studies which suggest a relationship between periodontal disease and emotional conditions. The studies include clinical case reports, correlational studies which look for a possible relationship between periodontal disease and personality characteristics or emotional disorders, quasi-experimental studies where individuals were assessed over time while exposed to naturally occurring stress, and experimental laboratory studies in animals.

The review quotes several case reports which note personality difficulties or emotional conditions in patients with periodontitis, gingivitis, and alveolar bone loss. De Marco,[81] for example, showed a disproportionally severe alveolar bone loss among a group of 11 veterans of the Vietnam War. The study presented a dramatic change in the alveolar bone height of one subject before and after military service. The author concluded that the alveolar bone loss was probably associated with stress and suggested naming the disease entity "periodontal emotional stress syndrome". Similarly, Krasner[82] presented seven case studies in which emotional stress caused increased caries activity, periodontitis, or ridge resorption.

The correlational studies reveal evidence of increased emotional and/or personality disturbances in patients with clinical periodontal conditions, e.g., a relationship between pathological periodontal conditions and traits of neurotic tendency and introversion-extraversion,[83] a positive correlation between periodontal disease and the anxiety scale of MMPI,[84] and a positive relationship between periodontal pathology and the MMPI hysteria scale.[85]

Studies which correlate periodontal status and naturally occurring stressful life situations point toward a relationship between emotional conditions and periodontal disease. Most of these studies refer to ANUG. A possible causal correlation was also suggested by several laboratory animal studies.[3]

A more recent study relating periodontal disease to chronic stress originating from life events was conducted by Green et al.[88] The study limited its focus to subjects prone to develop somatic symptoms (those most likely to manifest stress through somatic symptoms). Stressful life events were quantified with the Life Experience Survey (LES). Subjects rated the desirability and impact of each event they personally experienced during the past year (e.g., bereavement, divorce, job loss, illness) and their periodontal status was recorded. Evidence of somatic symptomatology was assessed with the Somatization (SOM) sub-scale of the Brief Symptom Inventory (BSI) which reflects distress originating from perceptions of bodily dysfunction.

Although the study did not use individual periodontal disease measurements (such as pocket depth or gingival index), and related only to general periodontal conditions, life events stress measurements were significantly correlated with periodontal disease. The general periodontal disease was found to be more severe and widespread as stressors increased. It was concluded that human periodontal disease is related to life events and that those with higher scores on the SOM sub-scale of the BSI are particularly prone to manifest periodontal disease as a stress-related condition.

1. Possible Mechanisms Mediating Stress and Periodontal Disease

The most possible mediator of stress and periodontal disease acts through the effect of stress on salivary flow and composition (see also Chapter 9.I).

Some suggest that stress-associated changes in the level of corticosteroid hormones in saliva and in the circulatory system affect changes in the periodontium. Others propose stress-induced changes in vasculization which influence the flow of nutrients or metabolic by-products to and from cells (see Rugh et al.[3] for a literature review).

Recently, newly-discovered neuropharmacological substances have been reported as possible mediators of the interrelationship between stress and periodontal disease.[87] Apparently, peptide hormones, such as substance P and bombesin affect not only the neurological system but also such behavior as drinking, eating, sexual drive, pain, and pleasure.[88] These aspects of mood can, therefore, influence behaviors such as diet (nutrition) or change in oral hygiene habits. Peptide hormones can also induce changes in lymphocyte cells which lead to the production of other hormones (i.e., growth hormones) and vasoactive intestine peptides. As lymphocytes are a common inflammatory cell of the periodontium, mood can presumably affect the periodontal condition in this manner.[87]

III. STRESS AND CARIES SUSCEPTIBILITY

Most of the research proposing a possible connection between stress and caries activity has been conducted on animals. Caries incidence has been shown to increase when the animals were subjected to different "stressors," such as separation of mother from the newborn litter, withholding of food, loud noises, electric shock, etc.[3]

In an initial epidemiological study conducted on humans, Manhold and Manhold[89] found a significant correlation between DMF ratings in 50 subjects and their personality scores on the Bernreuter Personality Inventory. These findings were not fully replicated in a study conducted on 266 naval aviation cadets,[90] but the overall findings pointed toward a possible relationship between personality variables and dental caries.

Although anxiety and DMFT scores did not correlate,[91] a possible connection between emotional factors and caries activity continued to intrigue the dental community. In 1962, Sutton attempted to correlate acute dental caries with circumstances of stressful life events in 661 patients.[92] The data indicated that 96% of patients who suffered from acute caries had undergone some severe mental stress. In most cases, stress was said to have been several months old.

A continuing study confirmed these findings.[93] The delay between the onset of mental stress and the development of acute dental caries was considerably less than 1 month. Case reports of patients in whom increased caries activity was preceded by periods of increased personal stress were also described by Krasner.[82]

A. POSSIBLE MECHANISMS MEDIATING STRESS AND CARIES ACTIVITY

The mechanism which apparently mediates most of the effects of stress on caries activity acts through saliva. The effect of saliva on bacterial adherence and colonization in the oral cavity, its buffering activity, and regulation of the ionic environment are some of the saliva-dependent processes affecting caries activity.[94]

Stress can potentially affect both the quantity (flow) and quality (pH, cortisol, IgA) of saliva. These changes can concomitantly lead to increased adherence and generation of plaque-forming bacteria on tooth surfaces and to increased caries susceptibility.[30]

Recently, Sutton[95] raised a new hypothesis regarding the mechanisms which mediate the association between mental stress and acute dental caries. He referred to the findings which demonstrate a flow of fluid and an active passage of ions, from the pulp through the dentin and enamel to the tooth surface. According to this hypothesis, the active movement of ions through the tooth is accompanied by a passage of lymphokines. The occurrence of chronic stress affects the pulpal tissues and disturbs this passage, thus reducing the reparative processes in enamel and the efficacy of the immune system at the tooth surface. The result would be a decrease in the enamel's defense against bacterial attack and a possible development of acute dental caries soon after the onset of stress.

IV. EFFECT OF STRESS ON LOCAL ANESTHESIA

The dentist's dedication to preventing pain is his/her most important concern regarding the patient.[96] The imminence of immediate physical harm, namely possible pain associated with dental treatment, is a primary factor causing stress in the dental situation. Indeed, many patients expect treatment to be painful in some way and report fear of pain as a major factor in their anxiety of dental treatment.[97]

Pain and anxiety are closely related. While the existence of acute pain usually leads to anxiety, the presence of anxiety can also influence the experience of pain (see Chapter 3).[98-106] In a double-blind human study, the degree of anxiety immediately before a performed pain test had a considerable and highly significant effect on the pain-intensity time curve.[100] The greater the increase of anxiety, the shorter time lapse before a certain pain level was reached.

Acute stress of any kind can profoundly influence the experience of pain. It can lead to stress-induced analgesia or hyperalgesia, depending on the "stressor" and emotional and cognitive variables.

Most animal and human studies concerning the interrelationship between stress and pain suggest that a variety of noxious and nonnoxious stressors can cause an increased pain threshold.[107] This phenomenon is generally referred to as stress-induced analgesia and has been regarded as a model for the environmental activation of endogenous pain-control mechanisms.

For example, in animal studies a mild physical stressor (15 min of vibration) caused stress-induced analgesia in some rats and hyperalgesia in others.[108] In another study, merely the anticipation of the painful stimulus acted as a specific stressor.[109] Male rats which were exposed repeatedly to a painful stimulus developed analgesia almost immediately after transferring to the conditioning box even if the physical stressor was absent. Furthermore, stress-induced analgesia was also influenced by emotions such as depression (chronically-stressed rats were significantly more analgesic than controls)[110] and by a past history of stress (animals exposed to shock 10 d before the experiment showed a significant attenuation of shock-induced analgesia).[111]

In humans, stress-induced analgesia among Vietnam veterans suffering from posttraumatic stress disorder has been reported. Among this population, a 30% decrease in pain intensity ratings of standardized heat stimuli was found after watching a combat videotape (a stressful stimulus).[112]

A. PROBLEMS IN ACHIEVING LOCAL ANESTHESIA IN THE DENTAL SETTING

Dental clinicians are familiar with cases where proper local anesthesia is difficult or impossible to achieve. Some patients pose a major problem, as they continually complain of pain despite all efforts to anesthesize the area being treated.

The percentage of clinical failures in achieving adequate local anesthesia during treatment ranges between 2 and 20%. The percentages are highest when failures occur after an initial attempt (e.g., 20% for mandibular block). Failure to achieve proper anesthesia after repeated injections is about 1.5%.[113] These results are similar to those reported by Cowan[114] regarding maxillary infiltration and mental block.

The factors mentioned as possible reasons for failure to achieve sufficient local anesthesia include anatomic variation, positive aspirations, and infection.[113,115,116] However, in view of the possible hyperalgetic effects of anxiety and stress, their influence on the effectiveness of local anesthesia cannot be overlooked.

An initial observation that highly fearful and apprehensive patients experience more difficulty in obtaining sufficient anesthesia was presented by Scheutz[117] with regard to drug addicts. This group is characterized by high general anxiety and high fear and aversion to intraoral injections. Drug addicts were more difficult to anesthesize and experienced a higher proportion of unwanted side effects (pallor, palpitations) than a control group. Although the results are difficult to interpret (the difficulty in achieving local anesthesia may be due to the drug concentration present in the blood, rather than the stress due to anxiety), it is possible that apprehension during dental treatment influences the ability to achieve proper local anesthesia.

A different approach has been adopted by Kaufman et al.[115] The study surveyed 93 general dental practitioners, as to their experience with patients who failed to feel numb after being administered local anesthesia. The majority of dentists (90%) reported some anesthetic failure during restorative visits 5 years prior to the survey. Unlike the authors' original hypothesis, no association was found between years of experience and percentage of failure reported. Furthermore, a similar percentage of at least one anesthetic failure was also found among dental students in a continuing study.[118] The dentists indicated that a high percentage (47%) of patients who did not experience numbness were fearful or anxious.[115]

A positive association between fear of dental treatment and the probability of unsuccessful dental anesthesia was also found by Weinstein et al.[119] The patient's perception of failure to achieve optimal local anesthesia was evaluated. The probability of unsuccessful local anesthesia was greater in those who were afraid of treatment.

Stress caused by fear and anxiety from dental treatment can adversely affect one's ability to achieve local anesthesia and can cause other undesired responses (drop in blood pressure, tachycardia, hyperventilation, and even hysterical blindness).[120,121]

B. POSSIBLE MECHANISMS MEDIATING STRESS AND PAIN

Recent research suggests that the mechanism which mediates stress and pain results from activation of an endogenous opioid peptide system. The evidence that stress induces endogenous opioid activity, which concomitantly leads to stress-induced analgesia, is primarily based on animal studies that use opioid antagonists (especially Naloxone) to block the analgesic effects of the opioid system. Antagonist drugs have been shown to neutralize the analgesia induced by stressful stimuli in animal studies.[107,109,122-127]

Several studies suggest that the mechanisms mediating stress and pain in humans are based on the same pharmacological pathways. For example, the stress-induced analgesia induced in Vietnam veterans by a combat videotape was not recorded when subjects were under the effect of Naloxone.[112]

Bandura et al.[128] showed that the endogenous opioid system can also be activated by perceived inefficacy in exercising control over cognitive stressors. (Perceived self-efficacy is concerned with beliefs in one's capability to mobilize the motivation, cognitive resources, and course of action needed to meet given situational demands.) The study was based on psychological stress resulting from a condition in which perceived environmental demands strain or exceed individual perceived coping capabilities.

Subjects were asked to perform mathematical operations under conditions in which they could exercise full control over the cognitive task demands, or under conditions in which the cognitive demands strained or exceeded their cognitive capabilities. Changes in perceived mathematical self-efficacy, their level of autonomic arousal during the cognitive stressor task, and subjective distress, mental strain, and perceived performance impairment were measured. Following induction of high and low levels of perceived mathematical self-efficacy, subjects at each level of self-efficacy were administered with either an inert saline solution or Naloxone.

Subjects who perceived themselves as unable to exercise control over the cognitive demands experienced a high stress level, whereas subjects who had a strong sense of controlling efficacy were relatively unperturbed by the cognitive task. When painfully stimulated, the self-inefficacious stressed subjects showed stress-induced analgesia (were able to withstand increasing amounts of pain stimulation) under the effect of saline. However, when the endogenous opioid mechanisms were blocked by Naloxone, the same subjects were unable to endure much pain stimulation. On the other hand, the self-efficacious, nonstressed subjects showed no evidence of opioid activation. Their pain tolerance did not change across repeated tests, either under saline or Naloxone treatments.

V. SYNCOPE IN THE DENTAL CHAIR

Syncope in the dental chair is a relatively rare occurrence. Approximately 2.5% of patients who receive anesthesia report some side effects, such as pallor, nausea, sweating, dizziness and fainting.[129] In spite of its relative rareness, syncope and even cardiac arrest can occur in the dental operatory, causing severe stress to both patient and dentist.

Several cases of cardiac arrest have been presented in the dental literature.[130,131] Three cases of death under local anesthetic were reported in England and Wales between 1963 and 1968.[130] Another report[131] described an apparently healthy 52-year-old man who collapsed under local anesthetic and suffered cardiac arrest. Successful resuscitation saved his life.

The occurrence of syncope in the dental chair is usually blamed on the intravascular injection of local anesthetic or on some previously undetected pathology; however, in many cases, fainting is a consequence of emotional factors.

Psychological stress has been reported to be a risk factor in sudden cardiac death in individuals without underlying structural heart disease. Brodsky et al.[132] identified 6 patients (out of a group of 80) who experienced life-threatening tachyarrhythmia without underlying structural heart disease. Of these patients, 5 experienced marked psychological stress. Cases have been described in which sudden and rapid death were attributed to psychological stress (e.g., loss of status or self-esteem, situations which present real or symbolic personal danger, etc.).[133]

Apprehensive individuals who experience or face injury, only seldom develop cardiac arrest. The usual reaction is a collapse followed by a quick recovery, generally referred to as vasodepressor (or vasovagal) syncope or fainting. Fainting can occur at any phase of treatment — on first entering the office or even sitting in the dental chair. The most predisposing factors usually comprise some kind of emotional stress evoked by fear of treatment; sudden, unexpected pain; sight of blood; threatening instruments; etc.[134]

Engel[135] summarized the psychological determinants implicated in vasodepressor syncope. In all cases physical injury, or threat of injury, was a major factor in fainting. However, psychological and social factors are crucial. Vasodepressor syncope is more likely to occur when one is relatively unfamiliar with the physical injury or threat, or when one is unable to cope with previous events. The likelihood of fainting increases even more when the injury or threat occurs under circumstances that one feels (rightly or not) expected to face with equanimity or courage.

Developmental factors, personal and cultural, render some individuals highly susceptible to vasodepressor fainting and others virtually immune. The need to exaggerate bravery, strength, and aggressiveness, and to deny or minimize fear, are classic reasons for vasodepressor syncope. Fainting is likely to occur when the individual feels there is no escape from the situation provoking the dilemma. A classic example is the obligation to submit to frightening, possibly painful, and unfamiliar treatment procedures.

In a study by Schmidt,[136] volunteers who fainted during blood donation showed significantly higher scores on seven of the ten clinical scores of the MMPI, indicating emotional hyperactivity as a possible reason for the vasovagal syncope.

Sledge[137] conducted a study concerning the antecedent psychological factors in the onset of vasovagal syncope among a group of U.S. Air Force active duty personnel on flying status. In most fainting cases, the individuals were explicitly thinking of a situation (either in fantasy or reality) in which the outcome was potentially harmful to them. In some cases the sense of harm derived from a fear of bodily harm (dental visit, injection, suture removal, etc.) or psychological harm (harmed by the examination, fear of fainting and the ensuing embarrassment, etc.). Frequently, patients perceived harm as coming from foreign, incompetent, or untrustworthy individuals, particularly when the social context was a medical procedure. In all instances of psychological harm, the harm involved a feeling of public ridicule and mortification.

In Western culture, the vasodepressor syncope is more common among men than women, especially in settings where the man feels the surrounding is one of strong social disapproval of any display of weakness.[134,135] Society does not permit men to readily express fear. Fear that is repressed can often manifest itself in a higher incidence of vasodepressor syncope. Therefore, vasodepressor syncope is a relatively rare occurrence in pediatric patients. Children express their fears by yelling, crying, and moving about, unlike the more inhibited typical adult man. The most commonly encountered dental situation of vasodepressor syncope is probably the administration of a local anesthetic to an anxious man under the age of 35.[134]

Anticipated physical threat and social disapproval of fear manifestation is especially common in the dental setting. Although many patients view treatment as a threat, the general expectation is for the patient to submit to treatment with no apparent apprehension. Some patients choose to avoid the dilemma by developing individual coping mechanisms, such as gagging (see Chapter 5) or fainting. Once fainting has occurred, and has served as an adequate means to avoid the conflict, it may then serve as a reinforcment which increases the probability of fainting during subsequent confrontations. Patients develop a "fainting-prone" behavior that "protects" them from the need to face treatment. Reluctance from the dentist to treat patients with such a medical history further reinforces the negative pattern.

VI. FATIGUE AND ASSOCIATED SYMPTOMS AND THEIR POSSIBLE RELATION TO THE ORAL CAVITY

In several publications, Eidelman[138-142] attempted to relate some phenomena, generally perceived as a psychogenic origin (e.g., fatigue at rest, vertigo, tension, irritability), with physiological findings in the oral cavity.

A syndrome of "fatigue at rest" is described by Eidelman as the feeling of energy loss experienced during or after adequate rest. The patient complains of waking up feeling tired, of frequently having the desire to sleep, and of never feeling fresh, no matter how much rest. The sensation of fatigue vanishes as soon as the patient starts work or becomes actively engaged.[138] Fatigue and general weakness have been described in cases of suspected chronic mercury poisoning;[143] however, no correlation was found between fatigue and the mean number of amalgam surfaces in the patients' mouths.[144]

Eidelman presented several clinical cases in which locally asymptomatic, unerupted, impacted teeth were directly associated with "fatigue at rest."[138] Although the impacted teeth were generally asymptomatic, situations and factors that produced stress led to aggravation of symptoms. While relief of the stress factors resulted in the amelioration of associated symptoms, the "fatigue at rest" remained, and disappeared only after patients were surgically treated. After removal of the impacted teeth, conditions of stress no longer provoked the symptoms.

Other cases are described with regard to symptoms of vertigo, blurred vision, nausea, tension, and irritability.[140] Three cases were presented in which removal of a suspected dental pathology (e.g., periapical granuloma) resulted in rapid and permanent cure of symptoms earlier diagnosed as "psychogenic."

Eidelman pointed out that physicians investigating the etiology of headache, vertigo, and fatigue generally neglect examining the mandible and maxilla.[141,142] Although some symptoms are generally referred to as having a psychogenic origin, the possible impact of pathophysiological features should not be overlooked.

VII. THE MULTI-ALLERGIC PATIENT

Occasionally, a patient enters the dental surgery and presents the dentist with a history of hypersensitivity to all local anesthetic agents. The history may include reports of immediate reactions to the application of the anesthetic (dizziness, shortness of breath, tachycardia, etc.) or delayed reactions (swelling, urticaria, etc.).[120,145-147]

In most cases, such a history includes apprehension on the part of the patient with regard to the use of the drug in question, and even greater apprehension from the dentist to treat the "problematic" patient.

The true incidence of local anesthetic allergy is low,[134,148-150] most being delayed reactions, such as contact dermatitis.[151] Barer and McAllen[152] expressed serious doubts as to whether true allergy to lidocaine had ever been shown. Tests *in vitro* were found unreliable and the proportion of false positive skin tests could be as high as 25% among atopic patients. deShazo and Nelson[153] claimed that most patients labeled as "allergic to local anesthetics" were, in fact, not allergic.

When carefully evaluated, most adverse reactions to local anesthetic are found to be psychogenic in nature. Fear of injection, or of dental treatment in general, may lead to some of the most frightening "allergic" reactions — tachycardia and vasodepressor syncope. Even a patient with a former diagnosis of allergy may often turn out to be nonallergic[120,145,153-157]

Babajews and Ivanyi[154] investigated 37 patients with a previous history of "allergy" to local anesthetic drugs by *in vivo* (intradermal injection) and *in vitro* (lymphocyte transformation) tests. Of these, 34 patients did not respond to either test, suggesting that the clinical diagnosis of "allergy" was not justified.

A false diagnosis of "allergy to local anesthetic," classifying the patient as unable to receive routine dental treatment, may lead to severe adverse consequences. Many apparently "allergic" patients are eventually able to receive routine treatment after their fear is properly addressed[120] However, if wrongly labeled as "allergic", their dental condition may deteriorate significantly due to their "inability" to receive appropriate dental care.[145]

Shapira and Rubinow[158] suggested treating these patients with progressively increasing concentrations of lidocaine, a procedure which both negates the presence of undesired reactions and reduces the patient's anxiety toward possible negative consequences of local analgesia.

Nevertheless, there are some cases where true hypersensitivity to local anesthetic agents does exist. Local injection may lead to catastrophic results (anaphylactic shock) or to unusual skin reactions, localized edema in the area of injection, development of joint pain, tenderness, and malaise.[153,159] In one case, multiple sensitivities to amide local anesthetics was described in a 70-year-old patient, including hypersensitivity to lidocaine, prilocaine, mepivacaine, and dibucaine.[160] In another case, a reproducible anaphylactic reaction to lidocaine was reported in a 43-year-old woman.[161]

If the presence of allergy has been confirmed and if the recommendations include prohibiting the use of local anesthetic agents, the patient can pose severe problems for the dentist. Even when the patient in question is not apprehensive, the prospect of treatment with no appropriate local anesthesia and the anticipation of unavoidable pain, generally lead to stress and physiological arousal. The need to treat a tense and suffering patient confronts the dentist with a stressful situation and often leads to rejection of the patient under a variety of excuses.

As treatment of these patients under deep sedation or general anesthesia is often contraindicated, nonpharmaceutical methods of analgesia can sometimes be used, such as electronic dental anesthesia, hypnosis, etc.[146,162] (see also Chapter 11).

VIII. SUMMARY

Stress affects many physiological conditions in the oral cavity. It influences the quantity and quality of saliva, the concentration of salivary cortisol and salivary IgA. It is positively correlated with various pathological conditions, such as ANUG, recurrent herpes labialis, recurrent aphthous ulcerations, and even periodontal disease and caries susceptibility.

The mutual effect between stress and psychophysiological mechanisms can lead to serious patient management problems (difficulty in achieving local anesthesia, or causing patient syncope in the dental chair).

REFERENCES

1. **Wolff, H. G.,** *Stress and Disease*, Charles C. Thomas, Springfield, IL, 1953, chap. 1.
2. **Giddon, D. B.,** Psychophysiology of the oral cavity, *J. Dent. Res.*, 45, 1627, 1966.
3. **Rugh, J. D., Jacobs, D. T., Taverna, R. D., and Johnson, R. W.,** Psychophysiological changes and oral conditions, in *Social Sciences and Dentistry, A Critical Bibliography*, Vol. 2, Cohen, L. K. and Bryant, P. S., Eds., Quintessence Publishing, Chicago, 1984.
4. **Brown, C. C.,** The parotid puzzle: a review of the literature on human salivation and its application to psychophysiology, *Psychophysiology*, 7, 66, 1970.
5. **Izutsu, K. T.,** Physiological aspects of salivary gland function, *Compendium Continuing Edu. Dent.*, Suppl. 13, S450, 1989.
6. **Ferguson, D. B.,** Current diagnostic uses of saliva, *J. Dent. Res.*, 66, 420, 1987.
7. **Mandel, I. D.,** Sialochemistry in diseases and clinical situations affecting salivary glands, *Crit. Rev. Clin. Lab. Sci.*, 12, 321, 1980.
8. **Sreebny, L. M.,** Salivary flow in health and disease, *Compendium Continuing Edu. Dent.*, Supplement 13, S461, 1989.
9. **Chauncey, H. H., Winer, R. A., and Barber, T. X.,** Influence of verbal suggestion on the parotid gland response to gustatory stimuli, in *Proc. Soc. Exp. Biol. Med.*, 116, 898, 1964.
10. **Jenkins, G. N. and Dawes, C.,** The psychic flow of saliva in man, *Arch. Oral Biol.*, 11, 1203, 1966.

11. **Hiramatsu, R.,** Direct assay of cortisol in human saliva by solid phase radioimmunoassay and its clinical applications, *Clin. Chim. Acta*, 117, 239, 1981.
12. **Riad-Fahmy, D., Read, G. F., and Walker, R. F.,** Salivary steroid assays for assessing variation in endocrine activity, *J. Steroid Biochem.*, 19, 265, 1983.
13. **Fox, P. C.,** Saliva composition and its importance in dental health, *Compendium Continuing Edu. Dent.*, Suppl. 13, S457, 1989.
14. **Morse, D. R., Schacterle, G. R., Furst, M. L., and Bose, K.,** Stress, relaxation, and saliva: a pilot study involving endodontic patients, *Oral Surg. Oral Med. Oral Pathol.*, 52, 308, 1981.
15. **Rice, B.,** The new truth machines, *Psychol. Today*, 12, 61, 1978.
16. **Winsor, A. L.,** The effect of mental effort on parotid secretion, *Am. J. Psychol.*, 43, 434, 1931.
17. **Lazarus, R. S.,** *Patterns of Adjustment and Human Effectiveness*, McGraw-Hill, New York, 1969.
18. **Bogdonoff, M. D., Bogdonoff, M. M., and Wolf, S. G., Jr.,** Studies on salivary function in man: variations in secretory rate as part of the individual's adaptive pattern, *J. Psychosom. Res.*, 5, 170, 1961.
19. **Hafner, R. J.,** Relationships between personality and autonomic nervous reactions to stress, *J. Psychosom. Res.*, 18, 181, 1974.
20. **Hafner, R. J.,** Physiological changes with stress in depression and obsessional neurosis, *J. Psychosom. Res.*, 18, 175, 1974.
21. **Corcoran, D. W. J.,** The relation between introversion and salivation, *Am. J. Psychol.*, 77, 298, 1964.
22. **Eysenck, S. B. and Eysenck, H. J.,** Salivary response to lemon juice as a measure of introversion, *Percept. Mot. Skills*, 24, 1047, 1967.
23. **Bates, J. F. and Adams, D.,** The influence of mental stress on the flow of saliva in man, *Arch. Oral Biol.*, 13, 593, 1968.
24. **Silverstein, L. and Iverson, M. A.,** Human salivary response to to interpersonal bargaining situations: a psycho-physiological investigation, *Psychol. Rep.*, 37, 771, 1975.
25. **Bricken, H.,** The effect of metal stress on the pH of the saliva: a preliminary study, *J. Dent. Med.*, 8, 96, 1953.
26. **Morse, D. R., Schacterle, G. R., Furst, M. L., Goldberg, J., Greenspan, B., Swiecinski, D., and Susek, J.,** The effect of stress and meditation on salivary protein and bacteria: a review and pilot study, *J. Hum. Stress*, 8(4), 31, 1982.
27. **Morse, D. R., Schacterle, G. R., Esposito, J. V., Furst, M. L., and Bose, K.,** Stress, relaxation and saliva: a follow-up study involving clinical endodontic patients, *J. Hum. Stress*, 7(1), 19, 1981.
28. **Morse, D. R., Schacterle, G. R., Eposito, J. V., Chod, S. D., Furst, M. L., DiPonziano, J., and Zaydenberg, M.,** Stress, meditation and saliva: a study of separate salivary gland secretions in endodontic patients, *J. Oral Med.*, 38, 150, 1983.
29. **Morse, D. R., Schacterle, G. R., Furst, L., Zaydenberg, M., and Pollack, R. L.,** Oral digestion of a complex-carbohydrate cereal: effects of stress and relaxation on physiological and salivary measures, *Am. J. Clin. Nutr.*, 49, 97, 1989.
30. **Morse, D. R., Schacterle, G. R., Furst, M. L., Esposito, J. V., and Zaydenburg, M.,** Stress, relaxation and saliva: relationship to dental caries and its prevention, with a literature review, *Ann. Dent.*, 42, 47, 1983.
31. **Morse, D. R., Schacterle, G. R., Martin, J. S., DiPonziano, J., Zaydenbrg, M., Esposito, J. V., Chod, S. D., and Furst, M. L.,** Stress and relaxation: evaluation by questionnaire, salivary changes and physiological responses in a trained meditator, *J. Oral Med.*, 39, 142, 1984.
32. **Morse, D. R., Schacterle, G. R., Furst, M. L., Brokenshire, J., Butterworth, M., and Cacchio, J.,** Examination-induced stress in meditators and non-meditators as measured by salivary protein changes, *Stress*, 2, 20, 1981.

33. **Morse, D. R., Schacterle, G. R., Furst, M. L., Mericle, P., Mendel, G., and Merrian, S.,** Examination-induced stress as measured by changes in total salivary protein and salivary glycoprotein, *Stress*, 3, 14, 1982.
34. **Riad-Fahmy, D., Read, G., Walker, R., and Griffiths, K.,** Immuno-assay of steroids in saliva, in *Ninth Tenovus Workshop*, Alpha Omega, Cardiff, 1984.
35. **Ferguson, D. B., Ed.,** Steroid hormones in saliva, in *Frontiers of Oral Physiology*, Vol. 5, S. Karger, Basel, 1984.
36. **Gunnar, M. R.,** Studies of the human infant's adrenocortical response to potentially stressful events, *New Dir. Child Dev.*, 45, 3, 1989.
37. **Grauer, T. T.,** Environmental lighting, behavioral state, and hormonal response in the newborn, *Scholary Inquiry Nursing Pract.*, 3, 53, 1989.
38. **Machac, M, Machacova, H., Starka, L., and Hampl, R.,** Changes in cortisol level in saliva following relaxation-activation autoregulative intervention, *Act. Nerv. Super. (Praha)*, 29, 159, 1987.
39. **Tarui, H. and Nakamura, A.,** Saliva cortisol: a good indicator for acceleration stress, *Aviat. Space Environ. Med.*, 58, 573, 1987.
40. **Kakimoto, Y., Nakamura, A., Tarui, H., Nagasawa, Y., and Yagura, S.,** Crew workload in ASDF C-1 transport flights. I. Change in heart rate and salivary cortisol, *Aviat. Space Environ. Med.*, 59, 511, 1988.
41. **Bassett, J. R., Marshall, P. M., and Spillane, R.,** The physiological measurement of acute stress (public speaking) in bank employees, *Int. J. Psychophysiol.*, 5, 265, 1987.
42. **Hubert, W. and de Jong-Meyer, R.,** Emotional stress and saliva cortisol response, *J. Clin. Chem. Clin. Biol.*, 27, 235, 1989.
43. **Kirschbaum, C. and Hellhammer, D.,** Response variability of salivary cortisol under psychological stimulation, *J. Clin. Chem. Clin. Biol.*, 27, 237, 1989.
44. **Rahe, R. H., Karson, S., Howard, N. S., Jr., Rubin, R. T., and Poland, R. E.,** Psychological and physiological assessments on American hostages freed from captivity in Iran, *Psychosomatic Medicine*, 52, 1, 1990.
45. **Ben-Aryeh, H., Roll, R., Kahana, L., Malberger, E. Szargel, R., and Gutman, D.,** Saliva as an indicator of stress, *Int. J. Psychosom.*, 32, 3, 1985.
46. **Yodfat, Y. and Silvian, I.,** A prospective study of acute respiratory tract infections among children in a kibbutz: the role of secretory IgA and serum immunoglobulins, *J. Infect. Dis.*, 136, 26, 1977.
47. **Rossen, R. D., Butler, W. T., Waldman, R. H., Alford, R. H., Hornick, R. B., Togo, Y., and Kasel, J. A.,** The proteins in nasal secretion. II. A longitudinal study of IgA and neutralizing antibody levels in nasal washings from men infected with influenza virus, *J. Am. Med. Assoc.*, 211, 1157, 1970.
48. **Butler, W. T., Waldman, T. A., Rossen, R. D., Douglas, R. G., Jr., and Couch, R. B.,** Changes in IgA and IgG concentrations in nasal secretions prior to the appearance of antibody during viral respiratory infection in man, *J. Immunol.*, 105, 584, 1970.
49. **Jemmott, J. B., III, Borysenko, J. Z., Borysenko, M., McClelland, D. C., Chapman, R., Meyer, D., and Benson, H.,** Academic stress, power motivation, and decrease in secretion rate of salivary secretory immunoglobulin A, *Lancet*, 1, 1400, 1983.
50. **Jasnoski, M. L. and Kugler, J.,** Relaxation, imagery, and neuroimmunomodulation, *Ann. N. Y. Acad. Sci.*, 496, 722, 1987.
51. **McClelland, D. C., Floor, E., Davidson, R. J., and Saron, C.,** Stressed power motivation, sympathetic activation, immune function, and illness, *J. Hum. Stress*, 6(2), 11, 1980.
52. **Jemmott, J. B., III and Magloire, K.,** Academic stress, social support, and secretory immunoglobulin A, *J. Pers. Soc. Psychol.*, 55, 803, 1988.
53. **Mouton, C., Fillion, L., Tawadros, E., and Tessier, R.,** Salivary IgA is a weak stress marker, *Behav. Med.*, 15, 179, 1989.
54. **Graham, N. M. H., Bartholomeusz, R. C. A., Taboonpong, N., and La Brooy, J. T.,** Does anxiety reduce the secretion rate of secretory IgA in saliva, *Med. J. Austr.*, 148, 131, 1988.

55. **Stone, A. A., Cox, D. S., Valdimarsdottir, H., Jandorf, L., and Neale, J. M.,** Evidence that secretory IgA antibody is associated with daily mood, *J. Pers. Soc. Psychol.*, 52, 988, 1987.
56. **Dillon, K. M., Minchoff, B., and Baker, K. H.,** Positive emotional states and enhancement of the immune system, *Int. J. Psychiatry Med.*, 15, 13, 1985.
57. **Martin, R. A. and Dobbin, J. P.,** Sense of humor, hassles, and immunoglobulin A: evidence for a stress-moderating effect of humor, *Int. J. Psychiatry Med.*, 18, 93, 1988.
58. **Graham, N. M. H., Douglas, R. M., and Ryan, P.,** Stress and acute respiratory infection, *Am. J. Epidemiol.*, 124, 389, 1986.
59. **Boyce, W. T., Jensen, E. W., Cassel, J. C., Collier, A. M., Smith, A. H., and Ramy, C. T.,** Influence of life events and family routines on childhood respiratory tract illness, *Pediatrics*, 60, 609, 1977.
60. **Broadbent, D. E., Broadbent, M. H. P., Phillpotts, R. J., and Wallace, J.,** Some further studies on the prediction of experimental colds in volunteers by psychological factors, *J. Psychosom. Res.*, 28, 511, 1984.
61. **Totman, R., Kiff, J., Reed, S. E., and Craig, J. W.,** Predicting experimental colds in volunteers from different measures of recent life stress, *J. Psychosom. Res.*, 24, 155, 1980.
62. **Miller, S. C. and Firestone, J. M.,** Psychosomatic factors in periodontal disease, *Am. J. Orthod.*, 33, 675, 1947.
63. **Roth, H.,** Psychosomatic and nutritional factors related to recurrent necrotizing ulcerative gingivitis, *J. Am. Dent. Assoc.*, 42, 474, 1951.
64. **Roth, H. and Weiss, M.,** Recurrent acute necrotizing ulcerative gingivitis, *N. Y. State Dent. J.*, 17, 89, 1951.
65. **Moulton, R., Ewen, S., and Thieman, W.,** Emotional factors in periodontal disease, *Oral Surg. Oral Med. Oral Pathol.*, 5, 833, 1952.
66. **Grupe, H. E. and Wilder, L. S.,** Observations of necrotizing gingivitis in 870 military trainees, *J. Periodontol.*, 27, 254, 1956.
67. **Goldhaber, P. and Giddon, D. B.,** Present concepts concerning the etiology and treatment of acute necrotizing ulcerative gingivitis, *Int. Dent. J.*, 14, 468, 1964.
68. **Giddon, D. B., Zackin, S. J., and Goldhaber, P.,** Acute necrotizing ulcerative gingivitis in college students, *J. Am. Dent. Assoc.*, 68, 381, 1964.
69. **Shannon, I. L., Kilgore, W. G., and O'Leary, T. J.,** Stress as a predisposing factor in necrotizing ulcerative gingivitis, *J. Periodontol.*, 40, 240, 1969.
70. **Formicola, A. J., Witte, E. T., and Curran, P. M.,** A study of personality traits and acute necrotizing ulcerative gingivitis, *J. Periodontol.*, 41, 36, 1970.
71. **Kaufman, A. Y.,** Aphthous stomatitis as a featuring syndrome of emotional stress in dental treatment, *Quintessence Int.*, 7(9), 75, 1976.
72. **Ship, I. I., Morris, A. L., Durocher, R. T., and Burket, L. W.,** Recurrent aphthous ulcerations and recurrent herpes labialis in a professional school student population. I. Experience, *Oral Surg. Oral Med. Oral Pathol.*, 13, 1191, 1960.
73. **Ship, I. I., Morris, A. L., Durocher, R. T., and Burket, L. W.,** Recurrent aphthous ulcerations and recurrent herpes labialis in a professional school student population. II. Medical history, *Oral Surg. Oral Med. Oral Pathol.*, 13, 1317, 1960.
74. **Ship, I. I., Morris, A. L., Durocher, R. T., and Burket, L. W.,** Recurrent aphthous ulcerations and recurrent herpes labialis in a professional school student population. III. Oral examinations, *Oral Surg. Oral Med. Oral Pathol.*, 13, 1438, 1960.
75. **Ship, I. I., Morris, A. L., Durocher, R. T., and Burket, L. W.,** Recurrent aphthous ulcerations and recurrent herpes labialis in a professional school student population. IV. Twelve-month study of natural disease patterns, *Oral Surg. Oral Med. Oral Pathol.*, 14, 30, 1960.
76. **Sircus, W., Church, R., and Kelleher, J.,** Recurrent aphthous ulceration of the mouth: a study of the natural history, aetiology, and treatment, *Q. J. Med. New Ser.*, 26, 235, 1957.
77. **Dalmau, C. J., Zegarelli, E. V., Kutscher, A. H., and Cattell, J. P.,** Psychogenic factors in recurrent ulcerative stomatitis and idiopathic orolingual paresthesia, *J. Periodontol.*, 32, 58, 1961.

78. **Katcher, A. H., Brightman, V., Luborsky, L., and Ship, I.,** Prediction of the incidence of recurrent herpes labialis and systemic illness from psychological measurements, *J. Dent. Res.*, 52, 49, 1973.
79. **Luborsky, L., Mintz, J., Brightman, V. J., and Katcher, A. H.,** Herpes simplex virus and moods: a longitudinal study, *J. Psychosom. Res.*, 20, 543, 1976.
80. **Friedmann, E., Katcher, A. H., and Brightman, V. J.,** Incidence of recurrent herpes labialis and upper respiratory infection: a prospective study of the influence of biologic, social, and psychologic predictors, *Oral Surg. Oral Med. Oral Pathol.*, 43, 873, 1977.
81. **DeMarco, T. J.,** Periodontal emotional stress syndrome, *J. Periodontol.*, 47, 67, 1976.
82. **Krasner, D.,** Stress on a distal factor in dental disease, *J. Prev. Dent.*, 5, 24, 1978.
83. **Manhold, J. H., Lt.,** Report of a study on the relationship of personality variables to periodontal conditions, *J. Periodontol.*, 24, 248, 1953.
84. **Miller, S. C., Thaller, J. L., and Soberman, A.,** The use of the Minnesota multiphasic personality inventory as a diagnostic aid in periodontal disease: a preliminary report, *J. Periodontol.*, 27, 44, 1956.
85. **Baker, E. G., Crook, G. H., and Schwabacher, E. D.,** Personality correlates of periodontal disease, *J. Dent. Res.*, 40, 396, 1961.
86. **Green, L. W., Tryon, W. W., Marks, B., and Huryn, J.,** Periodontal disease as a function of life events stress, *J. Hum. Stress*, 12(1), 32, 1986.
87. **Wilton, J. M. A., Griffiths, G. S., Curtis, M. A., Maiden, M. F. J., Gillett, I. R., Wilson, D. T., Sterne, J. A. C., and Johnson, N. W.,** Detection of high-risk groups and individuals for periodontal diseases: Systemic predisposition and markers of general health, *J. Clin. Periodontol.*, 15, 339, 1988.
88. **Schmitt, F. O.,** Molecular regulators of brain function: A new view, *Neuroscience*, 13, 991, 1984.
89. **Manhold, J. H. and Manhold, V.,** A preliminary report on the study of the relationship of psychosomatics to oral conditions: relationship of personality to dental caries, *Science*, 110, 585, 1949.
90. **Manhold, J. H. and Rosenberg, N.,** Study of the possible relationship of personality variables to dental cavities, *J. Dent. Res.*, 33, 357, 1954.
91. **Phipps, G. T. and Marcuse, F. L.,** Anxiety and dental caries, *J. Dent. Res.*, 36, 862, 1957.
92. **Sutton, P. R. N.,** Mental stress and acute dental caries, *Nature (London)*, 195, 254, 1962.
93. **Sutton, P. R. N.,** The early onset of acute dental caries in adults following mental stress, *N. Y. State Dent. J.*, 31, 450, 1965.
94. **Mandel, I. D.,** Impact of saliva on dental caries, *Compendium Continuing Edu. Dent.*, Supplement 13, S476, 1989.
95. **Sutton, P. R. N.,** Acute dental caries, mental stress, immunity and the active passage of ions through the teeth, *Med. Hypotheses*, 31, 17, 1990.
96. **Corah, N. L., O'Shea, R. M., Bissell, G. D., Thines, T. J., and Mendola, P.,** The dentist-patient relationship: perceived dentist behaviors that reduce patient anxiety and increase satisfaction, *J. Am. Dent. Assoc.*, 116, 73, 1988.
97. **Wardle, J.,** Fear of dentistry, *Br. J. Med. Psychol.*, 55, 119, 1982.
98. **Bowers, K. S.,** Pain, anxiety, and perceived control, *J. Consult. Clin. Psychol.*, 32, 596, 1968.
99. **Weisenberg, M.,** Pain and pain control, *Psychol. Bull.*, 84, 1008, 1977.
100. **Von Graffenried, B., Adler, R., Abt, K., Nuesch, E., and Spiegel, R.,** The influence of anxiety and pain sensitivity on experimental pain in man, *Pain*, 4, 253, 1978.
101. **Klepac, R. K., McDonald, M., Hauge, G., and Dowling, J.,** Reactions to pain among subjects high and low in dental fear, *J. Behav. Med.*, 3, 373, 1980.
102. **Kent, G.,** Anxiety, pain and type of dental procedure, *Behav. Res. Ther.*, 22, 465, 1984.
103. **Green, R. M. and Green, A.,** Adult attitudes to dentistry among dental attenders in South Wales, *Br. Dent. J.*, 159, 157, 1985.
104. **Kent, G.,** Memory of dental pain, *Pain*, 21, 187, 1985.
105. **Sternbach, R. A.,** Clinical aspects of pain, in *The Psychology of Pain*, 2nd ed., Sternbach, R. A., Ed., Raven Press, New York, 1986, 223.

106. **Robin, O., Vinard, H., Vernet-Maury, E., and Saumet, J. T.,** Influence of sex and anxiety on pain theshold and tolerance, *Functional Neurol.*, 2, 173, 1987.
107. **Amit, Z. and Galina, Z. H.,** Stress induced analgesia plays an adaptive role in the organization of behavioral responding, *Brain Res. Bull.*, 21, 955, 1988.
108. **Jørum, E.,** Analgesia or hyperalgesia following stress correlates with emotional behavior in rats, *Pain*, 32, 341, 1988.
109. **Sumová, A. and Jakoubek, B.,** Analgesia and impact induced by anticipation stress: involvement of the endogenous opioid peptide system, *Brain Res.*, 503, 273, 1989.
110. **Pignatiello, M. F., Olson, G. A., Kastin, A. J., Ehrensing, R. H., McLean, J. H., and Olson, R. D.,** MIF-1 is active in a chronic stress animal model of depression, *Pharmacol. Biochem. Behav.*, 32, 737, 1989.
111. **Caggiula, A. R., Antelman, S. M., Aul, E., Knopf, S., and Edwards, D. J.,** Prior stress attenuates the analgesic response but sensitizes the corticosterone and cortical dopamine responses to stress 10 days later, *Psychopharmacology*, 99, 233, 1989.
112. **van der Kolk, B. A., Greenberg, M. S., Orr, S. P., and Pitman, R. K.,** Endogenous opioids, stress induced analgesia, and post-traumatic stress disorder, *Psychopharmacol. Bull.*, 25, 417, 1989.
113. **Rood, J. P.,** Some anatomical and physiological causes of failure to achieve mandibular anesthesia, *Br. J. Oral Surg.*, 15, 75, 1977.
114. **Cowan, A.,** Minimum dosage technique in the clinical comparison of representative modern local anesthetic agents, *J. Dent. Res.*, 43, 1228, 1964.
115. **Kaufman, E., Weinstein, P., and Milgrom, P.,** Difficulties in achieving local anesthesia, *J. Am. Dent. Assoc.*, 108, 205, 1984.
116. **Najjar, T. A.,** Why can't you achieve adequate regional anesthesia in the presence of infection?, *Oral Surg. Oral Med. Oral Pathol.*, 44, 7, 1977.
117. **Scheutz, F.,** Drug addicts and local analgesia: effectivity and general side effects, *Scand. J. Dent. Res.*, 90, 299, 1982.
118. **Milgrom, P., Weinstein, P., and Kaufman, E.,** Student difficulties in achieving local anesthesia, *J. Dent. Educ.*, 48, 168, 1984.
119. **Weinstein, P., Milgrom, P., Kaufman, E., Fiset, L., and Ramsay, D.,** Patient perceptions of failure to achieve optimal local anesthesia, *Gen. Dent.*, 33, 218, 1985.
120. **Fiset, L., Milgrom, P., Weinstein, P., Getz, T., and Glassman, P.,** Psychophysiological responses to dental injections, *J. Am. Dent. Assoc.*, 111, 578, 1985.
121. **Clarke, J. R. and Clarke, D. J.,** Hysterical blindness during dental anaesthesia, *Br. Dent. J.*, 162, 267, 1987.
122. **Hemingway, R. B., III and Reigle, T. G.,** The involvement of endogenous opiate systems in learned helplessness and stress-induced analgesia, *Psychopharmacology*, 93, 353, 1987.
123. **Dalton, L. M. and Widdowson, P. S.,** The involvement of opioid peptides in stress-induced analgesia in the slug *Arion ater, Peptides*, 10, 9, 1989.
124. **Frischknecht, H. R. and Siegfried, B.,** Emergence and development of stress-induced analgesia and concomitant behavioral changes in mice exposed to social conflict, *Physiol. Behav.*, 44, 383, 1988.
125. **Van den Hoogen, R. H., Bervoets, K., and Colpaert, F. C.,** Enhancement by pain and stress of analgesia produced by epidural sufentanil in the rat, *Anesthesiology*, 69, 24, 1988.
126. **Takahashi, M., Tokuyama, S., and Kaneto, H.,** Distinctive implication of emotional factors in various types of stress-induced analgesia, *Jpn. J. Pharmacol.*, 46, 418, 1988.
127. **Tokuyama, S., Takahashi, M., and Kaneto, H.,** Blockade of the development of analgesic tolerance to morphine by psychological stress through benzodiazepine receptor mediated mechanism, *Jpn. J. Pharmacol.*, 51, 425, 1989.
128. **Bandura, A., Cioffi, D., Taylor, C. B., and Brouillard, M. E.,** Perceived self-efficacy in coping with cognitive stressors and opioid activation, *J. Pers. Soc. Psychol.*, 55, 479, 1988.
129. **Persson, G.,** General side effects of local dental anesthesia *Acta Odontol. Scand.*, 27, Supplement 53, 1969.
130. **Tomlin, P. J.,** Death in outpatient dental anaesthetic practice, *Anaesthesia*, 29, 551, 1974.

131. **Absi, E. G.,** A cardiac arrest in the dental chair, *Br. Dent. J.*, 163, 199, 1987.
132. **Brodsky, M. A., Sato, D. A., seri, L. T., Wolff, L. J., and Allen, B. J.,** Ventricular tachyarrhythmia associated with psychological stress: the role of the sympathetic nervous system, *J. Am. Med. Assoc.*, 257, 2064, 1987.
133. **Engel, G. L.,** Sudden and rapid death during psychological stress: folklore or folk wisdom, *Ann. Int. Med.*, 74, 771, 1971.
134. **Malamed, S. F.,** *Handbook of Medical Emergencies in the Dental Office*, 3rd ed., C. V. Mosby, St. Louis, 1987.
135. **Engel, G. L.,** Psychologic stress, vasodepressor (Vasovagal) syncope, and sudden death, *Ann. Int. Med.*, 89, 403, 1978.
136. **Schmidt, R. T.,** Personality and fainting, *J. Psychosom. Res.*, 19, 21, 1975.
137. **Sledge, W. E.,** Antecedent psychological factors in the onset of vasovagal syncope, *Psychosom. Med.*, 40, 568, 1978.
138. **Eidelman, D.,** "Fatigue on rest" and associated symptoms (headache, vertigo, blurred vision, nausea, tension and irritability) due to locally asymptomatic, unerupted, impacted teeth, *Med. Hypotheses*, 5, 339, 1979.
139. **Eidelman, D.,** Fatigue: towards an analysis and a unified definition, *Med. Hypotheses*, 6, 517, 1980.
140. **Eidelman, D.,** Vertigo of dental origin: case reports, *Aviat. Space Environ. Med.*, 52, 122, 1981.
141. **Eidelman, D.,** Pathology in the lower half of the functional face: its significance in clinical medicine, *Med. Hypotheses*, 8, 149, 1982.
142. **Eidelman, D.,** Logic in the study of headache, fatigue, vertigo and "psychogenic" illnesses, *Med. Hypotheses*, 31, 319, 1990.
143. **Swedish National Board of Health and Welfare,** Mercury/amalgam health hazards, 1987. 10.
144. **Michel, I., Norbäck, D., and Edling, C.,** An epidemiologic study of the relation between symptoms of fatigue, dental amalgam and other factors, *Swed. Dent. J.*, 13, 33, 1989.
145. **Doyle, K. A. and Goepferd, S. J.,** An allergy to local anesthetics? The consequences of a misdiagnosis, *J. Dent. Child.*, 56, 103, 1989.
146. **Malamed, S. F. and Quinn, C. L.,** Electronic dental anesthesia in a patient with suspected allergy to local anesthetics: report of case, *J. Am. Dent. Assoc.*, 116, 53, 1988.
147. **MacColl, S. and Young, E. R.,** An allergic reaction following injection of local anesthetic: a case report, *Can. Dent. Assoc.*, 55, 981, 1989.
148. **Neidle, E. A., Kroeger, D. C., and Yagiela, J. A.,** *Pharmacology and Therapeutics for Dentistry*, 2nd ed., C. V. Mosby, St. Louis, 1985.
149. **de Jong, R. H.,** Toxic effects of local anesthetics, *J. Am. Dent. Assoc.*, 239, 1166, 1978.
150. **Cawson, R. A., Cuson, I., and Whittington, D. R.,** The hazards of dental local anaesthetics, *Br. Dent. J.*, 154, 253, 1983.
151. **Adriani, J.,** Etiology and management of adverse reactions to local anesthetic, *Int. Anesthesiol. Clin.*, 10, 127, 1972.
152. **Barer, M. R. and McAllen, M. K.,** Hypersensitivity to local anaesthetics: a direct challenge test with lignocaine for definitive diagnosis, *Br. Med. J.*, 284, 1229, 1982.
153. **deShazo, R. D. and Nelson, H. S.,** An approach to the patient with a history of local anesthetic hypersensitivity: experience with 90 patients, *J. Allergy Clin. Immunol.*, 63, 387, 1979.
154. **Babajews, A. V. and Ivanyi, L.,** The relationship between *in vivo* and *in vitro* reactivity of patients with a history of allergy to local anaesthetics, *Br. Dent. J.*, 152, 385, 1982.
155. **Milam, S. B., Giovannitti, J. A., and Bright, D.,** Hypersensitivity to amide local anesthetics? Report of a case, *Oral Surg. Oral Med. Oral Pathol.*, 56, 593, 1983.
156. **Assem, E. S. K. and Punnia-Moorthy, A.,** Allergy to local anaesthetics: an approach to definitive diagnosis. A review with an illustrative study, *Br. Dent. J.*, 164, 44, 1988.
157. **Aldrete, J. A. and Johnson, D. A.,** Evaluation of intracutaneous testing for investigation of allergy to local anesthetic agents, *Anesth. Analg. (Cleveland)*, 49, 173, 1970.

158. **Shapira, J. and Rubinow, A.,** Evaluation and management of hypersensitivity to local anesthetics in pediatric dentistry *Anesth. Prog.*, 34, 191, 1987.
159. **Lederman, D. A., Freedman, P. D., Kerpel, S. M., and Lumerman, H.,** An unusual skin reaction following local anesthetic injection: review of the literature and report of four cases, *Oral Surg. Oral Med. Oral Pathol.*, 49, 28, 1980.
160. **Curley, R. K., Macfarlane, A. W., and King, C. M.,** Contact sensitivity to the amide anesthetics lidocaine, prilocaine, and mepivacaine: case report and review of the literature, *Arch. Dermatol.*, 122, 924, 1986.
161. **Kennedy, K. S. and Cave, R. H.,** Anaphylactic reaction to lidocaine, *Arch. Otolaryngol. Head Neck Surg.*, 112, 671, 1986.
162. **Morse, D. R., Schoor, R. S., and Cohen, B. B.,** Surgical and non-surgical dental treatments for a multi-allergic patient with meditation-hypnosis as the sole anesthetic: case report, *Int. J. Psychosom.*, 31, 27, 1984.

SECTION III

TREATMENT MODALITIES

Chapter 10

BEHAVIOR MODIFICATION

The terms behavior modification and behavior therapy describe clinical procedures in psychology where the therapist attempts to modify symptoms in the patient's behavior which interfere with his/her adaptive functioning.[1]

According to Wolpe,[2] the definition of behavior modification is straightforward: "Unadaptive habits that are learned can be unlearned...on the basis of knowledge of the learning process." The major assumption is that disordered behaviors result from faulty learning or insufficient motivation to change and can be modified by using the same principles in a controlled manner.[1]

Behavior modification is based on the principles of conditioning and learning, mainly classical conditioning,[2,3] operant conditioning,[4,5] general principles of learning,[6] and social learning.[7]

I. THEORETICAL BACKGROUND

A. THE THEORY OF LEARNING

Behavior is usually defined as "the ways people react to their environment and what they **do** in their environment" (accentuation in text).[1] These reactions and doings are the outcome of life-long learning processes of each individual.

Behavior patterns can be acquired in several ways:

1. Classical (Respondent) Conditioning

Classical conditioning emphasizes the importance of antecedents — the stimuli that precede behavior.[8] Pavlov[9] demonstrated the bond between stimulus and response by supplying positive reinforcement to dogs: the way in which an unconditioned stimulus (food) led to an unconditioned response (salivation). He observed that the unconditioned response often occurs in response to other stimuli temporarily associated with the unconditioned stimulus (sound of a bell). From this, he made the observation that a conditioned stimulus (the bell sound) could lead to the same physiological result (salivation), but this time as a learned, conditioned response.

Wolpe[2,3] used the classical conditioning model to explain the acquisition of different unadaptive habits, such as classically conditioned neurotic fears. Through a process of classical conditioning, a previously neutral stimuli (e.g., the smell of dental operatory, the sound of dental drill, etc.) can be transformed into conditioned stimuli which elicit a conditioned response (e.g., anxiety). This may originate from a single occurrence (single-trial learning) or be progressively built up in the course of a series of related events.

Examples among dental patients include those who, because of a single painful or traumatic encounter with a dentist, develop anxiety towards treatment, or individuals who, through the cumulative effect of pain, discomfort, or negative interpersonal experiences associated with the situation, feel a gradually increasing aversion to treatment. Classical conditioning is a common way of acquiring dental fear and anxiety[10-16] (see also Chapter 4). In most cases, the response is due not to a single trial learning but rather several consecutive adverse experiences.[11,15]

2. Operant (Instrumental) Conditioning

Unlike classical conditioning, in which the stimulus precedes behavior, operant conditioning focuses on the relationship between behavioral responses and their consequences.[8]

Skinner[4,5] suggested that it is often more important to understand the effect of the behavioral consequences on behavior itself than to perceive the original reasons for it. Consequences are generally contingent on behavior (i.e., wages are contingent on working, grades on studying for exams).[17] When a specific behavior leads to some reward (positive reinforcement), the likelihood of responding increases; when the consequence of behavior is an aversive stimulus (punishment), the likelihood of responding decreases. A yelling, uncooperative child may gain extra attention from his/her mother which then increases the probability of such behavior in the future. Similarly, when a desirable behavior is praised and rewarded, the behavior which initiated it is reinforced.

3. The SORKC Model

Kanfer and Phillips[18] combined the basic elements of the classical and operant conditioning models into a general model of learning which analyzes complex sequences of behavior occurring in the natural environment — the SORKC model.

This model is based on the following mutually connected variables:

S (prior stimulation) describes the relevant physical, social, or internal stimuli that have a functional relationship to the behaviorof the individual. For example, a toothache is a physical stimulus which can initiate the chain of responses that eventually brings the patient to the dental operatory. The same consequence can also be triggered by a social stimulus, such as the general acceptance that periodic examinations are a "must", or by an internal stimulation, such as fear of a possible damage to teeth, asthetics, etc.

O (biologic state of the organism) varies from individual to individual. For example, a handicapped person finding it difficult to travel to the dental operatory on his/her own; a person suffering from a systemic disease bearing immediate relevance to dental treatment, etc.

R (response repertoire) of the individual includes two classes of responses: (1) responses that are elicited by stimuli without training, most often involuntarily, and with little regard to the response consequences (e.g., holding or rubbing of the painful area with the hand); and (2) those conditioned by their consequences, that is, by reinforcement (operants), such as social approval from the environment for going to the dentist in spite of initial anxiety (positive reinforcement).

K (contingency relationship) describes the relationship between response and timing, magnitude, or frequency of the consequences it produces. In other words, it expresses the possibility that a particular response will be followed by a specific consequence. For example, in some societies, going to the dentist for treatment has a high probability of positive reinforcement. In others, dental treatment is considered unnecessary or "luxurious," and the probability of positive reinforcement is decreased.

C (consequence) is the eventual change in the environment or the consequence produced by the response, i.e., going to the dentist or avoiding treatment altogether.

This behavioral equation model stresses the effects of the response on the person and his/her environment, rather than the antecedents or causes of the behavior. It assumes that problematic behavior is learned and that it can be changed either by unlearning or by modification of the environment so that stimulus control of the symptomatic behavior is changed. Subjective experiences of the patient, including reports of his discomforts, thoughts, feelings, and other covert activities, are treated as behavior that both affect the listener to whom the report is made and serve as a response to internal stimulation.

4. Social Learning

Bandura[7] pointed out that although internal response-producing agents play a major role in the learning processes, one cannot disregard the effect of external variables. While actions are regulated by their consequences, the controlling environment is, in turn, often significantly altered by behavior. In social interactions, the behavior of one person exerts some degree of influence over the actions of others. The type of behavior that one exhibits partly determines environmental contingencies, which in turn influence that person's behavior.

Thus, learning can be achieved by processes of observation. A specific response may be acquired, not by a previous performance of a certain behavior, but by observing or imitating the behavior of others (vicarious learning or modeling).[7]

B. THE ROLE OF COGNITIONS

Several investigators emphasized the role of cognitions on human behavior.[7,18-21] Behavior is significantly affected by cognitive processes, such as thoughts, attitudes, beliefs, and expectations.

Basically, there are four cognitive processes and environmental events that influence human behavior:[7,17,20] attention (awareness of specific environmental events), mediation (coding or cognitive representation of events previously noticed), component behaviors (individual response repertoires), and motivational or incentive conditions (knowing the consequences associated with a particular behavior in a given environment).

In his theory of reason and emotion, Ellis[19] claimed that human thinking and emotion are not disparate or different processes; rather they significantly overlap and are in some respects the same thing. Fundamental life operations are not experienced in isolation. When an individual senses something (e.g., toothache) the tendency is to do something about it (touch the painful area), to have feelings about it (dislike or fear it), and to think about it (remember previous experiences with a dentist, imagine what the future treatment will be). Similarly, if the individual acts, emotes, or thinks, there will be conscious or unconscious involvement in other behavior processes.

II. GETTING TO KNOW THE PATIENT — THE INTERVIEW

To treat a patient with oro-related behavioral dysfunctions, the dentist must first become acquainted with the patient and his/her behavior. Several interviewing techniques can be selectively used in various situations to reach this objective.[22]

The direct approach is a procedure in which a series of questions are directed at obtaining specific information (e.g., when was the first time you remember being afraid of the dentist?). Generally, questions are those that require the patient to limit and restrict reactions and are defined as limited-response questions.

The nondirect approach is where the patient is asked a number of general questions, thus providing a variety of information (e.g., how do you generally feel about medical treatment?). Such questions are usually open-ended and enable elaboration in the patient's reply to give as much information as is necessary or desirable.

In some cases, the patient is willing and able to convey problems in a direct way. These patients find it easy, and sometimes comforting, to confess their fears to the dentist. Statements such as "You've never treated a patient as scared as I am," "I am so afraid it will hurt", "I can't stand the sound of the drill," are common expressions of anxious dental patients. In other patients, the problem is expressed in a less direct way (clenching of fists, restlessness, sweating, etc.). In either case, proper assessment of the patient (behaviorally and dentally) is an essential step of treatment.

The art of history-taking involves the ability to recognize the interrelationship between the details of the medical history and the patient's personal history.[23] Among behavioral psychologists, the interview is one of the most widely used assessment methods.[24] Although in dentistry proper assessment of dental patients requires use of specific manual skills, an efficient initial interview often reveals many important features.

In psychological treatment, the interview itself serves as therapeutic. The role of the behavioral interview is summarized by Keefe[8] as follows:

1. *Gather Background Information* — Medical and dental specialists usually focus on medical history that provides detailed information about the

pathophysiological processes responsible for the physical illness or disease. In behavioral medicine, the interviewer attempts to develop a behavioral learning history, the major task of which is to discover the habit patterns that constitute or contribute to the presenting problem. The interviewer is interested in how the specific patterns in question initially developed, how they modified over the years, and what the factors are that currently maintain them.

While interviewing the patient who suffers from an oro-related behavioral dysfunction, both aspects of the patient's personal history are equally important. Medical history is crucial to evaluate general health and to determine any related problems. A behavioral learning history is important to determine possible patterns of behavior which might have contributed to the current problem (respondent conditioning, e.g., former aversive encounters with a dentist, vicarious learning — a parent who was afraid of dental treatment, etc.).

2. *Specify and Define Problem* — Many complaints are expressed by patients in general terms ("I don't know why but I simply hate dentists..."; "I have always been afraid of the dentist..."). The interview should help define the complaints in more specific terms. For example: when exactly did the fear start? Was it initiated by a specific experience? What are the main objects of fear (pain, injection, drilling)? What is the magnitude of the fear? (Is routine dental examination tolerable or is the patient unable even to enter the operatory?).
3. *Identify Current Environmental Factors* — The need to examine possible relevant environmental antecedents and their consequences is quite clear. For example, an overprotective mother may convey her fears to her child; a social environment does not appreciate the importance of dental care; a patient comes to treatment only because his/her spouse insisted.
4. *Serve as a Sample of Behavior* — The interview provides an opportunity to observe the patient's behavior. Observation of nonverbal reactions to different aspects of the dental office (where most dental interviews are carried out) provides initial cues as to the origin of the patient's fears and anxiety. Mannerisms, gestures, and physical appearance may suggest problems which have not been initially reported. The patient who suffers from bruxism may show signs of muscular tension during the initial interview; extensive grinding of the anterior teeth may also be apparent at a superficial observation.
5. *Sharing Information* — It is most important for the patient to understand the kind of treatment to be expected. The anxious patient often feels so stressful that the very thought of an interview with a dentist is difficult to cope with. Careful explanation of the possible treatment modalities is important for future cooperation.

   The fact that most behavior modification strategies are applied on a long-term basis, must be clearly explained. Many patients expect a "magic solution" which will enable them to receive treatment quickly without pain or anxiety. Patients may find it difficult to meet the presented goal without a proper understanding of the full rationale which stands behind the behavioral approach.

6. *Social Reinforcement* — The first encounter with the dentist is often a crucial experience. In some cases, anxiety is so severe that the patient postpones treatment until pain overcomes the fear of treatment. If, at the first encounter, a positive interpersonal relationship is established, the chances of carrying through treatment increases.
   Many patients are ashamed of their situation due to their ugly, neglected teeth as well as from low self-esteem for being unable to overcome their fear. The initial interview should convey aspects of legitimation and acceptance. This serves as an initial reframing of the patient's attitudes and emotions toward the symptom and enables future cooperation.

III. TREATMENT APPROACHES BASED ON RESPONDENT CONDITIONING (EXTINCTION AND COUNTERCONDITIONING)

Behavioral treatments based on respondent conditioning include therapies aimed at breaking the stimulus/anxiety-response link by either extinction or counterconditioning procedures.

Extinction procedures are based on continually presenting the conditioned stimulus to the patient without it being paired with the unconditioned stimulus. For example, a dental patient who is afraid of an injection may be asked to imagine the process until such imagination no longer evokes anxiety. As a second step, the syringe might be shown from a safe distance, then the patient would be encouraged to touch it, hold it, feel it in his/her hand, then mouth, and finally, when anxiety is no longer present, attempt to receive the injection.

The process of counterconditioning involves the same principles, but attempts to condition a more adaptive response to the unpleasant situation rather than simply eliminating the maladaptive response. The principle of counterconditioning is widely applied in systematic desensitization, whereby the anxiety-evoking stimulus is shown in the presence of a pleasant experience, which gradually replaces the fear.[1]

A. SYSTEMATIC DESENSITIZATION (COUNTER-CONDITIONING)

One of the first cases of systematic desensitization was reported by Jones in 1924.[25,26] The case described the treatment of a small boy's fear of rabbits by bringing the feared object into association with a pleasant stimulus. The boy was exposed to a pleasant stimulus (receiving food) concomitantly with a gradual exposure to the object of his fears (a rabbit). At first the rabbit was kept at a safe distance from the boy, enough to not evoke the fearful reaction. Gradually, the rabbit was brought closer and closer until the boy no longer reacted with fear to its presence. The pleasant response from eating gradually replaced the fear associated with the presence of the rabbit.

Despite this early report, systematic desensitization was not a focus of attention until the 1950s. At that time Wolpe[3] presented his theory of "reciprocal inhibition", which used a response inhibitory to anxiety (deep muscle relaxation) in the presence of the anxiety provoking stimuli. According to Wolpe, the anxiety-suppressive features of deep muscle relaxation serve as a tool to weaken the bond between the anxiety-arousing stimulus and its response.

Systematic desensitization is based on the gradual exposure of the patient to anxiety-evoking stimulus during deep muscle relaxation. Wolpe strongly advises patients to reach the stage of a positive feeling of calm prior to confronting the stress-evoking stimulus.

The technique of systematic desensitization as a therapeutic mode involves four sets of operations:[2]

1. *Introduction of a subjective anxiety scale* — To carry out an efficient desensitization program, it is important to know the magnitude of the patient's anxiety response at each stage of treatment. In this respect, verbal descriptions are not very informative (how much is "very much"?). It is helpful to create, together with the patient, a subjective anxiety scale in which anxiety levels are reported on a private scale (i.e., highest terrifying anxiety may be ranked as 10, while complete relaxation is 0). In this way, the patient can communicate more efficiently with the therapist and convey feelings more accurately.
2. *Training in deep muscle relaxation* — Deep muscle relaxation is used as a pleasant situation which serves as an anti-anxiety stimulus. The assumption is that a person cannot be relaxed and tense simultaneously, and the relaxation of body musculature serves as an antagonist to the anxiety response. The technique of relaxation may vary among cases according to individual needs, but it is generally based on the gradual relaxation of the various body muscles.
3. *Construction of hierarchies* — To be able to expose the patient in a gradual manner to the anxiety-provoking stimuli, an individual list of anxiety-evoking stimuli has to be constructed (e.g., the stimulus that evokes the greatest anxiety is placed first on the list, while the stimulus that is the least anxiety-evoking is placed at the bottom of the list). The construction of hierarchies of anxiety is relatively simple in a dental office, where the patient is constantly confronted with objects of fear. Here, the hierarchy of fears can be constructed through direct communication with the patient or through observing the patient's behavior while facing the various aspects of the dental operatory.
4. *Counterposing the anxiety-evoking stimuli with relaxation-induced calmness* — This stage combines deep muscle relaxation with gradual exposure to the anxiety-evoking stimuli according to the hierarchy of the patient's fears.

B. GRADUAL EXPOSURE (EXTINCTION)

Gradual exposure to the stress-evoking stimuli, without necessarily counter-conditioning the anxiety by deep relaxation, has frequently been suggested as an efficient means to treat dental phobia in the dental setting. Here, gradual exposure to the stress-evoking stimuli may be carried out *in vivo*, by exposing the patient to the actual fear-producing situation.[1]

During the process, the anxious patient is gradually confronted with objects of fear according to the individual hierarchy of fears and subjective anxiety scale. The process and pace of progress are individually "tailored" according to each patient's needs, and can be carried out using relaxation as a counter-conditioning stimulus, or through a somewhat more simple extinction procedure where the conditioned stimulus (e.g., fear of the dental syringe) is gradually presented until it no longer elicits the conditioned response (e.g., anxiety).

Example of treatment through gradual exposure — A patient arrives at the clinic terrified of even the possibility of entering the dental operatory. An interview reveals that the patient's initial fear is the dental explorer ("sharp and pain-inflicting").

After construction of a subjective anxiety scale, the dentist can gradually begin with the extinction process, based on the patient's responses. Generally, the patient is instructed not to exceed an agreed-upon rate of anxiety (e.g., anxiety degree of 2 or 3 out of 10). Whenever a higher level is reached, the patient is asked to inform the dentist, who then returns to a lower hierarchy stimulus until anxiety decreases to an accepted level. Each step is repeated several times until there is no more anxiety beyond the agreed-upon rate.

A tentative scenario of a gradual exposure process may be conducted as follows: (1) the patient is advised to stay in the waiting room and gradually approach the door to the dental operatory; (2) the patient enters the operatory and gradually approaches the dental chair; (3) the patient sits in the chair; (4) the patient is shown the dental explorer from a safe distance; (5) the explorer is given to the patient, who is allowed to feel it on the palm of his/her hand; (6) the explorer is gradually moved near the oral cavity and inserted slowly in the patient's mouth, but with no contact with the teeth; (7) teeth are gently touched by the explorer with no application of pressure; (8) a more detailed examination of the tooth surfaces is carried out, etc.

A similar process may also be taken, if necessary, regarding other stress-arousing objects, such as the syringe (giving it to the patient to hold in his/her hand, gentle gradual insertion into the oral cavity, etc.), the dental drill, or any other specific anxiety-evoking objects.

In some cases anxiety is so deep that an *in vivo* exposure to the anxiety-evoking stimuli is not possible, even gradually. In these cases, initial steps of the extinction or counter-conditioning processes can be carried out in the patient's imagination. Instead of carrying out treatment in the dental operatory, the patient is instructed to imagine the stress-evoking situation in a neutral setting. The gradual exposure to stimuli according to their anxiety-evoking hierarchies is carried out in the patient's imagination (preferably under relaxation), and only at a later stage, transferred to the actual dental operatory.

The procedure of gradual exposure is also effective in cases where the patient cannot specify the exact object of his/her fear and relates generally to the situation as a whole. Gradual exposure to the dental operatory and all that it involves, together with the development of mutual trust, are efficient tools for treatment of many behavioral dysfunctions related to dentistry.

C. USE OF GRADUAL EXPOSURE AND SYSTEMATIC DESENSITIZATION IN TREATMENT OF ORO-RELATED BEHAVIORAL DYSFUNCTIONS

Systematic desensitization and gradual exposure are widely used in dental practice, primarily to treat dental fear, anxiety, and phobia. Reports published in the 1960s and 1970s included both child and adult patients whose behavior during treatment significantly improved after systematic desensitization

The use of desensitization to treat dental anxiety gained wide acceptance in the 1980s.[34-45] A desensitization method for fearful patients that combines progressive relaxation, bio-feedback training, and the use of videotaped dental scenes has been described.[37] In a series of controlled studies, the technique was shown to be effective in reducing dental fear and in enabling patients to undergo treatment.[35,38-40] When the technique was compared to treating anxious dental patients with general anesthesia, it was shown to be significantly more effective. People who had long avoided treatment because of severe dental fear and were treated according to the described desensitization protocol, completed their treatment programs and showed a higher reduction in their dental anxiety level.[40] The advantage of the behavioral treatment over using general anesthesia was also shown in the long term. When patients were followed up 2 and 10 years later, it was found that among those who had received behavioral therapy, the frequency of attendance for regular dental care was consistently higher than among those treated under general anesthesia.[38,39,46]

Systematic desensitization and gradual exposure have also been used to treat patients with excessive gagging[47-54] and vasovagal syncope.[55]

IV. TREATMENT APPROACHES BASED ON OPERANT CONDITIONING

Operant conditioning is modified by the consequences of the individual's behavior: pleasant consequences increase the probability of the specific behavior to recur in the future; unpleasant consequences decrease such probability. In the dental setting, the most popular treatment modes based on operant conditioning include positive and negative reinforcement and biofeedback.

A. POSITIVE REINFORCEMENT

Positive reinforcement provides the individual with pleasant rewards for performance of a requested behavioral pattern. The reinforcers may be naturally occurring and unlearned (e.g., food, water, or sex), but they are most often secondary reinforcers that have acquired their reinforcing properties through repeated associations with pleasant consequences (e.g., praise, attention, etc.).[1]

Barenie and Ripa[56] summarized possible reinforcers as material, social, and activity. Material reinforcers include small presents and are, in general, most effective with children. Social reinforcers include praise, facial expressions, nearness, and physical contact, and represent the majority of all reinforcers affecting human behavior. Activity reinforcers, include seeing a movie, watching TV, going out to play, etc.

Positive social reinforcements are often used intuitively by dentists to treat children and anxious adult patients. Praising the patient during treatment for excellent behavior is a common way of enhancing the patient's cooperation.

Positive reinforcement has been shown to be beneficial in treating children and adults.[57-63]

B. NEGATIVE REINFORCEMENT

Negative reinforcement is a procedure in which an aversive or unpleasant event is terminated or postponed contingent on the performance of a particular behavior.[1] In the dental office, learning by negative reinforcement can occasionally lead anxious patients to develop histories of syncope, dizziness, tachicardia, or "allergy" during treatment. In some of these patients, the symptom serves as a subconscious way of avoiding treatment. The common reaction of many dentists who avoid treating patients with such histories serves as a negative reinforcer which prevents patients from confronting the aversive stimulus (treatment) and increases the probability of such response in the future.

Negative reinforcement is used in some restraint techniques described for pediatric patients. One such controversial procedure is the "hand over mouth" technique which involves restraining an uncooperative child by covering his/her mouth, thus preventing continuous unpleasant actions.[64] Although this includes some features of negative reinforcement (the will to avoid the unpleasant restraint decreases the probability of the negative behavior which initiated it), the restraint also enables the dentist to gain the patient's attention as a first step for mutual communication and future cooperation.[65]

According to Weinstein et al.,[66] many dentists respond with negative responses (the use of rules, coercion, and coaxing) after a child has shown a fear-related behavior. Not only are these reactions ineffective in reducing fear, but they also tend to be followed by a substantial increase of fear-related responses by the child.

In a study by Melamed et al.,[58] the use of a punishment condition (in which verbal statements were used to correct noncompliance of children, and no positive reinforcement was given for positive behavior) had the most detrimental effect on cooperativeness and self-reported fear from children. Dentists who used only a punishment condition had the most uncooperative children. However, when a punishment condition was used together with positive reinforcement of desired behaviors, most children learned and exhibited the desired behaviors during treatment.

In another study concerning the effect of a punishment technique based on loud voice commands, Greenbaum et al.[67] reported that such techniques reduced the child's disruptive behavior during dental treatment.

C. BIOFEEDBACK

Operant conditioning affects not only gross, observable behavior, but can also be used to intervene with physiological autonomic responses, once considered involuntary. This principle is popular with the use of biofeedback, a process "in which a person learns to reliably influence physiological responses of two kinds: either responses which are not ordinarily under voluntary control, or responses which ordinarily are easily regulated but for which regulation has broken down due to trauma or disease."[68]

Biofeedback training is based on monitoring the physiological response one wishes to influence (blood pressure, heart rate, galvanic skin response, muscle tension, etc.) and presenting it in a continuous way to the patient. Concomitantly, the patient is asked to try to change the particular response in a predetermined manner. When the patient succeeds in achieving the desired change, the result is immediately presented as an auditory or a visual signal. The signal serves as a positive reinforcer to help the patient maintain the desired pattern of response.

Biofeedback devices are numerous and used to treat chronic pain, modify heart rate and blood pressure, and reduce muscle tension. Many articles and reviews cover the clinical and basic aspects of its use, and the interested reader is referred to some of these sources.[68-72]

In dentistry, biofeedback is used primarily to control muscle activity and reduce benign chronic orofacial pain originating in the musculoskeletal system (e.g., treatment of temporomandibular pain and dysfunction syndrome, treatment of nocturnal bruxism).[73-79] It may also be used to treat anxiety and to induce deep muscle relaxation during systematic desensitization.[37-40,80-83]

V. TREATMENT APPROACHES BASED ON SOCIAL LEARNING

Learning occurs not only through personal experience, but by observing the behavior of others.[7] Learning by observation or imitation (vicarious learning or modeling) is an important process in acquiring behavior and is often used as a therapeutic mode.[1]

A. MODELING

During the process of modeling, the patient is presented with a model acting in a certain manner in a given situation. In dentistry, modeling can be carried out *in vivo* (by observing other patients who receive treatment) or *in vitro* (through film presentations of such treatment). Both procedures have been shown to be effective in reducing dental fear among adults and children.[31,45,84-103]

For example, White and Davis[101] presented 15 children, who had demonstrated disruptive behavior during dental treatment, with the behavior of an 8-year-old model. Results clearly supported the efficacy of modeling as a means of curtailing the negative behavior of the subjects.

In a series of studies, Melamed et al.[84,99,100,102] showed how viewing a film of appropriate dental behaviors reduced anxiety-related disruptive behaviors. In one study, conducted with 16 city children attending a pedodontic clinic, a film of a child model cooperatively undergoing treatment significantly reduced the disruptive behavior during restorative care.[99] Similar results were found when the approach was used on other populations of pedodontic patients.[84,100] In a study aimed at identifying critical factors that influence successful modeling, Melamed[102] concluded that film modeling is more effective when the film presents the behavior of a peer model rather than showing a purely demonstrative one (describing and demonstrating the procedures but without a model).

Greenbaum and Melamed[98] summarized the variables that affect the efficiency of modeling as a method of reducing stress and increasing cooperation:

1. *Patient characteristics* — Generally, modeling is effective in reducing fear behavior among children in a wide age range (usually more effective in children with no previous dental experience).
2. *Model characteristics* — The modeling situation involves two distinct components: a vicarious experience of rewards (the patient observes the model receiving reinforcement for appropriate behavior), and presentation of relevant information about the forthcoming treatment (knowledge about procedures, etc.). Both components are equally important for effective modeling.

As for the type of model used, the authors concluded that both models that are similar to the patient, as well as those of high prestige (e.g., parent, older sibling, dentist), are effective. Generally, coping models (who initially present a fearful behavior but gradually replace it with nonfearful, positive coping behavior) are more effective with adults. Mastery models (who do not display fearful behavior whatsoever) are as effective as coping models in preparing children with no previous experience. Both live and film models are effective in this context.

VI. TREATMENT APPROACHES BASED ON COGNITIONS

Human behavior is affected largely by cognitive processes such as thoughts, expectations, and beliefs. For example, a patient believes that because of an unreasonable "allergy", he/she might die if local anesthetic is administered. That patient will avoid treatment even if this involves suffering, pain, and deterioration of dental health.

The relationship between cognitions and behavior can be used in a therapeutic process — one can influence behavior merely by affecting a person's cognitions concerning a certain matter. Ellis[19] suggested a treatment strategy based on identification of the patient's irrational ideas and replacement by rational ones (the Rational Emotive Therapy). During treatment, the therapist directly contradicts and denies the self-defeating notions of the patient, while encouraging, persuading, cajoling, and occasionally even insisting that the patient engage in the activity in question (something he/she is afraid of doing), which in itself serves as a counter against what the patient believes. In other words, by uncovering the elements of irrationality in the patient's thinking, the therapist leads the individual into more reasonable channels of behavior.

The Rational Emotive Therapy has many components, including patient self-instruction as to the desired behavior ("I know I can do it,…I can enter the dentist's office and not be afraid,…I am able to receive an injection,…It will not hurt at all,…I will not move and I will remain calm,…I am doing just fine,…" etc.).

Cognitive strategies are often used spontaneously by dental patients to cope with the stress involved with treatment. Chaves and Brown[104] found that among 75 patients undergoing extractions or mandibular block injections, 44% used cognitive strategies designed to minimize pain and stress, such as attention diversion (focus on something other than the stressful situation) or self-statements (positive self-verbalizations).

A. IATROSEDATION

Friedman and associates[105-108] described an interpersonal-cognitive process, termed "iatrosedation", to treat fearful dental patients. Iatrosedation is defined as "the act of making calm by the doctor's behavior" and is based on a broad spectrum of verbal and nonverbal communication cues from the doctor. The process includes the following steps:

1. An iatrosedative interview whereby the dentist attempts to recognize and acknowledge the problem, interpret, and explain it to the patient. During the interview, the dentist offers a solution in which the patient accepts a verbal commitment that the feared procedure will be performed with minimal pain or discomfort and that the patient will be in complete control of the situation.
2. An iatrosedative clinical encounter designed to address the specific fear stimuli (and the fear of losing control), by performing the procedure associated with these fears before any other treatment is considered.

During both interview and treatment, the dentist communicates to the patient feelings of attentiveness, concern, acceptance, supportiveness, and involvement with intention to help. All of this is conveyed either through verbal or nonverbal channels, such as eye contact, facial expressions, vocal characteristics, body orientation, trunk lean, proximity, etc.

The major advantage of the iatrosedative process lies in its systematization. Although many of its procedures are often used intuitively by dentists and physicians, the process enables a systematically structured approach which can readily be learned and used by everyone. The iatrosedative process is relatively short and effective in calming anxious patients as well as helping those who are unable to adapt to dentures because of fear, anxiety, and/or depression.[105,107]

B. DISTRACTION

Broadly defined, distraction is directing one's attention away from the sensations or emotional reactions produced by the noxious stimulus.[109] Although popular in different clinical settings (listening to music during treatment), little research exists as to its precise effect in alleviating stress during dental treatment.

Corah et al.[110] attempted to assess several methods of stress reduction in dental patients, among which was "active task" distraction. Patients were asked to play a video ping pong game "against the house" while undergoing treatment. The television monitor was mounted near the ceiling and the patient was given a joy stick to control the game. The game could be played throughout the procedure. Patients' responses were recorded through questionnaires (Corah Dental Anxiety Scale, Rotter Locus of Control Scale and Need for Social Approval Scale), and by recording electrodermal responses and heart rates. The results indicated that distraction (as well as relaxation) were effective in reducing anxiety and stress during treatment. Similar results were found in a follow-up study.[111] Men seemed to prefer the video game and women the relaxation technique, however, both procedures were found equally effective.

In an attempt to compare the effect of different distraction techniques, Seyrek et al.[112] presented 80 dental patients with three distraction methods: an audio-comedy program, a video-comedy program, and a video game. Anxiety was measured through completion of the Corah Dental Anxiety Scale and recording electrodermal responses of the patients. The video comedy and the video game were both efficient in reducing stress.

Aside from its effect on the reduction of anxiety and stress during treatment, distraction can also be used to cope with pain-producing distress[110] (see also Chapter 3) to treat excessive gagging reflex[47,113-115] and to treat those who find it difficult to adapt to dentures.[114]

VII. SUMMARY

Dentists are showing an increasing interest in various modes of behavior modification. The relative simplicity of behavior modification enables an effective use by even the general dental practitioner with no training in psychology.

The behavioral interview enables the dentist to collect medical and learning histories of patients together with establishing proper communication patterns and initial reframing of the patient's feelings and attitudes. Use of desensitization, gradual exposure, reinforcement, modeling, iatrosedation, and distraction helps to reduce the main cause of most oro-related behavioral dysfunctions — stress — and enables treatment.

Behavior modification techniques are not performed in isolation. Acting as both the dentist and as the patient's "psychologist," the dental practitioner usually uses a synthesis of various behavioral modes, such as gradual exposure *in vivo* (at the actual place), positive reinforcement of desired responses, iatrosedation through cognitive approach, etc.

It is important to remember that each patient is an individual and must be treated as such. Therefore, providing the dentist with a rigid "plan of action" may be counterproductive. It is far more important to be sensitive to the patient's verbal and nonverbal communication cues and be open-minded to possible application of behavior modification modes in the dental office.

Furthermore, individual patients may react differently to various treatment modes. Thus, while one patient finds systematic desensitization effective, another may find modeling more suitable. Therefore, an individual plan tailored for each patient, based on their needs, wishes, and abilities, is highly recommended.

REFERENCES

1. **Melamed, B. G. and Siegel, L. J.,** Practical applications in health care, in *Behavioral Medicine*, Springer-Verlag, New York, 1980.
2. **Wolpe, J.,** *The Practice of Behavior Therapy*, 3rd ed., Pergamon Press, New York, 1982.
3. **Wolpe, J.,** *Psychotherapy by Reciprocal Inhibition*, Stanford University Press, Stanford, CA, 1958.
4. **Skinner, B. F.,** *Science and Human Behavior*, Macmillan, New York, 1953.
5. **Skinner, B. F.,** *Beyond Freedom and Dignity*, Knopf, New York, 1971.
6. **Ullmann, L. P. and Krasner, L.,** *A Psychological Approach to Abnormal Behavior*, Prentice-Hall, Englewood Cliffs, NJ, 1969.
7. **Bandura, A.,** *Principles of Behavior Modification*, Holt, Rinehart and Winston, New York, 1969.
8. **Keefe, F. J.,** Assessment strategies in behavioral medicine, in *Behavioral Approaches to Medicine: Application and Analysis*, McNamara, J. R., Ed., Plenum Press, New York, 1979, 101.
9. **Pavlov, I. P.,** *Conditioned Reflexes*, transl. by Anrep, G. V., Liveright, New York, 1927.
10. **Kleinknecht, R. A., Klepac, R. K., and Alexander, L. D.,** Origins and characteristics of fear of dentistry, *J. Am. Dent. Assoc.*, 86, 842, 1973.
11. **Bernstein, D. A., Kleinknecht, R. A., and Alexander, L. D.,** Antecedents of dental fear, *J. Public Health Dent.*, 39, 113, 1979.
12. **Cohen, L. A., Snyder, T. L., and LaBelle, A. D.,** Correlates of dental anxiety in a university population, *J. Public Health Dent.*, 42, 228, 1982.

13. **Berggren, U. and Meynert, G.,** Dental fear and avoidance: causes, symptoms, and consequences, *J. Am. Dent. Assoc.*, 109, 247, 1984.
14. **Forgione, A. G. and Clark, R. E.,** Comments on an empirical study of the causes of dental fear, *J. Dent. Res.*, 53, 496, 1974.
15. **Lautch, H.,** Dental phobia, *Br. J. Psychiatry*, 119, 151, 1971.
16. **Green, R. M. and Green, A.,** Adult attitudes to dentistry among dental attenders in South Wales, *Br. Dent. J.*, 159, 157, 1985.
17. **Craighead, W. E., Kazdin, A. E., and Mahoney, M. J.,** *Behavior Modification: Principles, Issues, and Applications*, Houghton Mifflin, Boston, 1976.
18. **Kanfer, F. H. and Phillips, J. S.,** *Learning Foundations of Behavior Therapy*, John Wiley & Sons, New York, 1970.
19. **Ellis, A.,** *Reason and Emotion in Psychotherapy*, Lyle Stuart, Secaucus, NJ, 1975.
20. **Mahoney, M. J.,** *Cognition and Behavior Modification*, Ballinger, Cambridge, MA, 1974.
21. **Meichenbaum, D.,** *Cognitive Behavior Modification*, General Learning Press, Morristown, NJ, 1974.
22. **Protell, M. R., Krasner, J. D., and Fabrikant, B.,** The dental interview — clinical observations, in *Psychodynamics in Dental Practice*, Charles C Thomas, Springfield, IL, 1975, 122.
23. **Trieger, N.,** The art of history taking, *J. Oral Surg.*, 36, 118, 1978.
24. **Keefe, F. J., Kopel, S. A., and Gordon, S. B.,** *A Practical Guide to Behavioral Assessment*, Springer-Verlag, New York, 1978.
25. **Jones, M. C.,** The elimination of children's fears, *J. Exp. Psychol.*, 7, 382, 1924.
26. **Jones, M. C.,** A laboratory study of fear: the case of Peter, *J. Genet. Psychol.*, 31, 308, 1924.
27. **Cherches, M. L. and Blackman, S.,** Alleviating the anxiety of children in dental treatment, *J. Am. Dent. Assoc.*, 66, 824, 1963.
28. **Gale, E. N. and Ayer, W. A.,** Treatment of dental phobias, *J. Am. Dent. Assoc.*, 78, 1304, 1969.
29. **Gordon, D. A., Terdal, L., and Sterling, E.,** The use of modeling and desensitization in the treatment of a phobic child patient, *J. Dent. Child.*, 41, 102, 1974.
30. **Machen, J. B. and Johnson, R.,** Desensitization, model learning, and the dental behavior of children, *J. Dent. Res.*, 53, 83, 1974.
31. **Shaw, D. W. and Thoresen, C. E.,** Effects of modeling and desensitation in reducing dentist phobia, *J. Counseling Psychol.*, 21, 415, 1974.
32. **Sawtell, R. O., Simon, J. F., Jr., and Simeonsson, R. J.,** The effects of five preparatory methods upon child behavior during the first dental visit, *J. Dent. Child.*, 41, 367, 1974.
33. **Klepac, R. K.,** Successful treatment of avoidance of dentistry by desensitization or by increasing pain tolerance, *J. Behav. Ther. Exp. Psychiatry*, 6, 307, 1975.
34. **Milgrom, P., Weinstein, P., Kleinknecht, R., and Getz, T.,** *Treating Fearful Dental Patients*, Reston Publishing Co., Reston, VA, 1985.
35. **Harrison, J. A., Carlsson, S. G., and Berggren, U.,** Research in clinical process and outcome methodology: psycho-physiology, systematic desensitization and dental fear, *J. Behav. Ther. Exp. Psychiatry*, 16, 201, 1985.
36. **Lindsay, S. J. E., Humphris, G., and Barnby, G. J.,** Expectations and preferences for routine dentistry in anxious adult patients, *Br. Dent. J.*, 163, 120, 1987.
37. **Berggren, U. and Carlsson, S. G.,** A psychophysiological therapy for dental fear, *Behav. Res. Ther.*, 22, 487, 1984.
38. **Berggren, U. and Carlsson, S. G.,** Qualitative and quantitative effects of treatment for dental fear and avoidance, *Anesth. Prog.*, 33, 9, 1986.
39. **Berggren, U.,** Long-term effects of two different treatments for dental fear and avoidance, *J. Dent. Res.*, 65, 874, 1986.
40. **Berggren, U. and Linde, A.,** Dental fear and avoidance: a comparison of two modes of treatment, *J. Dent. Res.*, 63, 1223, 1984.

41. **Morse, D. R. and Cohen, B. B.,** Desensitization using meditation-hypnosis to control "needle" phobia in two dental patients, *Anesth. Prog.*, 30, 83, 1983.
42. **Carlsson, S. G., Linde, A., and Ohman, A.,** Reduction of tension in fearful dental patients, *J. Am. Dent. Assoc.*, 101, 638, 1980.
43. **Gatchel, R. J.,** Effectiveness of two procedures for reducing dental fear: group-administered desensitization and group education and discussion, *J. Am. Dent. Assoc.*, 101, 634, 1980.
44. **Bernstein, D. A. and Kleinknecht, R. A.,** Multiple approaches to the reduction of dental fear, *J. Behav. Ther. Exp. Psychiatry*, 13, 287, 1982.
45. **Smith, T., Getz, T., Milgrom, P., and Weinstein, P.,** Evaluation of treatment at a dental fears research clinic, *Spec. Care Dent.*, May-June, 130, 1987.
46. **Hakeberg, M., Berggren, U., and Carlsson, S. G.,** A 10-year follow-up of patients treated for dental fear, *Scand. J. Dent. Res.*, 98, 53, 1990.
47. **Ramsay, D. S., Weinstein, P., Milgrom, P., and Getz, T.,** Problematic gagging: principles of treatment, *J. Am. Dent. Assoc.*, 114, 178, 1987.
48. **Singer, I. L.,** The marble technique: a method for treating the "hopeless gagger" for complete dentures, *Quintessence Int.*, 6(2), 31, 1975.
49. **Murphy, W. M.,** A clinical survey of gagging patients, *J. Prosth. Dent.*, 42, 145, 1979.
50. **Morse, D. R., Hancock, R. R., and Cohen, B. B.,** *In vivo* desensitization using meditation-hypnosis in the treatment of tactile-induced gagging in a dental patient, *Int. J. Psychosom.*, 31, 20, 1984.
51. **Fleece, L., Linton, P., and Dudley, B.,** Rapid elimination of a hyperactive gag reflex, *J. Prosth. Dent.*, 60, 415, 1988.
52. **Eli, I. and Kleinhauz, M.,** Hypnosis: a tool for an integrative approach in the treatment of the gagging reflex, *International J. Clin. Exp. Hypn.*, 33, 99, 1985.
53. **Wilks, C. G. W. and Marks, I. M.,** Reducing hypersensitive gagging, *Br. Dent. J.*, 155, 263, 1983.
54. **Eli, I., Kleinhauz, M., and Bar-Gil, B.,** Extreme gag reflex: methods of treatment and control, *Isr. J. Dent. Sci.*, 1, 105, 1984.
55. **McGrady, A. V. and Argueta Bernal, G. A.,** Relaxation based treatment of stress induced syncope, *J. Behav. Ther. Exp. Psychiatry*, 17, 23, 1986.
56. **Barenie, J. T. and Ripa, L. W.,** The use of behavior modification techniques to successfully manage the child dental patient, *J. Am. Dent. Assoc.*, 94, 329, 1977.
57. **Weinstein, P., Getz, T., Ratener, P., and Domoto, P.,** The effect of dentists' behaviors on fear-related behaviors in children, *J. Am. Dent. Assoc.*, 104, 32, 1982.
58. **Melamed, B. G., Bennett, C. G., Jerrell, G., Ross, S. L., Bush, J. -P., Hill, C., Courts, F., and Ronk, S.,** Dentists' behavior management as it affects compliance and fear in pediatric patients, *J. Am. Dent. Assoc.*, 106, 324, 1983.
59. **Rosenberg, H. M.,** Behavior modification for the child dental patient, *J. Dent. Child.*, 41, 111, 1974.
60. **Kohlenberg, R., Greenberg, O., Reymore, L., and Hass, G.,** Behavior modification and management of mentally retarded dental patients, *J. Dent. Child.*, 39, 61, 1972.
61. **Horner, R. D. and Keilitz, I.,** Training mentally retarded adolescents to brush their teeth, *J. Appl. Behav. Anal.*, 8, 301, 1975.
62. **Allen, K. D., Stark, L. J., Rigney, B. A., Nash, D. A., and Stokes, T. F.,** Reinforced practice of children's cooperative behavior during restorative dental treatment, *J. Dent. Child.*, 55, 273, 1988.
63. **Allen, K. D. and Stokes, T. F.,** Use of escape and reward in the management of young children during dental treatment, *J. Appl. Behav. Anal.*, 20, 381, 1987.
64. **Craig, W.,** Hand over mouth technique, *J. Dent. Child.*, 38, 387, 1971.
65. **Levitas, T. C.,** HOME-hand over mouth exercise, *J. Dent. Child.*, 41, 178, 1974.
66. **Weinstein, P., Getz, T., Ratener, P., and Domoto, P.,** Dentists' responses to fear- and nonfear-related behaviors in children, *J. Am. Dent. Assoc.*, 104, 38, 1982.

67. **Greenbaum, P. E., Turner, C., Cook, E. W., III, and Melamed, B. G.,** Dentists' voice control: effects on children's disruptive and affective behavior, *Health Psychol.*, 9, 546, 1990.
68. **Blanchard, E. B. and Epstein, L. H.,** *A Biofeedback Primer*, Addison-Wesley, Reading, MA, 1978.
69. **Butler, F.,** *Biofeedback: A Survey of the Literature*, Plenum Press, New York, 1978.
70. **Blanchard, E. B. and Young, L. D.,** Clinical applications of biofeedback training: a review of evidence, *Arch. Gen. Psychiatry*, 30, 573, 1974.
71. **Blanchard, E. B.,** Biofeedback: a selective review of clinical applications in behavioral medicine, in *Behavioral Approaches to Medicine: Application and Analysis*, McNamara, J. R., Ed., Plenum Press, New York, 1979, 131.
72. **Turk, D. C., Meichenbaum, D. H., and Berman, W. H.,** Application of biofeedback for the regulation of pain: a critical review, *Psychol. Bull.*, 86, 1322, 1979.
73. **Lowenthal, U. and Pisanti, S.,** The syndrome of oral complaints: etiology and therapy, *Oral Surg. Oral Med. Oral Pathol.*, 46, 2, 1978.
74. **Gessel, A. H.,** Electromyographic biofeedback and tricyclic anti-depressants in myofascial pain-dysfunction syndrome: psychological predictors of outcome, *J. Am. Dent. Assoc.*, 91, 1048, 1975.
75. **Dahlström, L. and Carlsson, S. G.,** Treatment of mandibular dysfunction: the clinical usefulness of biofeedback in relation to splint therapy, *J. Oral Rehab.*, 11, 277, 1984.
76. **Rugh, J. D.,** Behavioral therapy, in *A Textbook of Occlusion*, Mohl, N. D., Zarb, G. A., Carlsson, G. E., and Rugh, J. D., Eds., Quintessence Publishing Co., Chicago, 1988, 329.
77. **Carlsson, S. G. and Gale, E. N.,** Biofeedback treatment for muscle pain associated with the temporomandibular joint, *J. Behav. Ther. Exp. Psychiatry*, 7, 383, 1976.
78. **Hudzinski, L. G. and Walters, P. J.,** Use of a portable electromyogram integrator and biofeedback unit in the treatment of chronic nocturnal bruxism, *J. Prosth. Dent.*, 58, 698, 1987.
79. **Pierce, C. J. and Gale, E. N.,** A comparison of different treatments or nocturnal bruxism, *J. Dent. Res.*, 67, 597, 1988.
80. **Elmore, A. M.,** Biofeedback therapy in the treatment of dental anxiety and dental phobia, *Dent. Clin. North Am.*, 32, 735, 1988.
81. **Clark, M. and Hirschman, R.,** Effects of paced respiration on affective responses during dental stress, *J. Dent. Res.*, 59, 1533, 1980.
82. **Hirschman, R. and Hall, C.,** Use of biofeedback to reduce anxiety, in *The President's Conference on the Dentist-Patient Relationship and the Management of Fear, Anxiety and Pain*, Moretti, R. and Ayer, W. A., Eds., American Dental Association, Chicago, 1983.
83. **Hirschman, R., Young, D., and Nelson, C.,** Physiologically based techniques for stress reduction, in *Clinical Research in Behavioral Dentistry*, Ingersoll, B. D. and McCutcheon, W. R., Eds., West Virginia University Foundation, Morgantown, 1979.
84. **Melamed, B. G., Weinstein, D., Hawes, R., and Borland, M.,** Reduction of fear-related dental management problems with use of filmed modeling, *J. Am. Dent. Assoc.*, 90, 822, 1975.
85. **Adelson, R. and Goldfried, M. R.,** Modeling and the fearful child patient, *J. Dent. Child.*, 6, 476, 1970.
86. **Chertock, S. L. and Bornstein, P. H.,** Covert modeling treatment of children's dental fears, *Child Behav. Ther.*, 1, 249, 1979.
87. **Gatchel, R. J.,** Impact of a videotaped dental fear-reduction program on people who avoid dental teatment, *J. Am. Dent. Assoc.*, 112, 218, 1986.
88. **Ginther, L. J. and Roberts, M. C.,** A test of mastery versus coping modeling in the reduction of children's dental fears, *Child Fam. Behav. Ther.*, 4, 41, 1982.
89. **Hermecz, D. A. and Melamed, B. G.,** The assessment of emotional imagery training in fearful children, *Behav. Ther.*, 15, 156, 1984.

90. **Kleinknecht, R. A. and Bernstein, D. A.,** Short term treatment of dental avoidance, *J. Behav. Ther. Exp. Psychiatry*, 10, 311, 1979.
91. **Klesges, R. C., Malott, J. M., and Ugland, M.,** The effects of graded exposure and parental modeling on the dental phobias of a four-year-old girl and her mother, *J. Behav. Ther. Exp. Psychiatry*, 15, 161, 1984.
92. **Klingman, A., Melamed, B. G., Cuthbert, M. I., and Hermecz, D. A.,** Effects of participant modeling on information acquisition and skill utilization, *J. Consult. Clin. Psychol.*, 52, 414, 1984.
93. **Klorman, R, Hilpert, P. L., Michael, R., LaGana, C., and Sveen, O. B.,** Effects of coping and mastery modeling on experienced and inexperienced pedodontic patients' disruptiveness, *Behav. Ther.*, 11, 156, 1980.
94. **Stokes, T. F. and Kennedy, S. H.,** Reducing child uncooperative behavior during dental treatment through modeling and reinforcement, *J. Appl. Behav. Anal.*, 13, 41, 1980.
95. **Tearnan, B. H. and Graziano, W. G.,** Covert modeling and children's fears: a methodological critique of Chertock and Bornstein, *Child Behav. Ther.*, 2, 73, 1980.
96. **Wroblewski, P. F., Jacob, T., and Rehm, L. P.,** The contribution of relaxation to symbolic modeling in the modification of dental fears, *Behav. Res. Ther.*, 15, 113, 1977.
97. **Williams, J. A., Hurst, M. K., and Stokes, T. F.,** Peer observation in decreasing uncooperative behavior in young dental patients, *Behav. Modification*, 7, 225, 1983.
98. **Greenbaum, P. E. and Melamed, B. G.,** Pretreatment modeling: a technique for reducing children's fear in the dental operatory, *Dent. Clin. North Am.*, 32, 693, 1988.
99. **Melamed, B. G., Hawes, R. R., Heiby, E., and Glick, J.,** Use of filmed modeling to reduce uncooperative behavior of children during dental treatment, *J. Dent. Res.*, 54, 797, 1975.
100. **Melamed, B. G., Yurcheson, R., Fleece, E. L., Hutcherson, S., and Hawes, R.,** Effects of film modeling on the reduction of anxiety-related behaviors in individuals varying in level of previous experience in the stress situation, *J. Consult. Clin. Psychol.*, 46, 1357, 1978.
101. **White, W. C., Jr. and Davis, M. T.,** Vicarious extinction of phobic behavior in early childhood, J. *Abnorm. Child Psychol.*, 2, 25, 1974.
102. **Melamed, B. G.,** Behavioral approaches to fear in dental settings, in *Progress in Behavior Modification*, Vol. 7, Hersen, M., Eisler, R. M., and Miller, P. M., Eds., Academic Press, New York, 1979, 171.
103. **Ghose, L. J., Giddon, D. B., Shiere, F. R., and Fogels, J. R.,** Evaluation of sibling support, *J. Dent. Child.*, 36, 35, 1969.
104. **Chaves, J. F. and Brown, J. M.,** Spontaneous cognitive strategies for the control of clinical pain and stress, *J. Behav. Med.*, 10, 263, 1987.
105. **Friedman, N., Landesman, H. M., and Wexler, M.,** The influences of fear, anxiety, and depression on the patient's adaptive responses to complete dentures, Part III, *J. Prosth. Dent.*, 59, 169, 1988.
106. **Friedman, N.,** Psychosedation, Part 2. Iatrosedaton, in *Emergencies in Dental Practice*, McCarthy, F. M., Ed., W. B. Saunders, Philadelphia, 1979, 236.
107. **Friedman, N., Cecchini, J. J., Wexler, M., and Pitts, W. C.,** A dentist oriented fear reduction technique: the iatrosedative process, *Compendium Continuing Educ. Dent.*, 10, 113, 1989.
108. **Friedman, N.,** Iatrosedation: the treatment of fear in the dental patient, *J. Dent. Educ.*, 47, 91, 1983.
109. **McCaul, K. D. and Malott, J. M.,** Distraction and coping with pain, *Psychol. Bull.*, 95, 516, 1984.
110. **Corah, N. L., Gale, E. N., and Illig, S. J.,** Psychological stress reduction during dental procedures, *J. Dent. Res.*, 58, 1347, 1979.
111. **Corah, N. L., Gale, E. N., and Illig, S. J.,** The use of relaxation and distraction to reduce psychological stress during dental procedure, *J. Am. Dent. Assoc.*, 98, 390, 1979.

112. **Seyrek, S. K., Corah, N. L., and Pace, L. F.,** Comparison of three distraction techniques in reducing stress in dental patients, *J. Am. Dent. Assoc.*, 108, 327, 1984.
113. **Krol, A. J.,** A new approach to the gagging problem, *J. Prosth. Dent.*, 13, 611, 1963.
114. **Stoffelmayr, B. E.,** The treatment of a retching response to dentures by counteractive reading aloud, *J. Behav. Ther. Exp. Psychiatry*, 1, 163, 1970.
115. **Kovats, J. J.,** Clinical evaluation of the gagging denture patient, *J. Prosth. Dent.*, 25, 613, 1971.

Chapter 11

HYPNOSIS

In spite of its ancient roots, hypnosis has been accepted only recently as a scientific and medical tool. It has been surrounded by myths and mystery for so long that even today various popular misconceptions regarding hypnosis exist.

The exact nature of hypnosis is not fully understood. Zimbardo et al. [1] defined hypnosis as "(a) a state in which the effects of cognitive processes on bodily functioning are amplified; (b) enables the subject to perceive the focus of causality for mind and body control as more internally centered and volitional; (c) is often accompanied by a heightened sense of visual imagery; and (d) can lead to intensive concentration and elimination of distractions."

Hypnosis as defined by Orne [2] is "...a state or condition which exists when appropriate suggestions will elicit hypnotic phenomena"; in other words, "a state or condition in which subjects are able to respond to appropriate suggestions with distortions of perception or memory."

Waxman [3] defined hypnosis as "...not sleep nor the normal state of wakefulness but a condition somewhere in between the two. It may therefore be described as an altered state of awareness, resulting in psychological, physical and neurophysiological changes in which may be produced distortion of emotion, sensation, image and time."

Orne [2] pointed out that most definitions of hypnosis (including his) are descriptive rather than explanatory and that despite the superficial similarity of the hypnotized individuals' behavior, the underlying mechanisms are not identical.

Even though there is a diversity of theories as to the nature of hypnotic phenomena, there is no doubt that hypnosis is a powerful therapeutic tool for psychotherapy, medicine, and dentistry. Erickson and Rossi [4] viewed hypnotherapy as "a process whereby we help people utilize their own mental associations, memories and life potentials to achieve their own therapeutic goals." While this definition was initially meant to cover the utilization of hypnosis in psychotherapy, it also successfully conveys the principles of hypnotherapy in the medical and dental settings.

It is impossible to cover the many aspects of the nature of hypnosis, techniques of induction, and the utilization of hypnotic phenomena in hypnotherapy, medicine, and dentistry in this chapter. The field is rapidly growing and developing. Between 1982 and 1985 alone, more than 1000 articles were published in the scientific literature concerning hypnosis. [5] This indicates an enduring willingness on the part of the scientific community to accept hypnosis as a legitimate topic for clinical and research investigation. The present chapter summarizes the common phenomena of hypnosis and possible clinical applications in dentistry.

I. COMMON PHENOMENA IN HYPNOSIS[3]

A. ALTERATIONS IN VOLUNTARY MUSCLES

A common sign of hypnotic induction is the effect of hypnosis on the function of voluntary muscles. A typical induction method includes initiation of muscular relaxation. As relaxation frequently plays a major role in the process of systematic desensitization, this by itself serves as a therapeutic mode and is utilized to reduce stress and anxiety in patients (see Chapter 10).

The effect on voluntary muscles during hypnosis is not always directed toward muscular relaxation. Muscular activity under hypnosis can either inhibit or exhibit increased muscular performance and rigid catalepsies through the elicitation of phenomena such as automatic movements. These phenomena have often been used in the past in stage performances of hypnosis, and their use in the treatment of oro-related behavioral dysfunctions is limited.

B. ALTERATIONS IN INVOLUNTARY MUSCLES, ORGANS, AND GLANDS

Many bodily functions and activities are controlled and regulated involuntarily, by action through the thalamus and the autonomic nervous system. Some of these actions can be successfully affected under hypnosis, a phenomenon which is often used as a therapeutic mode in various fields of medicine.

During hypnosis the heart rate can be either accelerated or reduced, conditional on proper verbal cues. A similar effect can be achieved on the respiratory system, alimentary system, secretion of saliva, and perspiration. Proper suggestions can influence blood vessels and lead to a decrease in blood pressure, or decreased bleeding during surgical procedures. These phenomena gradually gain acceptance in the treatment of various medical problems such as hypertension, or performing bloodless dental extractions.

C. ALTERATIONS IN SENSE ORGANS

In deep hypnosis, sight, hearing, smell, taste, and touch can be influenced by suggestion, and the subject's perception through any senses affected. Probably the most dramatic effect, that most often used in medicine, is on the perception of pain. Under deep hypnosis, sensations of hypoalgesia and analgesia can be induced without pharmaceutical agents. The patient's ability to experience numbness and a sensation of anesthesia in a specific region has been used to perform nonpainful surgical and dental treatments (e.g., in patients suspected of suffering from hypersensitivity to local anesthetic agents).

D. ALTERATIONS IN MENTAL ACTIVITY

In deep hypnosis, the subject's attention is primarily directed toward the hypnotist, a fact which affects some aspects of the subject's mental activity.

1. *Rapport* — The rapport between patient and hypnotist tends to prevent the subject from responding to any stimuli other than those arising from the hypnotist. This causes the subject to respond more effectively to suggestions from the hypnotist than from others. The increased rapport, and the patient's heightened suggestibility, are used to elicit the desired responses, such as muscular relaxation, hypoalgesia, etc.
2. *Time Orientation Changes* — There is no definite answer as to whether a subject under hypnosis is able to judge the passing of time more or less accurately than in the waking state. It is known, however, that suitable suggestions can elicit phenomena of time distortion, such as time regression (going back in time, in place and in memory) and sensations of time extension or time shortening. While time regression is more often used in hypnotherapy than in dentistry, suggestions of time can be used in dentistry to enable the patient to experience treatment as "a long, pleasant, relaxation" or "short, nonsignificant, experience".
3. *Memory Changes* — Memory changes, such as hypermnesia, paramnesia or amnesia, can be induced under hypnosis. Unless other suggestions are given, the subject frequently experiences memory loss upon awakening (posthypnotic amnesia). This phenomenon can often be deepened by suggestion. Generally, paramnesia rather than total amnesia should be implied so that the patient forgets only specific things concerning the session (e.g., unpleasant aspects of the treatment). Hypermnesia (to remember things apparently forgotten) is sometimes used in hypnotherapy as well as in criminal investigations.
4. *Illusions and Hallucinations* — Although illusions and hallucinations are sometimes used in hypnotherapy, their use in the dental setting is limited. Nevertheless, the vivid imagery involved with deep hypnosis can sometimes be used to initiate systematic desensitization through the patient's imagination (in patients who are too anxious to initiate the process *in vivo*).

II. USE OF HYPNOSIS IN DENTISTRY

A. TREATMENT OF DENTAL FEAR, ANXIETY, AND PHOBIA

An important use of hypnosis in dentistry is in alleviating fear, anxiety, and phobia. Although relatively little research has been conducted in this field, an increasing number of theoretical and clinical reports are being published concerning this issue.

In the early 1970s, Golan reported several relevant cases. In the first, [6] a woman was described who was generally "frightened to death" of dental treatment but had an urgent need for dental care (acute alveolar abscess in one of her few remaining teeth). Hypnosis was used to reduce the patient's anxiety, and eventually the necessary treatment was performed.

The procedures used by Golan did not include any attempt to investigate the roots of the anxiety and were based mainly on relaxation, positive reinforcement during treatment, and posthypnotic suggestions regarding future treatments. In a later report,[7] a case was described in which hypnosis was effective in the treatment of a specific dental fear (the fear of the noise of the dental drill).

Since these early reports, a growing number of authors have suggested the use of hypnosis to treat different variants of dental fear, anxiety, or phobia.[3,8-13] Reports include cases of fear of the dentist in general or particular fears, such as fear of extraction, suffocation, sound of the drill, needle, etc. Such reports are continuously being published in the medical as well as dental literature.[14,15]

B. TREATMENT OF EXTENSIVE GAGGING REFLEX

Hypnosis has been widely used to achieve control over excessive gagging reflex.[3,8,16-22] It has also worked in association with systematic desensitization.

Eli and Kleinhauz[21] described several cases whereby hypnosis was used to alleviate gagging in dental patients. In two patients, gagging was identified as a learned avoidance reaction, originating from former aversive encounters with treatment. Hypnosis was used as a tool to achieve deep relaxation and incorporated in a process of systematic desensitization carried out *in vivo* at the dental office.

In two other patients, the symptomatic gagging was identified as a defense mechanism which served as an inadequate solution to a deep-seated psychodynamic conflict (in one patient the conflict was of a sexual nature in which intrusion of dental instruments into the mouth had a symbolic oral-sexual meaning; the other suffered from a dependence-independence conflict). Since the patients came to the clinic with a specific need for dental treatment, no attempt was made to use hypnosis for psychotherapy. Hypnosis was used only as a tool to achieve deep relaxation together with suggestive procedures which attempted to "split" the patients' psychodynamic conflicts from the gagging symptom. This implied that gagging could be separated from the psychodynamic conflict. The suggestions allowed the patients to feel "safe" and to cope with the dental treatment without having their psychological integrity threatened.

C. PAIN MANAGEMENT

Hypnosis is widely used in the management of both acute and chronic pain, such as the induction of local anesthesia during minor surgical procedures (i.e., dental treatment) or reduction of chronic pain in cancer patients.[23]

1. Hypnosis as a Means for Local Anesthesia in Dentistry

Many reports regarding the use of hypnosis in the dental setting describe its dramatic effect when used as a sole anesthetic. Hilgard and Hilgard[23] summarized several case reports in which dental procedures were performed under hypnosis, without other anesthetic agents. These include cases of extractions, pulpotomies, and pulpectomies. The cases cover a wide age-range, from 4 years to 65 years. Others presented the use of hypnosis in endodontics [24-26] and other dental treatment procedures [3,11] to allow treatment without stress or pain.

Chen et al. [27] described a young woman who had undergone extensive oral surgery under hypnosis (removal of four impacted third molars). In order to understand the nature of hypnosis-induced analgesia, the cortical power spectrum of the patient's brain potentials during the surgical procedure was recorded. Results indicated an overall cortical reduction in functioning during hypnosis in a nonsymmetrical manner across both cerebral hemispheres, suggesting that hypnosis was a cognitive state alteration.

Houle et al. [28] indicated that analgesia produced by either hypnosis or relaxation-induced suggestions varies as a function of the type of pain. In their study, both hypnosis and relaxation significantly reduced the strength and the unpleasantness of electrical tooth pulp stimulation, but only the unpleasantness (and not the strength) of cold pressor stimulation in the arm. Apparently, the quality of analgesia varies, not only with the patient's characteristics, but also according to the nature of the noxious stimulus.

The use of hypnosis to induce local anesthesia is especially effective in patients with specific fears of the dental syringe, needle, or injections. [29] It is also an effective method in treating patients with true (or suspected) hypersensitivity to local anesthetic agents.[11,26,30] In cases of real allergy, hypnosis is the only method in which dental treatment can be administered without pain. In cases of false allergy (the patient claims to be allergic although the condition has not been confirmed by adequate tests), the use of hypnosis, rather than pharmaceutical methods, diminishes the patient's anxiety and enables further cooperation.

2. Hypnosis in the Treatment of Benign Chronic Orofacial Pain

Prolonged chronic pain conditions, such as temporomandibular pain and dysfunction syndrome, atypical odontalgia, or glossodynia, are difficult clinical conditions to treat and cause immense suffering to the patient.

In some patients, the pain syndrome is initiated by destructive habits such as bruxism. [31-33] The use of hypnosis has been suggested as a tool to eliminate such habits and to reduce the pain syndrome. [17,34-36]

Aside from using hypnosis to eliminate habits, hypnosis has been used in the management of chronic pain in various medical settings. [3,23] Hypnosis can be used to relieve symptoms of benign chronic orofacial pain not necessarily associated with destructive habits. It can be used not only to remove the presenting symptoms, but also to address different aspects of the pain experience (anxiety, depression, low self-esteem, sick role behavior, learned helplessness, and pain games). Ultimately, it can increase the patient's ability to accept and cope with the pain and to accept responsibility for personal progress. [37]

D. ADAPTATION TO DENTURES

Occasionally, the patient's adaptation to full or partial dentures leads to unexpected problems. Some find it hard to adapt emotionally to the new situation and present the dentist with a problem that is difficult to handle.

Hypnosis has been suggested as a possible treatment mode for these patients.[3,11,17] This can be accomplished by positive suggestions as to the patient's ability to tolerate the denture, and/or suggestions to increase motivation for the required cooperation.

E. CONTROL OF HEMORRHAGE AND SALIVARY FLOW

Proper administration of hypnotic suggestions can be useful in reducing hemorrhage and/or salivary flow during dental treatment.[3,17,38-40] For example, Morse and Wilcko[26] described a clinical case in which both hemorrhage and salivary flow were reduced during dental treatment where hypnosis was used as the only anesthetic.

F. TREATMENT OF SYNCOPE

Hypnosis can be used to facilitate treatment in patients who faint in the dental chair (usually during the administration of local anesthesia).[3,8] In one case report,[8] a patient was described who had always fainted when given any injection. When the patient was treated under hypnosis, no injection was necessary and the patient cooperated completely.

In treating these patients the role of hypnosis is twofold: it serves as local anesthesia without the necessity of injections and it reduces anxiety which is often the main cause for the syncope.

G. OTHER APPLICATIONS

Since the very essence of hypnosis is a positive interpersonal relationship between the patient and the hypnotist, and on an increased suggestibility and rapport on the part of the patient, these phenomena may be used to increase cooperation in various aspects of dental care. Golan,[7] for example, suggested the use of hypnosis as a tool to increase patient cooperation on matters such as prophylaxis care and follow-up visits. Apparently, positive motivation for the required behavior can be achieved through suggestions by which the patient imagines how good he/she will look with properly cared for teeth. Some evidence as to the efficiency of hypnosis in promoting patients' compliance with routine dental flossing is presented by Kelly et al.[41]

III. CAUTION IN THE USE OF HYPNOSIS

Hypnosis is a powerful medical tool and as such must be used with knowledge and care. Special training and, in some countries, a special license is required. Hypnosis, when improperly used, may carry adverse deleterious effects.

Several potential complications may take place following hypnotic procedures.[42-46] Complications from hypnosis are rather rare in the dental setting since the patient's encounter is usually episodic and used merely as a technique to ease discomfort.[47] While this is true when the technique is only used to obtain local anesthesia, occasionally the dentist may face a patient who seeks nondental applications of hypnosis, such as antismoking suggestions.[46] Such an intervention would be a deviation from the original "contract" between patient and dentist, and may lead to unexpected problems.

Kleinhauz and Eli[46] presented several cases of potential deleterious effects of hypnosis carried out in the dental setting, which originated from problems such as improper utilization of suggestive procedures, improper handling of spontaneous reactions, faulty dehypnotization, and lack of adequate psychodynamic knowledge by the hypnotist. Several safeguards are proposed in the use of hypnosis in the clinical setting:

1. The professional using hypnosis should not stray from his area of expertise.
2. The clinician using hypnosis should have basic psychological and psychopathological training in order to be able to identify, assess, and cope with possible psychological reactions during the hypnotic intervention.
3. Attention should be given to the wording used in the suggestive procedures, taking into consideration their possible literal interpretation by the subject.
4. Generally, a permissive technique is preferable.
5. Special attention and reassurance should be noted for proper completion of the dehypnotization procedures.
6. Psychological services should be available in case of need.

IV. SUMMARY

Hypnosis is a potent medical tool. Phenomena such as alterations in voluntary muscles, sense organs, and mental activity can be efficiently used to enhance treatment in patients with various oro-related behavioral dysfunctions. The use of hypnosis in dentistry includes inducing relaxation in anxious patients, treating of patients with excessive gagging reflex, managing pain during treatment, increasing patient compliance to procedures such as adaptation to dentures and oral hygiene, and controling hemorrhage and salivary flow.

REFERENCES

1. **Zimbardo, P., Maslach, C., and Marshall, G.,** Hypnosis and the psychology of cognitive and behavioral control, in *Hypnosis: Research Developments and Perspectives*, Fromm, E. and Shor, R. E., Eds., Aldine-Atherton, Chicago, 1972, 539.
2. **Orne, M. T.,** The construct of hypnosis: implications of the definition for research and practice, in *Conceptual and Investigative Approaches to Hypnosis and Hypnotic Phenomena*, Vol. 296, Edmonston, W. E., Jr., Ed., Annals of the New York Academy of Sciences, New York, 1977, 14.
3. **Waxman, D.,** *Hartland's Medical & Dental Hypnosis*, 3rd ed., Bailliere Tindall, London, 1989.
4. **Erickson, M. H. and Rossi, E. L.,** *Hypnotherapy: An Exploratory Casebook*, Irvington Publishers, New York, 1979.
5. **Nash, M. R.,** Twenty years of scientific hypnosis in dentistry, medicine, and psychology: a brief communication, *Int. J. Clin. Exp. Hypn.*, 36, 198, 1988.
6. **Golan, H. P.,** Control of fear reaction in dental patients by hypnosis: three case reports, *Am. J. Clin. Hypn.*, 13, 279, 1971.
7. **Golan, H. P.,** Further reports from Boston City Hospital, *Am. J. Clin. Hypn.*, 18, 55, 1975.
8. **Penzer, V.,** Applied hypnodontics: a case report, *Am. J. Clin. Hypn.*, 15, 46, 1972.
9. **Bar-Gil, B., Eli, I., and Kleinhauz, M.,** A multidisciplinary approach to the treatment of dental phobia, *J. Am. Soc. Psychosom. Dent. Med.*, 30, 137, 1983.
10. **Eli, I., Kleinhauz, M., and Bar-Gil, B.,** Anxiety and other behavioral dysfunctions related to dentistry: a multidisciplinary approach, *Dent. Med.*, 1, 9, 1983.
11. **Kleinhauz, M., Eli, I., and Rubinstein, Z.,** Treatment of dental and dental-related behavioral dysfunctions in a consultative outpatient clinic: a preliminary report, *Am. J. Clin. Hypn..*, 28, 4, 1985.
12. **Gerschman, J. A., Burrows, G. D., and Reade, P. C.,** Hypnotiz-ability and dental phobic disorders, *Int. J. Psychosom.*, 34, 42, 1987.
13. **Forgione, A. G.,** Hypnosis in the treatment of dental fear and phobia, *Dent. Clin. North Am.*, 32, 745, 1988.
14. **Manusov, E. G.,** Clinical applications of hypnotherapy, *J. Fam. Pract.*, 31, 180, 1990.
15. **Rodolfa, E. R., Kraft, W., and Reilley, R. R.,** Etiology and treatment of dental anxiety and phobia, *Am. J. Clin. Hypn.*, 33, 22, 1990.
16. **Weyandt, T. A.,** Three case reports in dental hypnotherapy, *Am. J. Clin. Hypn.*, 15, 49, 1972.
17. **Moss, A. A.,** Hypnodontics: hypnosis in dentistry, in *Clinical and Experimental Hypnosis in Medicine, Dentistry, and Psychology*, 2nd ed., Kroger, W. S., Ed., J. B. Lippincott, Philadelphia, 1977, 321.
18. **Rootenberg, A.,** Hypnosis as a means of treating a very difficult gagger, *J. Dent. Assoc. S. Afr.*, 529, 1979.
19. **Eli, I., Kleinhauz, M., and Bar-Gil, B.,** Extreme gag reflex: methods of treatment and control, *Isr. J. Dent. Sci.*, 1, 105, 1984.
20. **Morse, D. R., Hancock, R. R., and Cohen, B. B.,** *In vivo* desensitization using mediation-hypnosis in the treatment of tactile-induced gagging in a dental patient, *Int. J. Psychosom.*, 31, 20, 1984.
21. **Eli, I. and Kleinhauz, M.,** Hypnosis: a tool for an integrative approach in the treatment of the gagging reflex, *Int. J. Clin. Exp. Hypn.*, 33, 99, 1985.
22. **Clarke, J. H. and Persichetti, S. J.,** Hypnosis and concurrent denture construction for a patient with a hypersensitive gag reflex, *Am. J. Clin. Hypn.*, 30, 285, 1988.
23. **Hilgard, E. R. and Hilgard, J. R.,** *Hypnosis in the Relief of Pain*, William Kaufmann, Los Altos, CA, 1975.
24. **Morse, D. R.,** Hypnosis in the practice of endodontics, *J. Am. Soc. Psychosom. Dent. Med.*, 22, 17, 1975.

25. **Morse, D. R.,** Use of a meditative state for hypnotic induction in the practice of endodontics, *Oral Surg. Oral Med. Oral Pathol.*, 41, 664, 1976.
26. **Morse, D. R. and Wilcko, J. M.,** Nonsurgical endodontic therapy for a vital tooth with meditation-hypnosis as the sole anesthetic: a case report, *Am. J. Clin. Hypn.*, 21, 258, 1979.
27. **Chen, A. C. N., Dworkin, S. F., and Bloomquist, D. S.,** Cortical power spectrum analysis of hypnotic pain control in surgery, *Int. J. Neurosci.*, 13, 127, 1981.
28. **Houle, M., McGrath, P. A., Moran, G., and Garrett, O. J.,** The efficacy of hypnosis- and relaxation-induced analgesia on two dimensions of pain for cold pressor and electrical tooth pulp stimulation, *Pain*, 33, 241, 1988.
29. **Bernick, S. M.,** Relaxation, suggestion and hypnosis in dentistry, *Pediatr. Dent.*, 11, 72, 1972.
30. **Morse, D. R., Schoor, R. S., and Cohen, B. B.,** Surgical and non-surgical dental treatments for a multi-allergic patient with meditation-hypnosis as the sole anesthetic: case report, *Int. J. Psychosom.*, 31, 27, 1984.
31. **Rugh, J. D. and Ohrbach, R.,** Occlusal parafunction, in *A Textbook of Occlusion*, Mohl, N. D., Zarb, G. A., Carlsson, G. E., and Rugh, J. D., Eds., Quintessence Publishing Co., Chicago, 1988, 249.
32. **Rugh, J. D. and Lemke, R. R.,** Significance of oral habits, in *Behavioral Health: A Handbook of Health Enhancement and Disease Prevention*, Matarazzo, J. D., Weiss, S. M., Herd, J. A., Miller, N. E., and Weiss, S. M., Eds., John Wiley & Sons, New York, 1984, 947.
33. **Rugh, J. D.,** Psychological factors in the etiology of masticatory pain and dysfunction, in *The President's Conference on the Examination, Diagnosis and Management of Temporomandibular Disorders*, Laskin, D., Greenfield, W., Gale, E., Rugh, J., Neff, P., Alling, C., and Ayer, W., Eds., American Dental Association, Chicago, 1983, 85.
34. **Graham, G.,** Hypnoanalysis in dental practice, *Am. J. Clin. Hypn.*, 16, 178, 1974.
35. **Crasilneck, H. B. and Hall, J. A.,** *Clinical Hypnosis: Principles and Applications*, Grune & Stratton, New York, 1975, 295.
36. **Golan, H. P.,** Temporomandibular joint disease treated with hypnosis, *Am. J. Clin. Hypn.*, 31, 269, 1989.
37. **Finer, B.,** Mental mechanisms in the control of pain, in *Pain and Society*, Kosterlitz, H. W. and Terenius, L. Y., Eds., Dahlem Konferenzen, Weinheim, 1980.
38. **Lucas, O. N., Finkelman, A., and Tocantins, L. M.,** Management of tooth extractions in hemophiliacs by combined use of hypnotic suggestion, protective splint and packing of sockets, *J. Oral Surg. Anesth. Hosp. Dent. Serv.*, 20, 488, 1962.
39. **Lucas, O. N. and Tocantins, L. M.,** Problems in hemosthasis in hemophilianes undergoing dental extraction, *Ann. N. Y. Acad. Sci.*, 115, 470, 1964.
40. **Newman, M.,** The role of amnesia in dentistry: a case report, *Am. J. Clin. Hypn.*, 14, 127, 1971.
41. **Kelly, M. A., McKinty, H. R., and Carr, R.,** Utilization of hypnosis to promote compliance with routine dental flossing, *Am. J. Clin. Hypn.*, 31, 57, 1988.
42. **Meares, A.,** An evaluation of the dangers of medical hypnosis, *Am. J. Clin. Hypn.*, 4, 90, 1961.
43. **Kleinhauz, M. and Beran, B.,** Misuses of hypnosis: a medical emergency and its treatment, *Am. J. Clin. Hypn.*, 29, 148, 1981.
44. **Kleinhauz, M. and Beran, B.,** Misuse of hypnosis: a factor in psychopathology, *Am. J. Clin. Hypn.*, 26, 283, 1984.
45. **Kleinhauz, M., Dreyfuss, D. A., Beran, B., Goldberg, G., and Azikri, D.,** Some after effects of stage hypnosis: a case study of psychopathological manifestations, *Am. J. Clin. Hypn.*, 3, 219, 1979.
46. **Kleinhauz, M. and Eli, I.,** Potential deleterious effects of hypnosis in the clinical setting, *Am. J. Clin. Hypn.*, 29, 155, 1987.
47. **Orne, M. T.,** Undesirable effects of hypnosis: the determinants and management, *J. Clin. Exp. Hypn.*, 4, 226, 1965.

Chapter 12

PHARMACEUTICAL APPROACHES

Many approaches for controlling pain, stress, and anxiety are based on the use of pharmaceutical agents. Both physicians and dentists use relevant drugs which block pain and help the patient relax. Pharmaceutical approaches are relatively popular in the treatment of oro-related behavioral dysfunctions. Although such treatment does not address the psychodynamic needs of the patient, it is, in many cases, effective in solving immediate dental problems.

Most oro-related behavioral dysfunctions prevent the patient from receiving routine dental care, resulting in poor oral health. The mean DMFS-rates among patients suffering from severe dental fear and avoidance are usually high and indicate an immediate need for profound dental care.[1,2]

When these patients finally seek professional help, their dental condition is often catastrophic. In many cases the final drive to initiate treatment arises from severe pain which can no longer be overlooked. An immediate solution is then necessary, a solution which can only be achieved through the use of pharmaceutical drugs.

Furthermore, pharmaceutical agents are often preferred by the patients themselves. In a survey conducted in England, 31% of the respondents, mainly those most anxious about treatment, stated that they would prefer to be relaxed by medication (sedation) or to be put to sleep (general anesthesia).[3]

The field of pharmacosedation in dentistry is a specialty in its own and this chapter by no means intends to cover its numerous aspects. The objective is to point out general views of such treatments.

I. CONSCIOUS SEDATION

The primary objective of conscious sedation is to reduce anxiety and restlessness while the patient remains conscious and cooperative. This can be achieved by a variety of methods.

A. ORALLY ADMINISTERED DRUGS

Orally administered anti-anxiolytic drugs are used to reduce anxiety in the anxious patient. The drugs of choice include

1. *Barbiturates* — sedative-hypnotic drugs, at different doses they produce relaxation or induce drowsiness. The drugs best suited for dentistry are the short-acting barbiturates, which have a clinical duration of 3 to 4 h. The most significant are pentobarbital, secobarbital, and hexobarbital.[4]
2. *Benzodiazepines* — these drugs possess anti-anxiety, anti-convulsant, muscle-relaxing, sedative-hypnotic, and amnesic properties.[4,5] Benzodiazepines administered orally may be indicated to avoid treatment stress,

alleviate mild anxiety before dental treatment, and facilitate sleep on the night before treatment.[6] Orally administered drugs from this group, which are common in dental treatment, are chlordiazepoxide, diazepam, and flurazepam.[4]

3. *Antihistamines* — most have side effects that produce a degree of central nervous system depression (sedation). The drug that is especially efficient in this respect is hydroxizine, which has sedative, antihistaminic, antiemetic, antispasmodic, and anticholinergic properties. It is available in two forms: hydrochloride (Atarax) and pamoate (Vistaril).[4]
4. *Cabamates* — e.g., Meprobamate, they are useful in the management of anxiety and tension.

Oral premedication is generally used to provide a level of light sedation prior to dental treatment. In most cases, local anesthesia should be used for substantial dental procedures.[7]

B. SEDATION THROUGH INHALATION

The most popular sedative inhalation agent in dental care is nitrous oxide (N_2O). Nitrous oxide/oxygen mixtures are safe, well-established, effective in producing sedation, and are quickly reversible.[7] The main indication for use is fear and anxiety regarding dental treatment.[8]

The numerous clinical reports, basic research, and reviews published concerning the use of this agent in dentistry point to its popularity and efficiency in treating both children and adults.[9-12] In a recent survey conducted by members of the American Board of Pediatric Dentistry, 85% of pediatric dentists reported using nitrous oxide.[13]

Nitrous oxide is often considered an effective sedative but only a weak anesthetic agent.[14,15] Nevertheless, there is evidence that N_2O increases the levels of pain threshold and pain tolerance. Using nitrous oxide in concentrations of 15 to 45%, Dworkin et al.[16] produced statistically significant and subjectively meaningful increases in sensation and pain thresholds and in pain tolerance during electric pulp stimulation.

Since N_2O induces sedation while the patient remains conscious, consideration of the cognitive processes of the patient must be taken into account. The expected analgesic action of nitrous oxide can be reversed by creating the expectation of heightened awareness of bodily sensations (telling subjects that the drug induces an altered state of consciousness which results in heightened sensitivity). Under this condition of altered expectation, expected responses to electric tooth stimulation were reversed: instead of demonstrating reduced pain perception, subjects showed heightened awareness and sensitivity to the stimulation.[17]

These results were further confirmed in a clinical setting.[18] When pain thresholds and pain tolerance of dental patients were compared with and without the administration of 33% nitrous oxide, they were found to be significantly elevated under the effect of the drug. However, when patients were previously prepared by the expectation of increased sensitivity, their pain threshold and pain tolerance showed no increase.

The effect of N_2O as a sedative/analgesic drug is also affected by the amount of information provided to the patient regarding the drug's action and use as an analgesic and sedative.[19] Providing subjects with such relevant information yields higher sensation and pain thresholds and higher pain tolerance.

It is, therefore, not surprising that a wide range of responses to N_2O among individual subjects exists.[20] Although N_2O has specific pharmacological effects, its effectiveness is also influenced by factors of behavior management. Weinstein et al.[21] found that the dentist's behavior influences the fear-related responses of children, even when N_2O is utilized. Distracting the child, for example, was especially effective when nitrous oxide was administered, but not when the patient received only air through the inhalation masks. In addition, the use of suggestion by dentists during the placement of the mask resulted in fewer fear-related behaviors than when no suggestion was given.

The use of nitrous oxide inhalation with other modes of behavior modification may thus be effective.[12,22] Systematic desensitization and appropriate levels of nitrous oxide, together with behavioral preparation of the patient for treatment, have been suggested as especially efficient in treating specific dental phobias (fear of needles or drills).[12,23]

Among the psychological effects attributed to nitrous oxide are aspects of classical and operant conditioning. In a longitudinal, double-blind study, Nathan et al.[24] found that anxious pediatric patients who received nitrous oxide showed significantly less disruptive behaviors than children who received placebo gas (oxygen). Discontinuation of the nitrous oxide on the fourth visit did not result in a substantial deterioration of the child's behavior. It was suggested that the induction of a relaxed state by nitrous oxide acts as a process of desensitization in which the subject is trained to pair the relaxed state with the anxiety-provoking stimuli. Furthermore, as the relaxed and cooperative child receives more positive reinforcements from the dentist, the situation also involves elements of operant conditioning.

In general, relaxation with nitrous oxide/oxygen mixtures serves as an important adjunct to anxiety control in the conscious patient as well as in the treatment of other oro-related behavioral dysfunctions, such as excessive gagging reflex.[11]

C. INTRAVENOUS SEDATION

The purpose of intravenous sedation (i.v.) is to achieve relaxation and cooperation without obtundation and compromise of vital functions. The aim is to diminish anxiety and apprehension rather than to dull protective reflexes.[25] During intravenous sedation, the patient remains conscious and appropriately responsive to questions or commands. In some dental and oral surgical procedures, local anesthesia is added to avoid possible pain involved with the treatment.

The main advantages of intravenous sedation over other methods of drug administration include short time effect (the full effect is seen within minutes), accuracy (the speed in which the clinical effect is seen enables an accurate titration of drug concentration in the patient's bloodstream), and fast recovery rate.[25]

The disadvantages of the procedure include the possibility of local complications (intra-arterial injection, extravascular injection, thrombophlebitis, and venous thrombosis) and systemic complications (including respiratory and circulatory depression due to overdose, allergic reactions, and muscle tremors).[26]

Various combinations of agents have been used for i.v. sedation in dentistry, including the Jorgensen technique, a combination of pentobarbital (Nembutal), meperidine (Demerol), and scopolamine; the Shane technique, a combination of alphaprodine (Nisentil), hydroxyzine (Vistaril, Atarax), atropine, and methohexital (Brevital), with local anesthesia and verbal conditioning by the operator; Diazepam (Valium), administered alone or in combination with other agents such as nitrous oxide, meperidine, or pentazocine;[26] Mediazolam (Versed), a water soluble, short-acting impidazobenzodiazepine with two to three times the potency of diazepam; and narcotics (meperidine, alphaprodine, fentanyl, nabuphine, butorphanol).

II. GENERAL ANESTHESIA

General anesthesia is occasionally used to treat children as well as adults with severe oro-related behavioral dysfunctions. The method is a quick solution to those who are otherwise unable to cooperate while in the dental chair.

While treatment under general anesthesia is efficient in solving the patient's immediate dental problems, it does not address the behavioral aspects of the dysfunction on a long-term basis. In many cases, the patient receives the dental treatment but retains the behavioral pattern which prevented the receipt of routine dental care. If this aspect is not properly addressed, the patient will be compelled to return for treatments under general anesthesia.

As a rule, both dentists and patients are reluctant regarding the use of general anesthesia in treating minor carious lesions. Therefore, in most cases more severe deterioration occurs before any treatment is attempted, a pattern which is not in the patient's best interest.

Undoubtedly, general anesthesia has its benefits. In some cases, it is the only way to administer complicated, and often prolonged, dental treatment to the patient suffering from an oro-related behavioral dysfunction. In some patients, the mere knowledge that most of the loci of potential pain have been taken care of, reduces anxiety and enables the initiation of emotional re-education concerning dental care. However, on a long-term basis, behavior therapy is significantly more effective than general anesthesia in the treatment of fearful dental patients.[27-30] It is, therefore, recommended to use this mode in conjunction with other, more behaviorally oriented, modes of addressing the patient's problems.

III. SUMMARY

Modes of pharmaceutical treatment, such as orally administered drugs, sedation, inhalation, intravenous sedation, and general anesthesia are commonly used to treat dental patients with oro-related behavioral dysfunctions. Although not directly connected, most of the pharmaceutical treatment modes are linked with various aspects of behavior therapy.

There is an increasing recognition that behavioral variables influence the effectiveness of pharmaceutical drugs such as nitrous oxide. Variables including the dentist's behavior before, during, and after treatment; suggestions given to the patient; and individual differences among subjects may influence the effect of pharmaceutical drugs, especially during conscious sedation. Therefore, behavioral methodologies should be integrated in dental pharmacological use and research.[31]

Dworkin[32] presents a multidimensional model which emphasizes the need for simultaneous consideration of pharmacological, psychological, and clinical dental factors in order to arrive at therapeutic decisions. The psychological dimension includes assessment of the status of the patient (e.g., anxiety) and refers to behavioral therapeutic modalities, such as cognitive-behavioral and psychophysiological interventions known to be effective in managing anxiety in clinical settings. The pharmacological dimension reflects the knowledge and experience of relevant pharmaceutical agents and their possible integration with the behavioral dimensions of the patient (e.g., conscious sedation with N_2O). The clinical dental dimension involves the immediate clinical needs of the patient and their possible urgency.

Thus, an anxious patient who suffers from acute pain may initially be treated with pharmacological agents that make immediate dental care possible. Only in a second stage of the patient's treatment is behavior modification used. On the other hand, a patient whose dental needs are less urgent may initially be treated by gradual exposure or systematic desensitization. The combination of more than one therapeutic modality (pharmacological and psychological) is an efficient method of solving the patient's problems.

REFERENCES

1. **Berggren, U. and Meynert, G.,** Dental fear and avoidance: causes, symptoms, and consequences, *J. Am. Dent. Assoc.*, 109, 247, 1984.
2. **Harrison, J. A., Carlsson, S. G., and Berggren, U.,** Research in clinical process and outcome methodology: psycho-physiology, systematic desensitization and dental fear, *J. Behav. Ther. Exp. Psych.*, 16, 201, 1985.
3. **Lindsay, S. J. E., Humphris, G., and Barnby, G. J.,** Expectations and preferences for routine dentistry in anxious adult patients, *Br. Dent. J.*, 163, 120, 1987.

4. **Hagen, J. and Malamed, S. F.,** Psychosedation. Part 3. Pharmacosedation: oral route, in *Emergencies in Dental Practice, Prevention and Treatment*, 3rd ed., McCarthy, F. M., Ed., W. B. Saunders, Philadelphia, 1979, 226.
5. **Oreland, L.,** The benzodiazepines: a pharmacological overview, *Acta Anaesthesiol. Scand. Suppl.*, 88, 13, 1988.
6. **Hallonsten, A.-L.,** The use of oral sedatives in dental care, *Acta Anaesthesiol. Scand.*, 32 (Suppl. 88), 27, 1987.
7. Premedication in Dentistry, Federation Dentaire Internationale, Techn. Rep. No. 32, International Dental Journal, 39, 55, 1989.
8. **Hallonsten, A.-L.,** Sedation by the use of inhalation agents in dental care, *Acta Anaesthesiol. Scand.*, 32 (Suppl. 88), 31, 1987.
9. **Trieger, N. and Carr, S.,** Psychosedation. Part 4. Pharmacosedation: inhalation route, in *Emergencies in Dental Practice, Prevention and Treatment*, 3rd ed., McCarthy, F. M., Ed., W. B. Saunders, Philadelphia, 1979, 280.
10. **Nathan, J. E., Venham, L. L., and Gaulin-Kremer, E.,** Reduction of childhood dental anxiety with nitrous oxide: a literature review, *J. Am. Analg. Soc.*, 21, 9, 1987.
11. **Kaufman, E., Weinstein, P., Sommers, E. E., and Soltero, D. J.,** An experimental study of the control of the gag reflex with nitrous oxide, *Anesth. Prog.*, 35, 155, 1988.
12. **Weinstein, P., Milgrom, P., and Ramsay, D. S.,** Treating dental fears using nitrous oxide oxygen inhalation and systematic desensitization, *Gen. Dent.*, 36, 322, 1988.
13. **Nathan, J. E.,** Management of the difficult child: a survey of pediatric dentists' use of restraints, sedation and general anesthesia, *J. Dent. Child.*, 56, 293, 1989.
14. **Ryder, W. and Wright, P. A.,** Dental sedation. A review, *British Dental Journal*, 165, 207, 1988.
15. **Jastak, J. T.,** Nitrous oxide in dental practice, *Int. Anesthiol. Clin.*, 27, 92, 1989.
16. **Dworkin, S. F., Chen, A. C. N., Schubert, M. M., and Clark, D. W.,** Analgesic effects of nitrous oxide with controlled painful stimuli, *J. Am. Dent. Assoc.*, 107, 581, 1983.
17. **Dworkin, S. F., Chen, A. C. N., LeResche, L., and Clark, D. W.,** Cognitive reversal of expected nitrous oxide analgesia for acute pain, *Anesth. Analg.*, 62, 1073, 1983.
18. **Dworkin, S. F., Schubert, M., Chen, A. C. N., and Clark, D. W.,** Psychological preparation influences nitrous oxide analgesia: replication of laboratory findings in a clinical setting, *Oral Surg. Oral Med. Oral Pathol.*, 61, 108, 1986.
19. **Dworkin, S. F., Chen, A. C. N., Schubert, M. M., and Clark, D. W.,** Cognitive modification of pain: information in combination with N_2O, *Pain*, 19, 339, 1984.
20. **Hallonsten, A.-L., Koch, G., and Schroder, U.,** Nitrous oxide oxygen sedation in dental care, *Community Dent. Oral Epidemiol.*, 11, 347, 1983.
21. **Weinstein, P., Domoto, P. K., and Holleman, E.,** The use of nitrous oxide in the treatment of children: results of a controlled study, *J. Am. Dent. Assoc.*, 112, 325, 1986.
22. **Wikström, P.-O.,** The combination of hypnosis and conscious sedation in dental practice: a clinical study, *Sven. Tidskr. Hypnos*, 3-4, 106, 1980.
23. **Moore, P. A., Ramsay, D. S., Finder, R. L., and Laverick, W.,** Pharmacologic modalities in the management and treatment of dental anxiety, *Dent. Clin. North Am.*, 32, 803, 1988.
24. **Nathan, J. E., Venham, L. L., West, M. S., and Werboff, J.,** The effects of nitrous oxide on anxious young pediatric patients across sequential visits: a double-blind study, *J. Dent. Child.*, 55, 220, 1988.
25. **Trieger, N.,** Intravenous sedation in dentistry and oral surgery, *Int. Anesthesiol. Clin.*, 27, 83, 1989.
26. **Foreman, P. A.,** Psychosedation. Part 5, Pharmacosedation: intravenous route, in *Emergencies in Dental Practice, Prevention and Treatment*, 3rd ed., McCarthy, F. M., Ed., W. B. Saunders, Philadelphia, 1979, 317.
27. **Berggren, U. and Linde, A.,** Dental fear and avoidance: a comparison of two modes of treatment, *J. Dent. Res.*, 63, 1223, 1984.
28. **Berggren, U.,** Long-term effects of two different treatments for dental fear and avoidance, *J. Dent. Res.*, 65, 874, 1986.

29. **Berggren, U. and Carlsson, S. G.,** Qualitative and quantitative effects of treatment for dental fear and avoidance, *Anesth. Prog.*, 33, 9, 1986.
30. **Hakeberg, M., Berggren, U., and Carlsson, S. G.,** A 10-year follow-up of patients treated for dental fear, *Scand. J. Dent. Res.*, 98, 53, 1990.
31. **Weinstein, P.,** Integrating behavioral methodological into dental pharmacological research, *Anesth. Prog.*, 33, 55, 1986.
32. **Dworkin, S. F.,** Integrating behavioral and pharmacological therapeutic modalities, *Anesth. Prog.*, 33, 29, 1986.

Chapter 13

MULTIDISCIPLINARY COOPERATION

I. SPECIALIZED, MULTIDISCIPLINARY DENTAL CLINICS

The high prevalence of fear, anxiety, and other oro-related behavioral dysfunctions among dental patients requires special consideration. The increasing awareness among dental practitioners of the behavioral aspects of oral care helps to prevent some problems, but it is not always sufficient to solve all the complicated psychophysiological aspects of dental treatment.

When treating a patient suffering from an oro-related behavioral dysfunction (e.g., anxiety), treatment by a psychologist is not always sufficient due to lack of a real dental clinical setting. On the other hand, not all dentists have the knowledge, skill, or desire to attempt behavior therapy in the dental clinic itself.

Unlike psychologists who are paid for time devoted to the patient, dentists are usually paid according to the "product" supplied (filling, crown, etc.). This fact leads many dentists (often unconsciously) to avoid modes of treatment which are generally viewed as time consuming (e.g., behavior modification, hypnosis).

The idea of multidisciplinary teams, operating in public institutions such as hospitals, community centers, or universities, is gradually gaining world-wide acceptance.[1-19] Most of the clinics are operated by multidisciplinary teams of dentists, psychologists, psychiatrists, physical therapists and social workers. The teams deal with the various needs of the patient, including problems such as fear, anxiety, and phobia, benign chronic orofacial pain, excessive gagging reflex; rejection of dentures, etc.

One such center has been operating for more than 12 years at the School of Dental Medicine, Tel Aviv University, Israel (The Clinic for Oral Psychophysiology — COP).[2,3,6,7,19] The COP is operated by a multidisciplinary professional team (seven dentists, three psychologists, and one psychiatrist). The psychiatric and psychological team screens the patients for gross psychopathology which might interfere with the therapeutic plan, supplies a general evaluation of the patient's personality and needs, and collaborates with the dental team to decide on a suitable treatment plan for each individual.

Treatment at the COP is based mainly on behavior modification combined with relaxation and hypno-relaxation techniques. In some cases, patients are initially treated with the aid of pharmaceutical agents (N_2O, i.v. sedation, general anesthesia), followed by behavior therapy to enable future cooperation.

Patients are referred to the clinic by dentists throughout the country. The patient's first contact with the clinic and its team takes place in a nondental setting. The initial interview is performed by one of the COP members in the presence of the rest of the team. The emphasis is on an open, relaxed atmosphere devoid of any formality. The presence of the team as one "caring" unit serves to create an atmosphere of acceptance and "legitimization" and enables the initial reframing of the patient's attitude.

The aim of the interview is multifold: to receive relevant information, to develop initial interpersonal relationships, to legitimize and accept, to reframe (change the patient's attitude toward his symptom), to evaluate patient personality, to initiate a treatment plan, and to select a treating dentist whose personality best suits the patient's expectations and needs.

The patient is then referred to one of the team dentists who initiates treatment following the defined outlines. Further personality evaluation is carried out with adequate questionnaires, concomitant to the treatment. When necessary, a personal interview with a psychologist is arranged to provide a more detailed psychodynamic evaluation or to diagnose a possible psychopathology.

Clinical treatment is based on a close interpersonal relationship between patient and dentist. The team represents different personalities and approaches, all within the basic treatment philosophy. The initial referral is to a dentist whose personality best suits the individual needs of the patient, e.g., male or female, young or old, vigorous or fatherly, permissive or firm. During all stages of treatment, care is taken to establish mutual trust and a close interpersonal relationship. Treatment usually combines relaxation with behavioral techniques aimed at desensitizing the patient's anxiety from the dental situation.

To avoid developing patient dependence on one dentist and to promote exposure to different "dental" personalities, the patient is referred to other dentists in the team as soon as initial cooperation is achieved. This neutralizes the patient's need for a dentist with a specific personality and enables referral of the patient for treatment outside of the clinic. Treatment is considered successful when the patient is able to receive dental treatment not only from the initial dentist, but also from a subsequent one, and can be further referred for treatment in an outside setting.

Treatment includes behavior modification techniques such as desensitization, gradual exposure, and modeling. Deep muscle relaxation is used in the clinic as part of systematic desensitization. In some cases, hypno-relaxation and hypnotic suggestive techniques are used as a tool for anxiety and pain control. In patients with true (or false) hypersensitivity to local anesthetic agents, hypno-analgesia enables treatment without pain or discomfort. Proper suggestions also permit the use of the hypnotic stage for desensitization and positive reinforcement.

At the COP, integration of professionals from different fields encourages treatment planning that involves a combination of several therapeutic modalities. Thus, one patient may be assigned to a treatment routine which commences with conscious sedation and continues with behavior therapy, another is treated under hypnosis, and another is referred for systematic desensitization. The idea is to provide patients with multiple treatment disciplines, "tailor" specific treatment plans for each, and answer each individual's needs.

Operating under the roof of a community-oriented institution frees the team, and the patients, from the burden of financial considerations and promotes the administration of proper care without constraints irrelevant to the patient's psychological and dental needs.

II. PSYCHIATRIC/PSYCHOLOGICAL REFERRAL

In spite of all efforts, behavioral and/or pharmaceutical treatments are not always sufficient to help patients. Occasionally, the dental situation itself is not the origin of the patient's problems, but is a symbolic representation of other deep-seated psychological conflicts. In other cases, general emotional disturbances may be the main etiologic factor of the reported symptoms. In such instances, psychodynamic therapy may be necessary and patients should be referred for professional psychiatric and/or psychological treatment.

Improper treatment of a patient suffering from undiagnosed psychiatric pathology can be not only frustrating but also potentially deleterious to the patient. For example, Murphy[20] reported that more than half of the individuals who committed suicide by overdose of medication had received a prescription within the previous week or had an unlimited prescription for a lethal amount of the hypnotic substance ingested. Furthermore, more than two-thirds of patients who committed suicide had been under the care of a physician within six months or less before death, but a large majority of them were not recognized as representing a suicidal risk.[21]

Although these data may not be immediately relevant to the dental setting, they require some attention. In some patients, the oro-related behavioral dysfunction may involve deeper problems, which solutions cannot and should not be attempted in a dental office.

A common problem encountered in patients suffering from different variations of benign chronic orofacial pain is depression. Although depression is rather prevalent among the general population, it is often undetected by physicians.[22,23] Similarly, dentists have been unable to properly identify psychological problems in patients suffering from temporomandibular pain and dysfunction syndrome based on global clinical impressions.[24] Depression has a great impact on problems such as pain, anxiety, rejection of dentures, etc. Therefore, its proper diagnosis is important before attempting treatment. In serious cases, psychiatric treatment should be suggested.

Another problem that may be encountered in the dental office is patient avoidance of dental care, which originates from a deep-rooted psychopathology. In such cases, attempts at behavior modification are usually bound to fail. Proper consultation-liaison with a psychiatrist may shorten the time of involvement and allow the dentist to acknowledge susceptibility to frustration and a sense of failure. An ability to accept this reality helps to preserve the dentist's emotional equanimity and protect the patient from ineffective procedures.[25]

Although psychiatric consultations are rarely requested by dentists, they should be seriously considered. Blasberg et al.[26] outlined some of the problems of referring a dental patient to a psychiatrist: the patient may have a firm belief about the problem that does not include a psychiatric or emotional component, psychiatric referral may be perceived as a rejection or as a judgment that is negative, and the individual may believe that psychiatric therapy is not legitimate. The authors believe that successful referral is based on the relationship established between the dentist and patient. If the patient appreciates that the dentist's recommendation stems from an honest appraisal of what would be of greatest value, the patient is usually more likely to give it serious consideration.

III. SUMMARY

Treating oro-related behavioral dysfunctions is a complicated and often frustrating procedure. Although many of the mild problems can be avoided and/or solved simply by addressing the patient in a more "humane" way, and by establishing proper interpersonal relationships, some of the more severe cases require a multidisciplinary approach. Cooperation between professionals from the dental, psychological, and social fields are important in creating proper treatment frameworks for these patients. It is important, however, to bear in mind that some of the problems may originate in deeper psychodynamic conflicts which cannot be addressed properly in the dental setting. A consultation-liaison with professions from other fields (e.g., psychiatrists) is then recommended.

REFERENCES

1. **Gerschman, J. A., Reade, P. C., Burrows, G. W., and Wright, J.,** The management of chronic oro-facial pain at a multidisciplinary pain clinic, in *Advances in Pain Research and Therapy*, Vol. 3, Bonica, J., Ed., Raven Press, New York, 1979.
2. **Bar-Gil, B., Eli, J., and Kleinhauz, M.,** A multidisciplinary approach to the treatment of dental phobia, *J. Am. Soc. Psychosom. Dent. Med.*, 30, 137, 1983.
3. **Eli, J., Kleinhauz, M., and Bar-Gil, B.,** Anxiety and other behavioral dysfunctions related to dentistry: a multidisciplinary approach, *Dent. Med.*, 1, 9, 1983.
4. **Berggren, U. and Linde, A.,** Dental fear and avoidance: a comparison of two modes of treatment, *J. Dent. Res.*, 63, 1223, 1984.
5. **Seyrek, S. K., Corah, N. L., and Pace, L. F.,** Comparison of three distraction techniques in reducing stress in dental patients, *J. Am. Dent. Assoc.*, 108, 327, 1984.
6. **Eli, J. and Kleinhauz, M.,** Hypnosis: a tool for an integrative approach in the treatment of the gagging reflex, *Int. J. Clin. Exp. Hypn.*, 33, 99, 1985.
7. **Kleinhauz, M., Eli, I., and Rubinstein, Z.,** Treatment of dental and dental-related behavioral dysfunctions in a consultative out-patient clinic: a preliminary report, *Am. J. Clin. Hypn.*, 28, 4, 1985.
8. **Milgrom, P., Weinstein, P., Kleinknecht, R., and Getz, T.,** *Treating Fearful Dental Patients*, Reston Publishing Co., Reston, VA, 1985.
9. **Berggren, U.,** Long-term effects of two different treatments for dental fear and avoidance, *J. Dent. Res.*, 65, 874, 1986.

10. **Berggren, U. and Carlsson, S. G.,** Qualitative and quantitative effects of treatment for dental fear and avoidance, *Anesth. Prog.*, 33, 9, 1986.
11. **Gatchel, R. J.,** Increasing dental patients' access to measures for anxiety, fear and phobia management: perspectives from a community-based research program, *Anesth. Prog.*, 33, 67, 1986.
12. **Rubin, J. G. and Kaplan, A.,** Increasing dental patients' access to measures for anxiety, fear and phobia management: perspectives from a hospital-based program, *Anesth. Prog.*, 33, 65, 1986.
13. **Fricton, J. R., Hathaway, K. M., and Bromaghim, C.,** Interdisciplinary management of patients with TM and craniofacial pain: characteristics and outcome, *J. Craniomandibular Disorders*, 1, 115, 1987.
14. **Makkes, P. C., Schuurs, A. H. B., Thoden van Velzen, S. K., Duivenvoorden, H. J., and Verhage, F.,** Effect of a special dental program upon extreme dental anxiety, *Community Dent. Oral Epidemiol.*, 15, 173, 1987.
15. **Smith, T., Getz, T., Milgrom, P., and Weinstein, P.,** Evaluation of treatment at a dental fears research clinic, *Spec. Care Dent.*, May-June, 130, 1987.
16. **Fricton, J. R. and Hathaway, K. M.,** Interdisciplinary management: address complexity with teamwork, in *TMJ and Craniofacial Pain: Diagnosis and Management*, Fricton, J. R., Kroening, R. J., and Hathaway, K. M., Eds, Ishiyaku Euro-America, St. Louis, 1988, 167.
17. Dental phobia: conquering fear with trust (an interview), *J. Am. Dent. Assoc.*, 119, 593, 1989.
18. **Hakeberg, M., Berggren, U., and Carlsson, S. G.,** A 10-year follow-up of patients treated for dental fear, *Scand. J. Dent. Res.*, 98, 53, 1990.
19. **Eli, I. and Kleinhauz, M.,** Oro-related behavioral dysfunctions: a disabling factor in dental care, (in press).
20. **Murphy, G. E.,** The physician's responsibility for suicide. I. Errors of commission, *Ann. Int. Med.*, 82, 301, 1975.
21. **Murphy, G. E.,** The physician's responsibility for suicide. II. Errors of omission, *Ann. Int. Med.*, 82, 305, 1975.
22. **Nielsen, A. C., III and Williams, T. A.,** Depression in ambulatory medical patients: prevalency by self-report questionnaire and recognition by nonpsychiatric physicians, *Arch. Gen. Psychiatry*, 37, 999, 1980.
23. **Knights, E. B. and Folstein, M. F.,** Unsuspected emotional and cognitive disturbance in medical patients, *Ann. Int. Med.*, 87, 723, 1977.
24. **Oakley, M. E., McCreary, C. P., Flack, V. F., Clark, G. T., Solberg, W. K., and Pullinger, A. G.,** Dentists' ability to detect psychological problems in patients with temporomandibular disorders and chronic pain, *J. Am. Dent. Assoc.*, 118, 727, 1989.
25. **Lipsitt, D. R.,** Pain in the neck, face, and head: role of the consultation liaison psychiatrist, *Psychiatr. Clin. North Am.*, 10, 69, 1987.
26. **Blasberg, B., Remick, R. A., and Miles, J. E.,** The psychiatric referral in dentistry: indications and mechanics, *Oral Surg. Oral Med. Oral Pathol.*, 56, 368, 1983.

INDEX

A

B

C

D

L

M

N

O

P

SEPARATION AND DIVORCE IN NORTH CAROLINA

Answers
to the Most
Commonly Asked
Questions
About Your
Legal Rights

Mary K. Nicholson

Second Printing, August, 1994

ISBN 1-878086-16-2

Library of Congress Card Number 92-072659

Printed in the United States of America

Cover and book design by Elizabeth House

Down Home Press
P.O. Box 4126
Asheboro, N.C. 27204